The Effects of Genetic Hearing Impairment in the Family

The Effects of Genetic Hearing Impairment in the Family

Edited by

DAFYDD STEPHENS AND LESLEY JONES

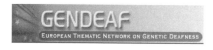

GENDEAF
EUROPEAN THEMATIC NETWORK ON GENETIC DEAFNESS

John Wiley & Sons, Ltd

KH

Other Wiley Editorial Offices

John Wiley & Sons, Inc., 111 River Street, Hoboken, NJ 07030, USA

Jossey-Bass, 989 Market Street, San Francisco, CA 94103-1741, USA

Wiley-VCH Verlag GmbH, Boschstr. 12, D-69469 Weinheim, Germany

John Wiley & Sons Australia Ltd, 42 McDougall Street, Milton, Queensland 4064, Australia

John Wiley & Sons (Asia) Pte Ltd, 2 Clementi Loop #02-01, Jin Xing Distripark, Singapore 129809

John Wiley & Sons Canada Ltd, 6045 Freemont Blvd, Mississauga, ONT L5R 4J3

Wiley also publishes its books in a variety of electronic formats. Some content that appears in print may not be
available in electronic books.

Library of Congress Cataloging-in-Publication Data

The effects of genetic hearing impairment in the family / edited by Dafydd
    Stephens and Lesley Jones.
        p. ; cm.
    Includes bibliographical references and index.
    ISBN-13: 978-0-470-02964-0 (pbk. : alk. paper)
    ISBN-10: 0-470-02964-1 (pbk. : alk. paper)
    1. Deafness–Genetic aspects.   2. Ear–Abnormalities–Genetic aspects.
3. Hearing disorders–Patients–Family relationships   I. Stephens, Dafydd.
II. Jones, Lesley, 1947-   .
    [DNLM: 1. Hearing Disorders–genetics. 2. Attitude to Health.   3. Family
Health. 4. Genetic Counseling.   5. Genetic Predisposition to Disease.
6. Hearing Disorders–psychology.   WV 270 E265 2006]
RF292.E354 2006
617.8′042–dc22

                                                                2006006471

British Library Cataloguing in Publication Data

A catalogue record for this book is available from the British Library
ISBN-13: 978-0-470-02964-0
ISBN-10: 0-470-02964-1

Typeset by SNP Best-set Typesetter Ltd., Hong Kong
Printed and bound in Great Britain by TJ International Ltd, Padstow, Cornwall
This book is printed on acid-free paper responsibly manufactured from sustainable forestry in which at least
two trees are planted for each one used for paper production.

8/17/11

Contents

PART V   RESEARCH NEEDS

Contributors

Patrick Axon, Department of Otolaryngology, Addenbrookes Hospital, Cambridge, England

Garry Barton, Division of Primary Care, University of Nottingham, Nottingham, England

Rachel Belk, Department of Genetic Conselling, University of Manchester, Manchester, England

Per-Inge Carlsson, Swedish Institute for Disability Research, Örebro University, Örebro, Sweden

Sylviane Chéry-Croze, Neurosciences and Sensory Systems Laboratory, UMR CNRS UMR 5020, Lyon, France

Lionel Collet, Neurosciences and Sensory Systems Laboratory, UMR CNRS UMR 5020, Lyon, France

Lotta Coniavitis Gellerstedt, Swedish Institute for Disability Research, Örebro University, Örebro, Sweden

Sarah Coulson, Department of Medical Genetics, Leeds, England

Peter and Cynthia Crawshaw, Department of Radiology, Furness General Hospital, Barrow-in-Furness, England

Graeme Crossland, Department of Otolaryngology, Addenbrookes Hospital, Cambridge, England

Adrian Davis, Department of Audiology, University of Manchester, Manchester, England

Berth Danermark, Swedish Institute for Disability Research, Örebro University, Örebro, Sweden

Angeles Espeso, Welsh Hearing Institute, University Hospital of Wales, Cardiff, Wales

Gareth Evans, Department of Medical Genetics, University of Manchester, Manchester, England

Heather Fortnum, Trent Research and Development Support Unit, Nottingham University Medical School, Queen's Medical Centre, Nottingham, England

Lesley Jones, Centre for Research in Primary Care, University of Leeds, Leeds, England

Roland Jouvent, CNRS UMR 7593, Hôpital de la Salpêtrière, Paris, France

Veronica Kennedy, Welsh Hearing Institute, University Hospital of Wales, Cardiff, Wales

Rehana Khan, Department of Genetic Counselling, University of Manchester, Manchester, England

Sophia E. Kramer, Department of Audiology, Vrije University, Amsterdam, Netherlands

Nele Lemkens, Department of Otolaryngology, University of Antwerp, Antwerp, Belgium

Peter Lewis, Department of Mathematical Sciences, University of Bath, Bath, England

Anna Middleton, Institute of Medical Genetics, University Hospital of Wales, Cardiff, Wales

Ghazalla Mir, Centre for Research in Primary Care, University of Leeds, Leeds, England

Paul Mitchell, Department of Ophthalmology, University of Sydney, Australia

Ioannis Moumoulidis, Department of Otolaryngology, Addenbrookes Hospital, Cambridge, England

Wanda Neary, Department of Paediatrics, Warrington Hospital, Warrington, England

Philip Newall, Department of Linguistics, Macquarie University, New South Wales, Australia

Fernando Perez-Diaz, CNRS UMR 7593, Hôpital de la Salpêtrière, Paris, France

Mallappa Raghu, Department of Otolaryngology, Addenbrookes Hospital, Cambridge, England

Richard Ramsden, Department of Otolaryngology, University of Manchester, Manchester, England

Anna-Carin Rehnman, Department of Human Development, Learning and Special Education, Stockholm Institute of Education, Stockholm, Sweden

Evan Reid, Department of Medical Genetics, Addenbrookes Hospital, Cambridge, England

Christophe Saglier, Neurosciences and Sensory Systems Laboratory, UMR CNRS UMR 5020, Lyon, France

Doungkamol Sindhusake, Centre for Health Services Research, School of Public Health, University of Sydney at Westmead, New South Wales, Australia

Pranay Kumar Singh, Department of Otolaryngology, Addenbrookes Hospital, Cambridge, England

Paula Stacey, Department of Psychology, University of York, England

Dafydd Stephens, Welsh Hearing Institute, University Hospital of Wales, Cardiff, Wales

A. Quentin Summerfield, Department of Psychology, University of York, York, England

Hung Thai-Van, Neurosciences and Sensory Systems Laboratory, UMR CNRS UMR 5020, Lyon, France

Claire Wilson, Welsh Hearing Institute, University Hospital of Wales, Cardiff, Wales

Adriana A. Zekveld, Department of Audiology, Vrije University, Amsterdam, Netherlands

Preface

RATIONALE FOR BOOK ON FAMILIAL HEARING IMPAIRMENT

What is to be gained by the study of a family history of hearing impairment? This book and our desire to pursue this question arose from the psychosocial working group (WP6) of the European Gendeaf Thematic Network (Stephens & Jones, 2005). During the course of this it became apparent that there were some significant effects of having a genetic hearing impairment compared with having an acquired disorder. With the increasing impact of genetics in health and medicine we felt it worthwhile to try to see whether or not the significance of family histories had an impact on people's decision-making about their lives and on clinicians' practice as well as on policy.

The first book revealed that, although the significance was not enormous, there did indeed seem to be some positive aspects of having a family history (e.g. Stephens, 2005; Stephens & Kramer, 2005). This could perhaps be explained in terms of having positive role models, a ready supply of help and advice or early anticipation of problems leading to solutions being sought in good time. There were a number of explanations, which have emerged in this collection of writing.

Such a family history may not always have a direct genetic aetiology. It may be due to a predisposition to noise-induced hearing impairment or to chronic otitis media. In some cases it may be merely due to a chance occurrence. However, whatever the aetiology, the fact of having a clear role model in the family appears to be a key factor.

We begin in Part I by looking at retrospective studies on the impact of hearing loss in elderly people, using secondary analyses. In Chapter 1, Stephens, Lewis and Davis in the UK found that those people in a population survey who reported a family history of hearing impairment, reported a greater impact of their own impairment in terms of hearing, tinnitus and hyperacusis, extending their earlier analyses (Stephens et al., 2003). In a parallel analysis of an Australian project, the Blue Mountains Survey, Sindhusake et al. (Chapter 2) report effects of a family history in elderly people resulting in greater hearing impairment and also the impact of such impairment, but no real effect on tinnitus.

A large-scale study on childhood hearing impairment in the UK by Fortnum and colleagues from Nottingham (Chapter 3) suggests that most of the somewhat limited effects, both positive and negative, reported of having a family history on hearing-impaired children are found in those with one or more profoundly deaf parents. Two studies in Sweden (Chapters 4 and 5) following up earlier investigations agree that, while there are some positive effects of such a family history, when the children become older, such effects are relatively small.

Part II looks at prospective studies of late onset hearing impairment, which do reveal differences, and generally positive aspects of the impairment. Building on the findings of earlier studies (e.g. Stephens & Kramer, 2005) we attempt to look at ways of determining these effects on people's perceptions (Kramer et al., Chapter 6; Stephens et al., Chapter 7; and Coulson, Chapter 8). These indicate a preponderance of positive effects which are found principally among those already aware of the familial nature of their hearing impairment. However, in terms of anxiety, depression and disabilities (Espeso and Stephens, Chapter 9) the effects, if any, are very small.

The ways in which people try to deal with their hearing impairment by seeking help is then examined in terms of help-seeking behaviour (Wilson and Stephens, Chapter 10) and on the effect of rehabilitative interventions by Saglier et al. (Chapter 11). Again, in these cases, effects of such a family history are minimal and dominated by other factors.

Part III looks at prospective studies on conditions associated with hearing impairment. It begins with a French study on the impact of tinnitus and the influence of a family history in self-help groups (Chéry-Croze and Thai-Van, Chapter 12), followed by a UK study of the same topic in a clinic population (Kennedy and Stephens, Chapter 13). Generally speaking there was a positive effect of having a family history of tinnitus, and hence a role-model, but that effect was less in the clinical population than in the self-help group.

Neary et al. look at the psychosocial effects of neurofibromatosis type 2 firstly at the effect on those with the condition (Chapter 14) and then on those closest to them (Chapter 15). Hearing impairment seems to have the largest effect on the individuals and, surprisingly, most of the patients and their partners are able to identify positive experiences associated with the condition.

Otosclerosis is the next topic and its relationship to genetics. Middleton et al. (Chapter 16) were unable to define any difference between the attitudes of those who had a family history of the condition and those who did not, but Stephens and Lemkens (Chapter 17) found that most had a positive experience associated with having a family history.

Part IV examines the pragmatic way in which everyday life is affected by a family history. It also concentrates on genetic counselling and how it deals with the issues and ways in which it may be improved. A forthcoming booklet by Middleton et al. will develop this further. In the present book Middleton (Chapter 18) begins by an examination of genetic counselling which is appropriate to national Sign Language users and those with a family history of deafness. She emphasises the need to work with interpreters and to avoid value-laden terms, such as 'abnormal', and negative words about deafness in general.

Belk (Chapter 19) continues this through the use of National Sign Language and the translation of genetic information. This may well be a complicated concept such as risk and transmission of genes. Belk develops some interesting ways in which these difficulties can be overcome in a culturally sensitive way.

Jones, Mir and Khan (Chapter 20) write about ethnicity, spirituality and genetic counselling. This chapter explores the contested ways of describing and measuring ethnicity and its relationship to spirituality and religion. It also looks at the ways in which people's beliefs affect how they view having a child born with a hearing impairment or discovering that their family history may be involved. Decisions about whether or not to have genetic testing or whether or not to terminate are all influenced by people's beliefs. Clinicians have to find their way through this complex picture of expressed and unexpressed views. The notion of informed consent is one which requires both parties to understand each other well, so this chapter, like the earlier two about the Deaf community, discusses interpreting and translation of terms.

Chapter 21 is a personal account by Peter Crawshaw and his wife, Cynthia, of living with NF2 from the point of the view of the person with the condition. Anna-Carin Rehnman (Chapter 22) writes about her own family history of hearing impairment over 200 years in a fascinating account including changes in technology and societal attitudes over that time.

We conclude, in Part V, with Chapter 23 by Danermark (with contributions from others) which looks at future developments in the field and attempts to provide a model of family history and the psychological and social consequences. This acknowledges the incompleteness of our data and the complexity of the social processes involved. The chapter summarises the technological, demographic and aetiological changes affecting this area of research as well as those in medicine and socio-economics.

We are seeking to identify the impact of a family history of hearing impairment on people's lives. This is obviously an area which needs more work and to which we would want to make a contribution by changing practice. In order to do this we have tried to bring together a multi-disciplinary group from several countries writing from very different perspectives. The authors in this book have been working independently and with great commitment in related fields and their research and experience have been brought together to try to broaden the scope of the study of familial hearing impairment.

Lesley Jones and Dafydd Stephens

REFERENCES

Stephens D (2005) The impact of hearing impairment in children. In D Stephens, L Jones (eds) *The Impact of Genetic Hearing Impairment.* London: Whurr, pp. 73–105.

Stephens D, Jones L (eds) (2005) *The Impact of Genetic Hearing Impairment.* London: Whurr.

Stephens D, Kramer S (2005) The impact of having a family history of hearing problems on those with hearing difficulties themselves: an exploratory study. *International Journal of Audiology* 44: 206–12.

Stephens D, Lewis P, Davis A (2003) The influence of a perceived family history of hearing difficulties in an epidemiological study of hearing problems. *Audiological Medicine* 1: 228–31.

Acknowledgements

This book is published with the support of the European Commission, Fifth Framework programme, Quality of Life and Management of Living Resources programme. The authors and editors are solely responsible for this publication. It does not represent the opinion of the Community. The Community is not responsible for any use that might be made of the data appearing therein.

The studies described in Chapters 7 and 9 were also supported in part by the European Commission FP5 Quality of Life project, ARHI QLK6-CT-2002-00331.

I Retrospective Studies

1 The Impact of Having a Family History of Hearing Loss in Elderly People

DAFYDD STEPHENS, PETER LEWIS AND ADRIAN DAVIS

INTRODUCTION

The UK Medical Research Council's Survey of Ear, Nose and Throat Problems asked one member of a household (the respondent) to report various hearing problems for all the adults in the household. An analysis of these data in a previous report suggested that having a family history of early-onset hearing loss made respondents more likely to report hearing problems themselves, and be more likely to be disturbed by such problems (Stephens et al., 2003). In addition, they were more likely to be sensitive to loud noises and be disturbed by any tinnitus which they experienced.

In a subsequent study on a clinical sample in whom we explored the specific impacts of having such a family history (Stephens & Kramer, 2005), we found conversely that those with a family history reported more positive than negative experiences related to having relatives with hearing problems. There were many differences between the approach of these two studies, one epidemiological and one clinical, which may explain the differences between these overall results. These differences include the definition of a family history, which was quite strict in the MRC–ENT study and more lax in the clinical study, and also the age breakdown of the subjects. Thus the median age of the subjects in the epidemiological study was 50 years (IQ range 36–63), but in the clinical study we were dealing with a predominantly elderly population with a median age of 61 years (IQ range 56–77 years).

Within the present study we have therefore split the population into younger and older subjects, with a cut-off point of 60 years to explore the possible effect of age on the results. In addition, in the next chapter in this book (Sindhusake et al.), we explore the effects of using a more liberal definition of a family history of hearing impairment in a separate epidemiological study conducted in Australia.

The Effects of Genetic Hearing Impairment in the Family. Edited by D. Stephens and L. Jones.
Copyright © 2006 by John Wiley & Sons, Ltd.

For the purpose of the present study, we considered only the replies from the respondents relating to themselves. Elsewhere (Stephens et al., 2004), we have found that such respondents are more likely to report hearing difficulties in themselves than in other members of their households. Thus they report a prevalence of 22.3% of hearing difficulties for themselves, but only 15.0% in other household members. It was also difficult to determine the reliability of the responses to the family history question (Q12) when applied to other household members who were not necessarily from the same family.

METHOD

This work is a secondary analysis of the MRC National Study of Ear, Nose and Throat problems which was administered to 22,000 households in Wales, Scotland and England randomly selected according to their postal code. The respondent was asked to complete the questionnaire for all members of their household over 14 years of age. Three mailings were undertaken.

The questionnaire comprised 33 questions covering different aspects of ear, nose and throat problems, of which 13 concerned hearing, hearing aids and tinnitus. Question 12 on the family history was worded: '*Did any of your parents, children, brothers or sisters have great difficulty in hearing before the age of 55 years?*' The wording of this question enabled first-degree relatives to be tapped, and mild to moderate age-related hearing impairment was excluded. However, it includes those individuals with first-degree relatives experiencing hearing difficulties related to acquired causes such as otitis media, ototoxicity and noise exposure.

We examined the association between the responses to this question and the demographic variables age and gender, the presence of tinnitus (a functional impairment) and questions on Activity Limitation (Disability) and Participation Restriction/Emotional Problems (Handicap) relating to the impact of the hearing and/or tinnitus on the individual.

The specific questions which form the basis of this study are listed below (Table 1.1).

RESULTS BY AGE AND SEX

There were responses from 15,796 households. Of these there were 14,878 answers to the initial question about hearing difficulty (Q4), representing a response rate of 68%. Among these, 4821 were aged 60 years or older, of whom 2418 were males and 2403 females. Of all the elderly subjects, 453 had a family history of hearing loss.

In all further analyses, categories will be excluded in which the total within such a category is less than 100 respondents. This applies, in particular, to groups reporting great difficulty hearing the television.

Table 1.1 MRC–ENT questions forming the basis of the present analysis

Q4	*Do you have difficulty with your hearing?* (Activity Limitation)
Q6a	*Do you have difficulty following TV programmes at a volume others find acceptable without any aid to hearing?* (Activity Limitation)
Q6b	*Do you have any difficulty hearing a conversation with several people in a group?* (Activity Limitation)
Q7	*Do very loud sounds annoy you?* (Psychosocial)
Q8	***Nowadays** how much does any difficulty in hearing worry, annoy or upset you?* (Psychosocial)
Q13a	***Nowadays,** do you **ever** get noises in your head or ears (tinnitus) which usually last longer than five minutes* (Functional Impairment)
Q13b	***Nowadays,** how much do these noises worry, annoy or upset you when they are at their worst?* (Psychosocial)
Q13c	***Nowadays** how much do these noises affect your ability to lead a normal life?* (Psychosocial)

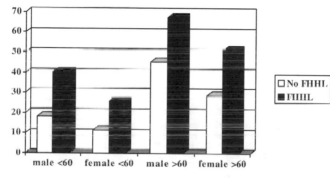

Figure 1.1 Percentage of respondents reporting hearing difficulty by gender, age band (under and over 60 years of age) and whether or not they have a family history of hearing loss.

Figure 1.1 addresses the general question of reported hearing loss (Q4), which we had initially used in the Cardiff Health Survey (Stephens et al., 1990) by reported family history of hearing loss (FHHL), by age, by sex.

Figure 1.2 shows the graded response to difficulty hearing the television set at a level which other people find acceptable (Q6a) in males by FHHL and age. A similar pattern of responses was obtained for the female respondents, of both age bands, with and without a family history.

The consistency of these results with assessments of Activity Limitation indicates that elderly subjects follow the same pattern of effects of having a family history of hearing loss as young subjects. Therefore, in the following analyses, we shall present only the results for the elderly subjects. In addition, as male and female respondents both showed the same pattern of effects, we shall present results lumped across the genders.

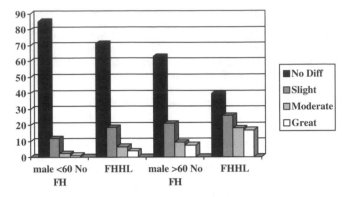

Figure 1.2 Percentage of male respondents reporting various levels of difficulty in hearing the TV by FHHL and age band (under and over 60 years of age).

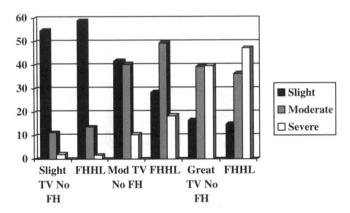

Figure 1.3 Percentage of annoyance caused by the reported difficulty with hearing the television as a function of FHHL. All responses for those aged over 60 years and reporting hearing difficulties.

RESULTS FOR OVER-60s WITH SEXES COMBINED

Figure 1.3 examines how disturbed the individual was by their hearing loss (Q8) adjusted for the degree of hearing difficulty the individual was experiencing (Q6a) by FHHL.

Reports of phonophobia or hyperacusis (Q7) in subjects who had reported no difficulty hearing the television are shown in Figure 1.4.

Next we considered reported hypersensitivity as a function of the degree of reported hearing difficulty for those reporting slight and moderate difficulties hearing the television. The results of this analysis are shown in Figure 1.5.

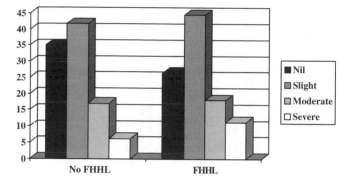

Figure 1.4 Effect of FHHL on the level of annoyance caused by loud sounds. Percentage of different levels of annoyance for all respondents aged over 60 years who reported no difficulty hearing the television.

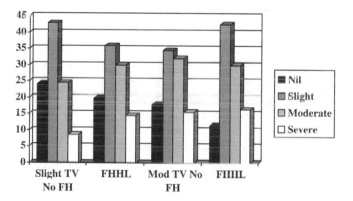

Figure 1.5 Levels of annoyance caused by loud sounds reported by individuals aged over 60 years with slight and moderate levels of hearing difficulty with and without a FHHL.

Finally we examined the presence, annoyance and life-effects caused by tinnitus in elderly subjects with and without a family history of hearing difficulties. Figure 1.6 compares tinnitus occurring sometimes or most of the time in subjects younger and older than 60 years of age with and without such a family history.

Among those respondents indicating tinnitus being present sometimes or most of the time, we examined the annoyance reported as being caused by such tinnitus as a function of the presence or absence of a family history of

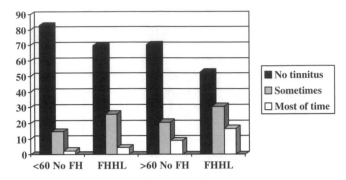

Figure 1.6 Prevalence of tinnitus in younger (<60 years) and older (>60 years) respondents with and without a family history of hearing difficulties.

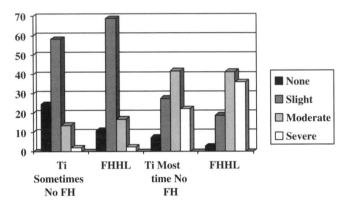

Figure 1.7 Degree of annoyance caused by tinnitus reported by older subjects with tinnitus present sometimes or most of the time, as a function of the presence of a FHHL.

hearing difficulties in the elderly subjects. These results are shown in Figure 1.7. This shows that, with a family history, no annoyance occurs less frequently and severe annoyance more frequently than in those subjects without such a family history.

Figures 1.8 and 1.9 examine the annoyance caused by the tinnitus as a function of the reported hearing difficulties. Figure 1.8 shows the results for subjects with no reported hearing difficulty.

Figure 1.9 shows the results for subjects with hearing difficulties and tinnitus.

The reported effects of tinnitus on the individual's life by whether the individual's tinnitus is present 'some of the time' or 'most of the time' is shown in Figure 1.10. Figure 1.11 shows the results for subjects with hearing difficulties and tinnitus.

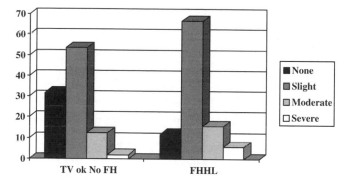

Figure 1.8 Percentage tinnitus annoyance in those with no hearing difficulties but tinnitus, as a function of family history, in elderly subjects.

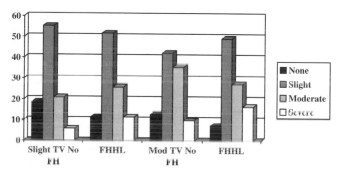

Figure 1.9 Percentage tinnitus annoyance in those with slight or moderate difficulties hearing the television by FHHL. Elderly respondents.

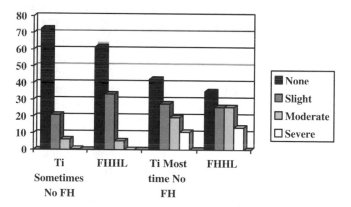

Figure 1.10 Degree of effect on life caused by tinnitus reported by older subjects with tinnitus present sometimes or most of the time, as a function of the presence of a FHHL.

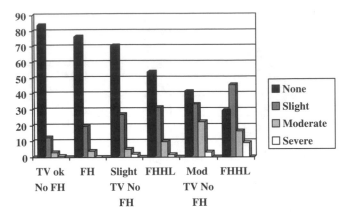

Figure 1.11 Percentage of different categories of the reported effect of the tinnitus on the respondent's life by hearing difficulty and FHHL, in elderly subjects.

DISCUSSION

The results show a markedly greater percentage of people reporting a FHHL also reporting hearing problems themselves in both the young and old and both males and females (Figure 1.1). The ageing effect is similar between the sexes with about 25% more reporting hearing problems in the older groups. The percentage of respondents indicating a difficulty hearing the television increases in both male age bands when there is a FHHL. This result is repeated for females.

In addition similar results (not presented here) were obtained in response to question 6b concerning difficulty hearing in a group conversation. This again applied to both younger and older groups and to males and females, all of whom indicated increased levels of difficulty if they had a FHHL.

Such results are not surprising and could be explained by the fact that those with a family history of hearing problems are more likely to have hearing problems and, if they do, that those problems are more likely to be severe. An alternative explanation is that individuals with such a family history will be more conscious of hearing difficulties, more sensitive to them, and hence more likely to report them and consider them to be severe. This would be particularly true if other family members had had negative experiences as a result of their hearing problems. Within the present study, based on a secondary analysis of an earlier study, it is not possible to differentiate between these two hypotheses, the pathophysiological and the psychological/experiential. In order to make such a differentiation, auditory thresholds or another measure of impaired function would be necessary.

For the older subjects with the sexes combined, for each level of reported hearing difficulty, the annoyance or worry stemming from it is greater if the individual has a family history of hearing loss (FHHL) than if they do not (Figure 1.3). As might be expected, the level of annoyance increases with the degree of hearing difficulty experienced. Despite this, however, there are consistent effects of FHHL increasing the level of annoyance. Thus, in those with slight hearing difficulty, the level of slight or moderate hearing loss is increased. In those with moderate hearing difficulty, the level of moderate and severe annoyance is increased, and in those with great hearing difficulty the level of severe annoyance is increased. By allowing for the level of hearing problems in this way, we have attempted to minimise any hearing level effects and these results point toward a psychological rather than a pathophysiological explanation.

Furthermore, Figure 1.4 suggests the intriguing possibility that individuals who report no hearing difficulties are more sensitive to loud external sounds if they have a family history of hearing problems. This again adds support to the 'psychological sensitisation' hypothesis.

Figure 1.5 shows reported hypersensitivity as a function of the degree of hearing difficulty for those reporting slight and moderate difficulties hearing the television. This is important, given that most hearing impairment in elderly individuals is cochlear and hence is associated with an abnormally rapid growth of loudness. Again, these show that those individuals with a family history of hearing difficulty report more annoyance caused by loud sounds than those without such a family history, although in this case there is a smaller effect of hearing level, as might be expected.

Figure 1.6 shows that tinnitus is found more commonly in those with a FHHL. This broad finding does not contribute to the differentiation between the two hypotheses as Coles et al. (1990) have shown that hearing level is the strongest single predictor of tinnitus. It is, however, interesting in itself that the impact of the presence of a family history of 'hearing difficulty' extends across into this domain.

Among those respondents indicating tinnitus being present sometimes or most of the time, the annoyance reported as being caused by such tinnitus is such that, with a family history, no annoyance occurs less frequently and severe annoyance more frequently than in those subjects without such a family history.

As mentioned earlier, there may be some concern that various studies (e.g. Coles et al., 1990) have indicated that tinnitus annoyance increases with increasing hearing loss, and that having a family history is associated with increased reported hearing difficulties. This has been addressed in Figures 1.8 and 1.9 which examined the annoyance caused by the tinnitus as a function of the reported hearing difficulties. The degree of annoyance caused by the tinnitus is greater when there is a family history of hearing difficulty, irrespective of the degree of hearing difficulty reported by the respondents for themselves.

Broadly similar results were found in terms of the effects of the tinnitus on the individual's life, and are shown in Figures 1.10 and 1.11. The question here arises as to whether or not such an effect is mediated via the annoyance experienced. This question is addressed in Figure 1.12. This figure shows that while there is an increasing likelihood of the tinnitus affecting the individual's life with the level of the annoyance reported, there is an additional component stemming from the presence of a family history. The impact of family history, however, becomes minimal with the greater levels of annoyance.

These results strengthen the argument that having a family history of hearing difficulties sensitises the individual to a range of hearing related difficulties or makes them more likely to report them. The question then arises as to whether this is a specifically auditory phenomenon or is generalised across to other complaints. To clarify this we analysed the annoyance caused by nose, throat and voice problems in terms of whether or not there was a family history of hearing loss. These questions are listed in Table 1.2. While there was a notable effect of those with a family history being more likely to be annoyed by their voice problems, this did not extend to throat or nose problems.

This might be related to knock-on effects within their family of a severe hearing loss on voice problems in general.

The results present a consistent picture of a FHHL predisposing some individuals to greater annoyance with a hearing problem. However, despite that,

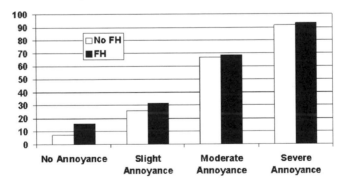

Figure 1.12 Presence of life effects of tinnitus of different levels of annoyance by presence of family history.

Table 1.2 MRC–ENT questions on nose, throat and voice investigated

Q15	*In the last 12 months, how much have ANY problems with your nose worried, annoyed or upset you?*
Q18	*In the last 12 months, how much have ANY voice problems worried, annoyed or upset you?*
Q21	*In the last 12 months, how much have ANY throat problems worried, annoyed or upset you?*

we found no evidence that those with a FHHL were more likely to have consulted their general practitioner (primary physician) or have been referred to hospital because of their hearing loss.

Furthermore, these results are from an observational study using self-reporting, so care should be taken in not over-interpreting these results. For example, subjects who are particularly sensitive to their hearing problems may be predisposed to look for a 'family effect'. Alternatively individuals with objectively mild hearing problems might view these problems as more serious as they have experienced the negative impact of hearing problems within their own family.

CONCLUSIONS

These results, obtained by secondary analysis of survey data, raise several intriguing possibilities which warrant a more thorough investigation using both objective and subjective methods. In particular we suggest that the following priority areas should be investigated:

1. A follow-up of the sample in this study or others should be undertaken to disentangle the reported activity limitation and the functional impairment in different age groups and family history groups.
2. The results with respect to hyperacusis are very interesting and could be followed through in a subsample.

REFERENCES

Coles R, Davis A, Smith P (1990) Tinnitus: its epidemiology and management. In JH Jensen (ed.) *Presbyacusis and Other Age Related Aspects.* Copenhagen: Jensen, pp. 377–402.
Stephens D, Kramer S (2005) The impact of having a family history of hearing problems on those with hearing difficulties themselves: an exploratory study. *International Journal of Audiology* 44: 206–12.
Stephens D, Lewis P, Davis A (2003) The influence of a perceived family history of hearing difficulties in an epidemiological study of hearing problems. *Audiological Medicine* 1: 228–31.
Stephens D, Lewis P, Davis A (2004) The epidemiology of hearing problems: how should we investigate it? *Acta Otolaryngologica* Suppl. 552: 11–15.
Stephens SDG, Lewis PA, Charny M (1991) Assessing hearing problems within a community survey. *British Journal of Audiology* 25: 337–43.

2 The Impact of a Family History of Hearing Loss in the Blue Mountains Study

DOUNGKAMOL SINDHUSAKE, DAFYDD STEPHENS, PHILIP NEWALL AND PAUL MITCHELL

INTRODUCTION

Recent reviews (Kramer, 2005; Danermark, 2005) have not been able to highlight any experimental data on the effects of having a family history of hearing problems on individuals' reaction to their hearing loss in either working age or elderly adults. In order to obtain some information on this matter, we investigated retrospectively the impact of a reported family history of hearing loss in the UK Medical Research Council Survey of Ear, Nose and Throat Problems (MRC–ENT, Stephens et al., 2003).

Within the retrospective analysis of the MRC–ENT survey from the UK, we had no measures of auditory impairment (i.e. hearing thresholds), and a fairly extreme measure of a family history of genetic hearing impairment (Stephens et al., 2003; this volume, Chapter 1). Despite this, we found that, for those individuals with a family history of moderate–severe hearing impairment of onset prior to the age of 50 years, there was a disproportionate impact on their reaction to their hearing loss. This occurred even when allowing for their level of Activity Limitation.

The occurrence of a family history had an impact not only on the annoyance resulting from their hearing loss, but also on their sensitivity to external noises and the impact of their tinnitus. In all these ways, having a family history of hearing loss resulted in a greater impact of the individual's own hearing loss.

These results appear to have been contradicted in a clinical population, in which we found that those patients seen with a family history of hearing impairment listed three times as many positive effects of having a family history of hearing impairment as negative effects (Stephens & Kramer, 2005).

We were thus anxious to test the validity of the initial findings in a further population study performed in a different country, with a different criterion of familial hearing impairment and, also, with a widely accepted measure of impairment. This opportunity was offered by the Blue Mountains Study, conducted in an urban area of New South Wales, Australia (e.g. Mitchell, 2002; Sindhusake et al., 2003). Within the present chapter, we shall present the results of the impact of the family history of hearing loss found in that study on the psychosocial effects of the hearing loss found in the targeted members. In addition, while the MRC–ENT study covered the whole age range of adults (17–99 years), the present study focused on older adults ≥50 years, in whom hearing impairment was likely to be more prevalent.

METHOD

STUDY POPULATION

The Blue Mountains Hearing Study (BMHS) was a population-based survey of age-related hearing loss in a representative older Australian community (Attebo et al., 1998). Data collection commenced in March 1997 and finished in April 2000. The BMHS was conducted in conjunction with the Blue Mountains Eye Study-2 (BMES-2), which was a follow-up to an initial eye study, the Blue Mountains Eye Study-1 (BMES-1).

The BMES-1, conducted during 1992–94, was the first population-based survey to provide information about the frequency, causes, risk factors and impacts of visual impairment in a representative older Australian community (Attebo et al., 1998). Subjects selected for the BMES-1 had to be a resident in postcode areas 2780 or 2782 for more than six months a year, a non-institutional resident, and born before 31 December 1942, thus aged 49 years or older at the time of examination. Experienced trained interviewers, most of whom had worked for the Australian Bureau of Statistics (ABS) population census in 1991 (conducted three months earlier), performed a sequential door knock of all dwellings in 38 ABS census collection districts (CCDs) in the areas west of Sydney, using the ABS Census 1991 maps and methods.

The census counted 5058 permanent residents aged 49 years or older, only six fewer than the ABS Census 1991; 625 nursing home residents were excluded and all other residents were invited to participate. Of 4433 eligible residents, 3654 aged 49–97 years (82.4%) were examined.

Five years later, this cohort was invited to participate in 5-year follow-up eye examinations (BMES-2), and subsequently, in the BMHS detailed assessment of hearing. Of the original 3654 participants, 575 (15.7%) died before taking part in the BMES-2, and 383 (10.5%) had migrated from the study area before the time of recruitment for the hearing examinations. This left 2696 subjects still living in the region and eligible to participate. Of these, 2015 (74.7%) agreed to take part in hearing examinations during 1999–2000 while 681 (25.3%) declined to participate (Sindhusake et al., 2003).

In 2001, a repeat door-to-door census of the area then identified further eligible permanent residents who had moved into the area and were aged 50 or older. At the time hearing examinations of this second group were conducted, 1218 were still alive and living in the area, of whom 941 (77.3%) participated in hearing examinations during 2001–03.

This gave an overall response of 2956/3914 (75.5%) for the cross-section of people aged 50 years or older. The Blue Mountains Hearing Study was approved by the University of Sydney Human Ethics Committee and written and informed consent was obtained from all participants at the interview stage, before any examinations were conducted.

BMHS participants were, on average, two years younger at the baseline examination than those who refused the hearing examination and an average 10 years younger than those who had died. Compared with those who refused, participants were slightly more likely to be male, to be living alone and to rate their health slightly worse. They were also slightly less likely to report hearing loss at the baseline examination, consistent with the age difference. Participants had relatively similar baseline characteristics to those who moved from the area prior to the study, but differed substantially from those who had died, in keeping with their older age at baseline. They were slightly better educated and reported slightly better general health.

Compared with the Australian population (ABS census data) aged 50+ years (Australian Bureau of Statistics, 1998), BMHS participants were on average slightly older and more likely to be female. There were only minor differences in the proportion born outside Australia or having a non-English-speaking background and in the occupation distribution between participants and the overall Australian population. Our sample therefore, appeared to be reasonably representative of the general Australian population.

RECRUITMENT AND DATA COLLECTION

During the BMES 1, all participants were told of the plan for a second examination after 5 years and none indicated a wish not to participate in the follow-up. A detailed letter describing examination findings and blood results was sent to each participant, with a copy sent to the medical practitioners of his/her choice. In August 1996, 4.5 years from the start of BMES-1 examinations, each participant was sent a report outlining the major findings, presented in lay language with a reply-paid letter requesting participation in both the follow-up eye study (BMES-2) and the hearing study (BMHS). A phone call followed to advise the suggested month and year for the examination, which was close to a 5-year interval from the first visit in BMES-1. We asked respondents to notify changes of address. Missing participants were traced using next-of-kin, general practitioner or neighbour contacts and deaths confirmed by death certificates.

Participants were offered two alternatives for the hearing study. Either a second visit would be scheduled after the eye examination (our recommended option), or both examinations would be scheduled consecutively on one day. An appointment was then arranged for each eligible person to attend a clinic at the Blue Mountains District Hospital in Katoomba. Seven rooms were set up at the hospital for the Eye and Hearing Studies during 1997–99. The BMHS examination sequence took an average of 105 minutes. An audiologist examined each participant by means of the comprehensive questionnaire and measures of hearing, middle ear and cochlear status and central auditory function. Details of the comprehensive questionnaire administered and hearing examinations are summarised in the next section.

BMHS COMPREHENSIVE QUESTIONNAIRE ABOUT HEARING

An audiologist administered the comprehensive hearing questionnaire, at the hearing examination. It included:

- The Hearing Handicap Inventory for the Elderly – Shortened (HHIE-S) (Ventry & Weinstein, 1982) – to determine the extent of perceived 'handicap' by a subject due to hearing loss in various situations.
- Questions on tinnitus adapted from questions used in the American Tinnitus Association (ATA) survey conducted in Portland, Oregon, USA.
- Questions documenting any history of subjective hearing loss or tinnitus, history of potential causes of hearing loss and tinnitus including medical information about recurrent colds, sinus conditions, allergies, ear infections, dizziness and balance, childhood illnesses associated with hearing loss, neurological conditions, radiation and chemotherapy, and handedness, as well as documentation of any past medical or surgical treatment of ENT (ear, nose and throat) conditions.
- Questions documenting detailed noise exposure adapted for Australian conditions covering occupational, leisure and military-related exposure, history of ototoxic drug exposure, family history of hearing loss and history of diseases and medical conditions which may affect hearing loss such as diabetes, stroke, cardiovascular diseases, cancer etc.
- Questions about whether a hearing assessment had been sought and a hearing aid provided, use of hearing aids or other amplification devices and the reasons for non-wearing of provided hearing aids, the effectiveness of follow-up after fitting, and the use of hearing rehabilitation services.

HEARING EXAMINATIONS

Measurements of hearing, middle ear and cochlear status and central auditory function included:

- Pure tone air-conduction audiometry was conducted in a standard sound-treated room by an audiologist, using a Madsen OB822 audiometer. Hearing thresholds at frequencies of 0.25, 0.5, 1, 2, 4, 6 and 8 kHz were measured, with 3 kHz added if a gap of 20 dB existed between 2 and 4 kHz thresholds.

* Bone-conduction audiometry was performed at frequencies of 0.5, 1, 2 and 4 kHz. Audiometer calibration was conducted regularly during the period of the study and complied with International Standards Organization (ISO) protocol 389:1991.
* Admittance audiometry which included tympanometry of both ears and testing for stapedial reflexes (both ipsilaterally and contralaterally) and the presence of acoustic reflex decay.
* Measures of transient evoked (TEOAE) and spontaneous (SOAE) oto-acoustic emissions.
* Speech recognition testing using the AB word lists presented to both ears at 30 and 50 dB above speech reception threshold in decibels hearing level (dB HL).
* Measures of central auditory function included the Synthetic Sentence Identification (SSI) test: Ipsilateral Competing Message with a 0 dB message to competition ratio and the Dichotic Sentence Identification (DSI) test.

METHOD

The BMHS comprehensive hearing questionnaire documented history of sub-jective hearing loss, Hearing Handicap Inventory for Elderly (HHIE) and exposure to potential risk factors which included family history of hearing loss and tinnitus.

We defined subjective hearing loss using the question: 'Do you feel you have a hearing loss?' It provided possible responses of 'yes', 'no' or 'don't know'. Missing and 'don't know' responses were excluded from the analysis. A ques-tion on the history of prolonged tinnitus was also included in the compre-hensive questionnaire administered by an audiologist. Questions also asked about any self-perceived hearing problem, including its severity, onset and duration.

The question 'Do (or did) any of your close relatives have a hearing loss?' was used to define parental or sibling family history of hearing loss. This ques-tion was repeated for father, mother, any brother(s) and any sister(s). The four possible responses were 'yes', 'no', 'unsure' and 'missing'. After excluding par-ticipants reporting 'missing' or 'unsure' responses for both father and mother from the analysis, those reporting either their father or mother had hearing loss were classified as having parental family history, otherwise no parental family history of hearing loss was recorded.

The HHIE-S was developed by Ventry and Weinstein (1982) as a diagnos-tic tool to identify older persons with hearing difficulties and was included as part of the hearing questionnaire administered by an audiologist to all participants. This instrument consists of 10 questions designed to assess perceived emotional and social problems associated with impaired hearing (e.g. frustration, embarrassment or difficulty in certain situations). One of three responses ('yes', 'sometimes' or 'no') was recorded for each question and scored as 4, 2 or 0, respectively. Missing values were excluded and scores from the 10 questions were totalled for a minimum score of 0 and a maximum score of 40. According to the American Speech-Language-Hearing Association, total HHIE-S scores > 8 indicated the presence of hearing handicap (Sindhusake et al., 2001).

Pure-tone audiometric hearing thresholds averaged over the commonly used four frequencies of 500, 1000, 2000 and 4000 Hz (4FA) and over three high frequencies of 4000, 6000 and 8000 Hz (3FA) were compared between persons with and without parental family history of hearing loss using analysis of variance. The results in the left, right, better, worse and both ears combined were assessed after adjusting for covariates (sex and age). We also tested significant effects of parental family history on subjective hearing loss, on individual items of the HHIE and on tinnitus and its severity using χ^2 statistics. The impact of sibling(s) family history of hearing loss on respondents' measures of impairment, activity limitation, participation restriction and tinnitus were also assessed. We used SPSS version 11.0 statistical software (SPSS Inc., 2002) for all analyses and p levels of 0.05 were used to denote statistical significance.

RESULTS

Within this report we present the effects of a family history of hearing loss on measures of impairment (audiogram), activity limitation (self-rated hearing), participation restriction (HHIE) and tinnitus. In the case of the last, we examine both its presence and the reported annoyance caused by the tinnitus. In all cases, we have compared the responses when one or both parents were reported to have hearing problems (n = 1079), with those when neither had hearing problems (n = 1767). In addition, for the latter group, we have compared those where one or more siblings report hearing problems (n = 214) with those in which no siblings are reported to have hearing problems (n = 1550).

IMPAIRMENT

Firstly we took the most widely used measure of hearing impairment (e.g. Davis, 1995), that of the averaged hearing level across the octave frequencies 500 Hz to 4 kHz. There was a significant effect of a history of parental hearing loss on the averages after adjusting for sex and age, in terms of left and right ears or better and worse ears. The mean results are shown in Table 2.1.

Next we performed the same comparison for those whose parents were reported as not having hearing problems, comparing those with one or more

Table 2.1 Mean hearing levels (500 Hz–4 kHz) for subjects with and without a parental history of hearing problems, adjusting for sex and age

Condition	Parent(s) hearing problems Mean (SE) HL (dB)	Parent(s) hearing Mean (SE) HL (dB)	F	Significance
Right ear	26.5 (0.5)	23.6 (0.4)	23.5	0.001
Left ear	28.3 (0.5)	25.0 (0.4)	30.6	0.001
Worse ear	30.7 (0.5)	27.6 (0.4)	21.2	0.001
Better ear	24.1 (0.4)	21.0 (0.3)	41.9	0.001
Ears combined	27.4 (0.4)	24.3 (0.3)	32.5	0.001

Table 2.2 Mean hearing levels (500 Hz–4 kHz) for subjects with and without a sibling history of hearing problems, adjusting for sex and age

Condition	Sibling(s) hearing problems Mean (SE) HL (dB)	Sibling(s) hearing Mean (SE) HL (dB)	F	Significance
Right ear	27.3 (1.0)	24.0 (0.4)	9.0	0.003
Left ear	27.7 (1.0)	25.7 (0.4)	3.3	0.07 (ns)
Worse ear	30.8 (1.2)	28.2 (0.4)	4.3	0.04
Better ear	24.2 (0.8)	21.5 (0.3)	9.9	0.002
Ears combined	27.5 (0.9)	24.9 (0.3)	7.3	0.007

Table 2.3 Mean hearing levels (4, 6 and 8 kHz) for subjects with and without a parental history of hearing problems, adjusting for sex and age

Condition	Parent(s) hearing problems Mean (SE) HL (dB)	Parent(s) hearing Mean (SE) HL (dB)	F	Significance
Right ear	49.1 (0.6)	45.9 (0.5)	17.0	0.001
Left ear	51.5 (0.6)	48.4 (0.5)	16.4	0.001
Worse ear	54.9 (0.6)	52.0 (0.5)	13.3	0.001
Better ear	45.7 (0.5)	42.3 (0.4)	24.0	0.001
Ears combined	50.3 (0.6)	47.1 (0.4)	19.9	0.001

siblings with a hearing problem with those with no siblings with hearing problems. These results are shown in Table 2.2, which indicates that, in every case, those with hearing-impaired sibling(s), had worse hearing levels after adjusting for sex and age.

We then examined the high-frequency hearing levels taken as the average across 4, 6 and 8 kHz. Again we examined the results in terms of both parental and sibling hearing problems for the various combinations of ears considered above. Table 2.3 indicates that there was a statistically significant effect of

Table 2.4 Mean hearing levels (4, 6 and 8 kHz) for subjects with and without a sibling history of hearing problems, adjusting for sex and age

Condition	Sibling(s) hearing problems Mean (SE) HL (dB)	Sibling(s) hearing Mean (SE) HL (dB)	F	Significance
Right ear	50.1 (1.3)	46.9 (0.5)	5.1	0.02
Left ear	52.9 (1.3)	49.3 (0.5)	6.3	0.01
Worse ear	56.5 (1.4)	52.9 (0.5)	5.8	0.02
Better ear	46.4 (1.2)	43.3 (0.4)	6.5	0.01
Ears combined	51.5 (1.2)	48.1 (0.5)	7.0	0.008

a history of parental hearing loss on the high-frequency averages after adjusting for sex and age, with a tendency for those with one or both parents with normal hearing to have significantly better hearing themselves. In terms of sibling hearing loss, results were similar to those found for the four-frequency average, with those with siblings with hearing difficulties having significantly worse hearing than those with hearing siblings. These results are shown in Table 2.4.

ACTIVITY LIMITATION

Within the questionnaire, this was assessed using the question '*Do you feel you have a hearing loss?*' When we examined the response to this question as a function of having a reported family history affecting either or both parents, we found that among those with such a family history 58.2% reported that they felt they had a hearing loss. This compares with 46.8% of those who had no parents with hearing difficulties (χ^2 = 33.8; P < 0.001).

We performed the same analysis for those without a parental family history, comparing those with one or more hearing-impaired siblings with those without such affected siblings. The difference here was smaller and not significant. Thus while 52.5% of those with hearing-impaired siblings reported a subjective hearing difficulty, this was reported by 46.0% of those without such a family history (χ^2 = 2.99; NS).

It may also be argued that while the majority of the questions in the Hearing Handicap Inventory for the Elderly (HHIE) represent what was known as 'Handicap' in the International Classification of Impairment, Disability and Handicap (ICIDH – WHO, 1980), certain questions represent Activity Limitation (WHO, 2001). These are questions 3, 8 and 10, concerned with difficulty hearing whispers (Q3), listening to the TV or radio (Q8), and hearing in a club or restaurant (Q10).

We therefore examined the impact of having a parental history of hearing problems on the responses to these, and in each case found the differences to be highly significant (P < 0.001), when Chi square tests were used to compare those with and without such a family history. Those with such a family history were more likely to report problems on these questions than those without. The responses are shown in Table 2.5, together with the Participation Restriction and Psychological problems.

Finally we examined the impact of a history of having one or more hearing-impaired siblings on these responses. The responses were in the same direction, with those with hearing-impaired siblings more likely to report difficulties in reply to these questions. However, the differences were smaller and, in the case of Q10, not significant.

PARTICIPATION RESTRICTION

We took the overall response to the ten HHIE questions as our best response of Participation Restriction/Emotional Impact. After adjusting for sex and age, the mean total score when there was a parental family history of hearing problems was 9.4 (SE 0.3) and that for individuals without such a family history 6.4 (SE 0.2) (F = 68.9; P < 0.001). Equivalent results for those with hearing-impaired siblings showed individuals with and without such affected siblings had means total HHIE score of 8.5 (SE – 0.6) and 6.3 (SE – 0.2) respectively (F = 12.2; P < 0.001).

Table 2.5 shows the differences for the individual questions between those with and without a parental family history of hearing difficulties. From this, it may be seen that there were significant differences in all questions except Q6 – 'Hearing problem causing the respondent to attend meetings and religious services less often than they would like' and Q7 – 'Hearing problem causing the respondent to have arguments with family members.' There are no clear differences between the differences found between the different types of questions, Activity Limitation, Participation Restriction and Psychological.

Table 2.5 Percentages responding 'yes' on the different questions of HHIE as a function of parental hearing problems

Question number	Parents hearing problems	Parents hearing	χ^2	P	Question type
1	9.8	6.7	21.1	<0.001	Psychological
2	13.1	8.9	15.0	0.001	Psychological
3	36.9	28.9	23.4	<0.001	Activity Limitation
4	11.8	6.7	40.9	<0.001	Participation Restriction
5	10.2	7.3	17.8	<0.001	Participation Restriction
6	6.5	4.9	5.3	NS	Participation Restriction
7	4.6	3.9	2.1	NS	Psychological
8	20.7	14.4	25.3	<0.001	Activity Limitation
9	8.2	5.9	9.8	<0.01	Participation Restriction
10	30.0	19.2	42.8	<0.001	Activity Limitation

When we examined the responses for those with hearing parents but hearing-impaired siblings, significant differences in the responses from those with hearing siblings were found only with questions 1 (χ^2 = 6.4; P < 0.05), 3 (χ^2 = 14.9; P = 0.001), 5 (χ^2 = 6.4; P < 0.05) and 8 (χ^2 = 13.3; P = 0.001). It is interesting to note that two of the four questions showing the biggest differences were questions addressing Activity Limitation.

TINNITUS

The first question on tinnitus was concerned with whether or not the individual had experienced any prolonged tinnitus within the past year. 35.6% of those with a parental history of hearing loss reported such tinnitus, compared with 29.2% of those without such a family history (χ^2 = 12.5; 1 df; P < 0.001). For those without parental history of hearing loss, there was no significant difference in tinnitus prevalence between respondents with and without sibling family history (28.5% vs 29.2% respectively, χ^2 = 0.04; 1 df; NS).

In terms of the annoyance caused by such tinnitus, 70.3% of those with a parental history reported mild to extreme annoyance, compared with 65.2% who reported no such family history (χ^2 = 2.5; 1 df; NS). Likewise, no difference was found between the two populations in response to the question 'Does your tinnitus get you down at times?' with 19.8% of those with a parental history of hearing loss and 19.7% of those without such a parental history responding affirmatively (χ^2 = 0.003; 1 df; NS). Finally, in response to the question 'Does your tinnitus keep you awake at night?', 83.5% of those with hearing-impaired parents said no, and 84.7% of those with hearing parents (χ^2 = 0.3; 1 df; NS).

In addition, when we examined the occurrence and the annoyance, getting down and sleep disturbance caused by such tinnitus in those with hearing parents with and without affected siblings, no significant difference was found in any measure.

DISCUSSION

The results of these analyses support and extend our earlier findings (Stephens et al., 2003) that hearing-impaired individuals with a family history of hearing problem are more affected than those individuals without such a family history. The generalisability of these results is enhanced by the fact that this study was performed completely independently of the MRC–ENT Study, in a different country, using different criteria for a family history and different measures of the impact of the hearing impairment.

Important new aspects of the present study concern the fact that audiometric measures were available and also that we were able to separate out the impact of having hearing-impaired parents from that of having hearing-impaired siblings. In addition the use of a broad definition of what comprises a family history may result in greater applicability of the results.

The defining question for a family history used in the MRC–ENT study, '*Did any of your parents, children, brothers or sisters have great difficulty in hearing before the age of 55 years?*' excludes those individuals with late onset and moderate hearing loss, concentrating on the severe congenital or early onset conditions. It does not exclude early severe acquired hearing loss, and in total 11% of the respondents answered that they had such a family history. Within the Blue Mountains Study the question asked was '*Do (or did) any of your close relatives have a hearing loss including ... your father, your mother, any brothers, any sisters, any children?*' – not specifying its severity. With each there was a supplementary question about the age of onset, but we have not examined that in the present analysis.

Within the present study 37.9% of respondents indicated that either their father, their mother, or both parents had a hearing loss. In addition 12.1% of those with hearing parents had one or more hearing-impaired siblings. Thus, in this study, half of the respondents reported one or more hearing-impaired parents or siblings. There are thus two differences in the criterion, the severity and the age of onset. MRC–ENT specifies before the age of 55 years, Blue Mountains has three categories, childhood, before the age of 50 years and after the age of 50 years.

If we compare the results for the impact of the 'General hearing problems' questions in the two studies ('*Do you feel you have a hearing loss?*' – Blue Mountains; '*Do you have difficulty with your hearing?*' – MRC–ENT), taking the > 60-year-old age band from MRC–ENT, we find a significant increase in affirmative responses in those with a family history in both studies. In the present study, those responding 'Yes' went up from 46.8% to 58.2%. In the MRC–ENT study, the increase was from 37.5% to 58.9%. This suggests that with the tighter definition, there is a greater effect. Unfortunately, however, while we know that the thresholds differ significantly from each other in the present study, we do not have that information for the MRC–ENT study. Thus it could be argued that the definition used in the MRC–ENT study resulted in a sampling of individuals with more severe impairments.

We further have information on the influence of having one or more hearing-impaired siblings in the present study. Having such a sibling in the absence of hearing problems in either parent suggests either an acquired or a recessive aetiology, whereas having a loss in one or both parents suggests an acquired or a dominant aetiology. Recessive aetiologies on the whole are associated with more severe hearing losses than dominant aetiologies (e.g. Parving et al., 1996). It is thus not surprising that those with a sibling history of hearing problems have a significantly greater hearing loss than those without such a history (Tables 2.2 and 2.4). It is, therefore, particularly interesting to note that this group did not show a significant difference in self-reported hearing loss from those without a sibling family history, despite having worse hearing. This was also broadly true for the Activity Limitation questions in the HHIE (Qs 3, 8 and 10), for which there was a significant effect of parental hearing loss, but a much smaller effect of sibling hearing loss.

For the overall HHIE scores after adjusting for effects of sex and age, a similar result was found, with a more significant effect on the mean score of a parental history than of a sibling history. When broken down by individual questions, those with hearing-impaired parents had significant differences on eight of the ten questions, whereas those with hearing-impaired siblings showed significant differences on only four. In is interesting to note that neither group showed a significant effect on Q7 *'Does a hearing problem cause you to have arguments with your family members?'*, as might have been anticipated, although having other affected family members may have led to more tolerance of hearing problems, despite a more severe hearing loss.

The one area in which there was a significant difference between the two studies concerned tinnitus, despite the questions used being broadly similar. While both those in the present study with a parental family history of hearing loss and those in the MRC–ENT study showed a significant effect in terms of increased prevalence of reported tinnitus, the effects of this tinnitus on the individual differed between the studies. In addition the effect on prevalence was greater in the MRC–ENT study (47.2% with a FH vs 29.7% without) reporting tinnitus with a family history, compared with 35.6% vs 29.2% in the present study. Again this might be attributable to those with the family history in the MRC–ENT survey having a more severe hearing impairment, which Coles et al. (1991), have shown to be the most important predictor of tinnitus.

In the MRC–ENT study, even when allowing for the tinnitus severity in terms of how much of the time it was present, the annoyance caused and its life effect were still greater in individuals with a family history of hearing problems. In the present study, no such effect was found on Annoyance, its Depressiveness and its effect on Sleep. There is no simple explanation for this difference except possibly the severity of the family history criterion. In addition, in the present study, whether or not the individual had one or more siblings with hearing difficulties did not influence the responses to any of the tinnitus questions.

Finally it is worth briefly considering the difference in the impact of a parental and sibling family history. Overall, the present study highlights the effects of a parental history on the individual's hearing loss and reaction to their hearing loss. The same is true for the influence of a sibling history.

It could be argued that, as is the case with children (e.g. Vernon & Koh, 1970; Conrad, 1979), what is important is the role model derived from the individual's parents. In individuals of this age, the management of hearing impairment in their parents' generation was often poor, with consequent negative effects on their parents. Thus, when they feel they have a hearing loss, they will react negatively to it and describe greater consequences of it than those without such a parental history.

REFERENCES

Attebo K, Mitchell P, Cumming R, Smith W, Jolly N, Sparkes R (1998) Prevalence and causes of amblyopia in an adult population. *Ophthalmology* 105: 154–9.

Australian Bureau of Statistics. Cdata96 (1998) Canberra. Ref Type: Audiovisual material.

Coles R, Davis A, Smith P (1990) Tinnitus: its epidemiology and management. In JH Jensen (ed.) *Presbyacusis and Other Age Related Aspects.* Copenhagen: Jensen, pp. 377–402.

Conrad R (1979) *The Deaf Schoolchild.* London: Harper & Row.

Davis A (1995) *Hearing in Adults.* London: Whurr.

Danermark B (2005) A review of the psychosocial effects of hearing impairment in the working age population. In D Stephens, L Jones (eds) *Impact of Genetic Hearing Impairment.* London: Whurr, pp. 106–36.

Kramer S (2005) The psychosocial impact of hearing loss among elderly people: a review. In D Stephens, L Jones (eds) *Impact of Genetic Hearing Impairment.* London: Whurr, pp. 137–64.

Mitchell P (2002) The prevalence, risk factors and impacts of hearing impairment in an older Australian community: the Blue Mountains Hearing study. The Libby Harricks Memorial Oration No 4. Brandon, Deafness Forum of Australia.

Parving A, France EA, Stephens SDG (1996) Factors causing hearing impairment in identical birth cohorts in Denmark and Wales. *Journal of Audiological Medicine* 5: 67–72.

Sindhusake D, Mitchell P, Newall P, Golding M, Rochtchina E, Rubin G (2003) Prevalence and characteristics of tinnitus in older adults: the Blue Mountains Hearing Study. *International Journal of Audiology* 42: 289–94.

Sindhusake D, Mitchell P, Smith W, Golding M, Newall P, Hartley D et al. (2001) Validation of self-reported hearing loss. The Blue Mountains Hearing Study. *International Journal of Epidemiology* 30: 1371–8.

SPSS Inc. SPSS version 11.0 for Windows, 2002 (computer program).

Stephens D, Kramer S (2005) The impact of having a family history of hearing problems on those with hearing difficulties themselves: an exploratory study. *International Journal of Audiology* 44: 206–12.

Stephens D, Lewis P, Davis A (2003) The influence of a perceived family history of hearing difficulties in an epidemiological study of hearing problems. *Audiological Medicine* 1: 228–31.

Ventry IM, Weinstein BE (1982) The hearing handicap inventory for the elderly: a new tool. *Ear and Hearing* 3: 128–34.

Vernon McK, Koh SD (1970) Early manual communication and deaf children's achievement. *American Annals of the Deaf* 115: 527–36.

WHO (World Health Organization) (2001) *International Classification of Functioning, Disability and Health – ICF.* Geneva: World Health Organization.

3 The Impact for Children of Having a Family History of Hearing Impairment in a UK-Wide Population Study

HEATHER FORTNUM, GARRY BARTON, DAFYDD STEPHENS, PAULA STACEY AND A. QUENTIN SUMMERFIELD

INTRODUCTION

A recent review of the psychosocial impact of hearing impairment in children highlighted a dearth of data on the specific impact of genetic disorders (Stephens, 2005). While a fair number of studies have considered the impact of the child having deaf parents, most studies have considered relatively small numbers of children, and failed to distinguish between different types of parental hearing impairment.

Two key studies in this area were by Vernon and Koh (1970) and by Conrad (1979). Vernon and Koh (1970) compared the academic achievements of 37 children with a genetic hearing impairment and 'deaf' parents with a genetic group of 32 children without deaf parents matched for performance scale IO and age. It was found that the children of 'deaf' parents had significantly better scores in Reading, Paragraph Meaning, and Word Meaning Scores on the Stamford Achievement Test, as well as higher ratings of their written language from teachers.

Conrad (1979) likewise compared the achievements of children with a genetic hearing disorder and 'deaf' parents, with the achievements of children with a genetic hearing disorder and hearing parents, and of children with acquired or unknown causes for their hearing impairment. He found that children with a hearing disorder and 'deaf' parents had a higher reading age than those whose parents had no hearing problems, and a higher speech comprehension ratio, although there was no difference in the intelligibility of their speech. There was no difference in academic performances between those with a genetic aetiology but hearing parents (recessive), and those with an acquired

The Effects of Genetic Hearing Impairment in the Family. Edited by D. Stephens and L. Jones.
Copyright © 2006 by John Wiley & Sons, Ltd.

or unknown cause for their hearing loss. However, there were small numbers (27) in some groups and analyses lacked multivariate control.

Kusché et al. (1983) found better vocabulary achievement and comprehension in hearing-impaired children with 'deaf' parents compared with those with hearing parents but deaf siblings. However, again there were only 19 or 20 children in their groups.

Powers (2003) examined the results of the GCSE examination taken by 344 hearing-impaired children in 1995 and by 403 hearing-impaired children in 1996, in mainstream schools. GCSE is an examination sat in England at about age 16. Having hearing-impaired parents had a significant beneficial effect on both English and Mathematics in the 1996 cohort but not in the 1995 cohort. In multiple regression analyses the effect of parents' socio-economic status was however also significant, with children whose parents were in a higher socio-economic group tending to perform better.

In addition a range of studies (see Stephens, 2005) have shown that hearing-impaired children with hearing-impaired parents are less disturbed, have fewer behavioural problems and psychiatric disorders than those with hearing parents. For example, in an extensive recent study of over 1000 deaf students in Turkey, Polat (2003) found that parental hearing status was one of the most important predictors of psychosocial adjustment, as assessed on the Turkish adaptation of the Meadow/Kendall Social and Emotional Adjustment Inventory (Meadow & Dyssegaard, 1983). Compared with the deaf children of hearing parents, the deaf children of deaf parents were found to have improved levels of overall adjustment, social adjustment, self-image and emotional adjustment.

Several of these studies included only small numbers of children and none was able to exercise multivariate control over potentially confounding variables. Not all included details of the degree of parental deafness nor the means by which it was determined. The reported results therefore indicate a possible effect which requires further investigation.

Recently, a large UK study (Stacey et al., 2006) compared the achievements on a range of outcome measures of hearing-impaired children whose parents reported that at least one parent had at least some degree of hearing difficulties, with those for hearing-impaired children whose parents reported no hearing difficulties. After controlling for average (unaided) hearing level (AHL), age at onset of hearing-impairment, possession of a cochlear implant, age, gender, the number of additional disabilities, parental occupational skill level, and ethnicity, the following results were found. Teachers judged that children who had at least one parent who had at least some hearing difficulties displayed poorer auditory receptive capabilities than children who had parents with no hearing difficulties, although the data reported by parents did not display the same association (Stacey et al., 2006). Children whose parents had at least some hearing difficulties were reported by teachers to be more likely to use British Sign Language (BSL) and their parents reported that they were more likely to use BSL and Signed Supported English (SSE). Parents and teachers both reported such children to have better understanding of BSL and SSE than the children of parents with no hearing difficulties. The children of parents with hearing difficulties were also reported to have higher levels of educational achievement as measured by academic abilities, Key-stage attainments, and participation and engagement in education. Finally, in terms of quality of life, children whose parents had at least some hearing difficulties were reported by parents to have less positive feelings about their lives, but to need less help with social activities such as shopping and inviting friends than children whose parents who had no hearing difficulties (Stacey et al., 2006).

These analyses included up to 338 children whose parents had at least some hearing difficulties who could be compared with 2519 children whose parents had no hearing difficulties. Within the group of 338 children, as in previous papers (e.g. Polat, 2003), children were not differentiated according to whether they had totally deaf parents or parents with some hearing difficulties. In order to assess whether the reported judgements were equally applicable to both these groups of children we re-analysed the data after creating a new parental hearing variable. Additionally, we assessed whether these judgements differed according to whether children had hearing-impaired siblings. The subsequent analysis thereby seeks to identify whether the outcome for a child on a range of communication, academic and quality of life measures (as judged by parents and/or teachers) varies systematically according to whether a child has a parent or sibling with hearing difficulties, and the extent of those hearing difficulties, while controlling for the effects of other characteristics of the child and family.

METHODS

PARTICIPANTS AND PROCEDURES

A questionnaire-based ascertainment study of hearing-impaired children (permanent bilateral impairment > 40 dBHL) in the United Kingdom in 1998 identified 17,160 children aged between 3 years and 18 years. (Fortnum et al., 2001). The data reported here come from a study of short- and medium-term outcomes in a sample of these children, which included all children with severe or profound impairment, all with cochlear implants and 1 in 9 of those with moderate impairments (N = 8876). The parents of these 8876 children were asked to provide consent for their child's audiologist, teacher and parent to be sent a questionnaire.[1] Together, the information requested provided a description of each child's clinical and demographic history and level of

---

[1] The questionnaires are available at www.ihr.mrc.ac.uk/publications/papers/nesodhic. Further details of the methods employed to obtain the sample and to test it for its representativeness have been described by Fortnum et al. (submitted).

performance over a variety of outcome measures. Responding parents were asked to indicate if they themselves had 'no hearing difficulties', had 'some hearing difficulties' or were 'totally deaf'. They were also asked to indicate if other members of the child's family had 'some hearing difficulties' or were 'totally deaf'. These responses were combined into a variable which described each child's family hearing status. Children were categorised into *one* of the following groups, which were designed to reflect the extent and degree of family hearing impairment:

I   1 or 2 parents with total deafness (any number of hearing-impaired siblings)
II 1 or 2 parents with some hearing difficulties (any number of hearing-impaired siblings)
III ≥1 sibling with total deafness, parent(s) with no hearing difficulties
IV ≥1 sibling with some hearing difficulties, parent(s) with no hearing difficulties
V   no parents and no siblings with total deafness or some hearing difficulties

Those children who could potentially be categorised into more than one group were categorised into the lowest numbered group, e.g. children who had one parent with total deafness and one parent with some hearing difficulty were categorised into group I. The analyses on the impact of having hearing-impaired siblings were based on those children with hearing parents, as we hypothesised that having parents with hearing problems would be the primary influence on the children under consideration, with siblings having a secondary influence.

After controlling for the eight explanatory variables listed in Table 3.1, we sought to identify whether children's family hearing status was associated with how they were judged to perform in terms of auditory receptive capabilities, communication skills, educational achievements, and quality of life (described further below).

We used the same analysis techniques as those used previously by Stacey et al. (2006), but replaced the previous parental hearing status variable (no hearing difficulties vs at least some hearing difficulties) with the new family hearing status variable. It should be noted that the number of children included in each analysis varies according to the extent of missing data, which is determined firstly by how many parents or teachers provided complete information about the outcome measure in question and, secondly, by the number of children for whom complete data on other explanatory variables were available.

OUTCOME MEASURES

Auditory receptive capabilities

As described by Stacey et al. (2006) each child's auditory receptive capabilities were assessed by both parents and teachers using a modified version of

Table 3.1 Explanatory variables controlled in analyses of association between family
hearing status and outcome measures

Variable	Values
Gender	(i) Male, (ii) female
Age	Age in years on date questionnaire was returned
Ethnicity	(i) White, (ii) other
Average unaided (pre-operative) hearing level (AHL)	Unaided pure-tone air-conduction thresholds in the better-hearing ear averaged across four frequencies, 0.5, 1, 2 and 4 kHz
Age at onset of hearing impairment	(i) At birth, (ii) between the ages of 0 and 3 years, (iii) after 3 years of age
Number of additional disabilities	(i) None, (ii) one, (iii) two or more
Parental occupational skill level	Classification of the level of skill entailed in the parent's job, ranging from lowest to highest (i) Level 1, (ii) Level 2, (iii) Level 3, (iv) Level 4

Cochlear implantation	Group	Age at implantation	Duration of use
	(1)	<5 years	≥4 years
	(2)	≥5 years	≥4 years
	(3)	<5 years	≥2, <4 years
	(4)	≥5 years	≥2, <4 years
	(5)	<5 years	<2 years
	(6)	≥5 years	<2 years
	(7)	not implanted	NA

the Categories of Auditory Performance Scale (CAP – Archbold et al., 1995). Ordinal logistic regression analysis was used to assess the strength of the association between a child's auditory receptive capabilities and the family hearing status variable. The results are presented in terms of odds ratios (ORs). An OR of > 1 indicates that possession of the particular level of the explanatory variable was associated with higher levels of auditory receptive capability. In addition, the association is significant when the 95% confidence interval (95% c.i.) of an odds ratio does not include one.

Communication skills

For each of three modes of communication, Spoken Language (Speech), British Sign Language (BSL) and Sign Supported English (SSE), parents and teachers were asked to rate the children in three respects. These were whether the child used the mode of communication (Use), how well the child could understand other people using it (Perception) and how well other people could understand the child when he/she was using it (Intelligibility). As with auditory receptive capabilities, ordinal logistic regression analysis was used to assess the strength of the association between the modes of communication and a child's family hearing status.

Educational achievements

As described by Stacey et al. (2006), Categorical Principal Components Analysis (Meulman & Heiser, 1999) was used to derive three summary outcomes of educational achievement. These were (i) academic abilities in reading, writing, number, time, money and measurement rated by parents and teachers using category-referenced scales, (ii) performance on Key Stages of the English National Curriculum in reading, writing, maths, and science, as reported by teachers, and (iii) participation and engagement in education. The last entailed the teacher's report of the ability of the child to pay attention in small classes, how much they understood, and how engaged they were in group discussions. Teachers were also asked to report a fourth measure of educational achievement – a child's reading age. Linear regression analysis was used to estimate the association between each of these four measures of educational achievement and family hearing status. Within linear regression analyses a positive parameter estimate for a particular level of an explanatory variable indicates an association with higher levels of educational achievement. That association is significant when the 95% c.i. does not include zero.

Quality of life

Parents and teachers were asked to rate different aspects of the quality of life of the child and family, derived in part from the Child Health Questionnaire (Landgraf et al., 1996) and in part from other questions devised in consultation with teachers and parents (Stacey et al., 2006). Categorical Principal Components Analysis was used to condense responses into ten summary measures – disruption to family life (Disruption), child's satisfaction with their lives (Satisfaction), positive feelings about their lives (Feelings), concern for the future (Future), concerns about friendships (Friends), concerns about behaviour (Behaviour), concerns about physical and emotional well-being (Well-being), amount of help required with the social activities of shopping and inviting friends (Help, Shop & Friend), the amount of help required when using the telephone and using public transport (Help, Phone & Travel) (all reported by parents), and socialisation at school (Socialisation) which was reported by teachers. As with educational achievements, linear regression analysis was used to estimate the association between each of these summary measures of quality of life and family hearing status.

RESULTS

Consent to participate in the study was provided by the parents of 3274 children, with questionnaires being returned by 2858 parents, 2709 audiologists and 2241 teachers of the children.

FAMILY HEARING STATUS

The questions concerning family hearing were completed by 2857 parents. The parent(s) of 2519 children (88% of responding parents) were reported to have no hearing difficulties (Table 3.2). Among parents who reported a hearing difficulty, it was unusual for both parents to be reported as having some hearing difficulties (N = 17), but relatively common for just one parent to be reported as having such problems (N = 228). However, the presence of total deafness among parents was almost as commonly reported for both parents (N = 41) as for one (N = 52), possibly reflecting the tendency of Deaf people to choose Deaf partners.

Of the 2857 responding parents, 374 reported that their child had at least one sibling at least some hearing difficulties (Table 3.3). Approximately twice as many children were reported to have a sibling or siblings with some hearing difficulties (N = 246), compared to the number of children with siblings who were reported to be totally deaf (N = 128).

Information on parental and sibling hearing status was combined to form the new family hearing status variable (Table 3.4), as previously described.

In all analyses, children with parents and/or siblings with hearing difficulties (each of Groups I to IV) are compared with children with hearing parents and siblings (Group V). Only statistically significant results (p < 0.05) are summarised in the text.

Table 3.2 Parental hearing status

	N	%
No hearing-impaired parents	2519	88.2
1 parent with some hearing difficulties	228	8.0
2 parents with some hearing difficulties	17	0.6
1 parent with total deafness	52	1.8
2 parents with total deafness	41	1.4
Total	2857	100.0
Not reported	417	

Table 3.3 Sibling hearing status

	N	%
No hearing-impaired siblings	2483	86.9
1 sibling with some hearing difficulties	210	7.3
≥2 siblings with some hearing difficulties	36	1.3
1 sibling with total deafness	112	3.9
≥2 siblings with total deafness	16	0.6
Total	2857	100.0
Not reported	417	

Table 3.4 Family hearing status variable (FHS)

	N	%	FHS
No parents and no siblings with total deafness or some hearing difficulties	2264	79.2	V
≥1 sibling with some hearing difficulties, parent(s) with no hearing difficulties	169	5.9	IV
≥1 sibling with total deafness, parent(s) with no hearing difficulties	86	3.0	III
1 or 2 parents with some hearing difficulty, with or without siblings with hearing difficulties	245	8.6	II
1 or 2 parents with total deafness, with or without siblings with hearing difficulties	93	3.3	I
Total	2857	100.0	
Not reported	417		

Table 3.5 Strength of association between child's auditory receptive capabilities and family hearing status (reported as odds ratios)

Groups compared (see Table 3.4)	Parents	Teachers
I vs V	0.621*	0.742
II vs V	1.002	0.868
III vs V	0.953	1.114
IV vs V	1.116	1.136
N	2361	1788

* $p < 0.05$; ** $p < 0.01$; *** $p < 0.001$

AUDITORY RECEPTIVE CAPABILITIES

The only statistically significant effect of family hearing status on the measure of auditory receptive capabilities is that parents reported that children with 1 or 2 totally deaf parents (Group I) perform worse (Table 3.5).

COMMUNICATION SKILLS

Parents and teachers both reported more use of BSL and SSE among children with 1 or 2 deaf parents (Group I). Teachers reported more use of BSL among children with 1 or 2 parents with some hearing difficulties (Group II), and parents reported more use of speech among children with 1 or more totally deaf siblings (Group III) (Table 3.6).

Among children with 1 or 2 deaf parents (Group I), teachers reported worse perception of speech, but better perception of BSL and SSE, and parents reported better perception of BSL. Parents also reported better perception of

Table 3.6 Strength of association between child's use of each of three communication modes and family hearing status (reported as odds ratios)

Groups compared (see Table 3.4)	Speech		BSL		SSE	
	Parents	Teachers	Parents	Teachers	Parents	Teachers
I vs V	0.556	0.908	6.423***	5.355***	2.175**	3.090***
II vs V	1.312	0.782	1.235	1.658*	1.044	0.862
III vs V	4.007*	3.914	1.096	1.477	1.002	1.136
IV vs V	1.097	0.750	0.807	0.658	0.853	0.691
N	2593	1820	2587	1697	2583	1610

* $p < 0.05$; ** $p < 0.01$; *** $p < 0.001$

Table 3.7 Strength of association between child's perception (understanding) of each of three communication modes and family hearing status (reported as odds ratios)

Groups compared (see Table 3.4)	Speech		BSL		SSE	
	Parents	Teachers	Parents	Teachers	Parents	Teachers
I vs V	0.916	0.506*	1.749*	3.205**	1.339	3.340**
II vs V	1.013	1.072	1.295	1.017	1.830*	1.360
III vs V	0.782	0.832	1.050	0.900	0.996	1.125
IV vs V	0.879	1.171	1.412	0.799	0.864	0.740
N	2245	1602	1057	460	966	533

* $p < 0.05$; ** $p < 0.01$; *** $p < 0.001$

Table 3.8 Strength of association between child's intelligiblity (being understood) when using each of three communication modes and family hearing status (reported as odds ratios)

Groups compared (see Table 3.4)	Speech		BSL		SSE	
	Parents	Teachers	Parents	Teachers	Parents	Teachers
I vs V	0.918	0.602	0.968	2.635*	0.928	2.315*
II vs V	1.092	1.068	0.771	1.121	1.149	1.111
III vs V	0.939	0.516*	0.426**	1.561	0.589	1.009
IV vs V	0.939	1.207	0.698	0.629	0.761	1.011
N	2223	1596	1041	453	944	522

* $p < 0.05$; ** $p < 0.01$; *** $p < 0.001$

SSE for children with 1 or more parents with some hearing difficulties (Group II) (Table 3.7).

Finally, teachers reported better intelligibility when children with 1 or 2 totally deaf parents (Group I) used BSL or SSE, and worse intelligibility when children with 1 or more deaf siblings (Group III) used speech. Parents reported worse intelligibility of BSL among children with 1 or more deaf siblings (Group III) (Table 3.8).

EDUCATIONAL ACHIEVEMENTS

Parents reported better academic abilities for children with at least one parent with at least some hearing difficulties (Groups I and II). Teachers reported no significant differences in academic abilities but did report better reading ages and engagement for children with at least one totally deaf parent (Group I) and better Key Stage achievements for children with at least one sibling with some hearing difficulties (Group IV) (Table 3.9).

QUALITY OF LIFE

Children with 1 or 2 totally deaf parents (Group I) were reported to need less help when shopping and inviting friends. Parents of children with 1 or 2 parents with some hearing difficulties (Group II) reported that their child's hearing impairment led to more disruption, as did the parents of children with totally deaf sibling(s) (Group III). Children with 1 or 2 parents with some hearing difficulties (Group II) were also reported to have less positive feelings about their lives. Finally, children with sibling(s) with some hearing difficulties (Group IV) were reported to experience less satisfaction with a range of aspects of their lives (Table 3.10).

DISCUSSION

This study reports associations between the hearing status of a child's family and the child's academic and communicative performance and quality of life. All comparisons were made with the group of children with no parent and no siblings with any hearing difficulties while controlling other explanatory variables for outcomes.

Comparing children of deaf parents (Group I) with children from hearing families (Group V) the following significant associations were found:

Table 3.9 Strength of association between child's academic abilities (rated by parents and teachers), reading age, Key Stage achievements, and engagement (rated by teachers) and family hearing status (reported as parameter values)

Groups compared (see Table 3.4)	Academic abilities Parents	Academic abilities Teachers	Reading Age	Key Stages	Engagement
I vs V	0.167*	0.091	1.037*	0.298	0.278*
II vs V	0.088*	0.082	0.342	0.190	0.099
III vs V	0.008	0.070	0.455	−0.020	0.155
IV vs V	−0.021	−0.018	0.247	0.321**	−0.106
N	2 209	1 631	908	697	1 541

* p < 0.05; ** p < 0.01; *** p < 0.001

Table 3.10 Strength of association between ten quality of life measures (9 reported by parents and 1 by teachers) and family hearing status (reported as parameter values)

Group compared (see Table 3.4)	Disruption	Satisfaction	Feelings	Future	Friends	Behaviour	Well-being	Help, Shop & Friend	Help, Phone & Travel	Socialisation
I vs V	0.055	0.052	-0.161	0.254	-0.132	0.046	-0.200	0.207*	0.247	-0.016
II vs V	-0.190*	0.087	-0.224**	0.102	0.100	0.069	-0.019	0.126	0.060	0.127
III vs V	-0.331*	-0.108	0.055	0.113	-0.098	0.025	0.118	0.171	-0.426	-0.082
IV vs V	-0.122	-0.224*	-0.030	0.020	0.084	-0.076	0.052	0.118	-0.146	-0.030
N	1672	1672	1672	1672	1672	1672	1672	2059	534	1429

* $p < 0.05$; ** $p < 0.01$; *** $p < 0.001$

Children with deaf parents:

1. perceive and produce BSL and SSE better (in the judgements of teachers);
2. exhibit poorer perception of speech (in the judgement of teachers);
3. have poorer auditory receptive abilities (in the judgements of parents);
4. exhibit increased use of BSL and SSE (in the judgement of both parents and teachers);
5. display slightly, but significantly, higher academic abilities (in the judgement of parents), together with an older reading age and more engagement in the process of education (in the judgements of teachers);
6. require less help to perform the social tasks of shopping and inviting a friend to visit (in the judgement of parents).

The first four results support the previous literature and, in doing so, suggest that the present data are systematic, and thus that other results not previously reported are valid.

The final two results summarised above (5 and 6) have not previously been found reliably. Point 5 may reflect the benefits of early identification and early commitment to a viable form of language. Point 6 may reflect good use of manual communication or increased confidence in general.

Results arising from comparisons of Groups II, III and IV with Group V are harder to interpret. Of 140 comparisons involving Groups II to IV, 8 are significant at the $p < 0.05$ level and 3 at the $p < 0.01$ level (Tables 3.6 to 3.10). The three associations that met the more stringent significance level are:

1. Children with one or more siblings with total deafness were reported by their (hearing) parents to have poorer intelligibility of BSL and to use speech more, although teachers reported poorer intelligibility when speaking. The extent of use of BSL within the family may be an explanation.
2. Children with one or more siblings with some hearing difficulties achieve better Key Stage Results. This could reflect the possibility that a second hearing-impaired child is identified at an earlier age, and receives more appropriate educational support from an early age, than does a first hearing-impaired child. We might assume that approximately half the children with a hearing-impaired sibling were the second hearing-impaired child in the family.
3. Children with one or two parents with some hearing difficulties have less positive feelings about their lives. This final very significant association requires further exploration than is possible within these analyses.

From a genetic standpoint, these data do not allow further interpretation although it is likely that children with deaf siblings and deaf parents would have a dominant genetic disorder, whereas children with deaf siblings and hearing parents would be more likely to have a recessive condition.

The large number of children included in these analyses enabled control over the influence of a wide range of explanatory variables thereby generating more robust evidence of the effect of family hearing status than has been achieved in previous studies. Even so, due to the relatively small numbers of children included in each analysis it is not possible to analyse beyond two descriptive levels of impairment and two levels of family relationship. In addition we are unable to break the groups down to distinguish children with hearing-impaired parent(s) who do and do not have hearing-impaired siblings nor can we separately analyse children with one or two totally deaf or hearing-impaired parents. More detailed information on family hearing status would therefore need to be gathered to further explore the association between family history and children's achievements.

In conclusion, although these data do not allow full interpretation of the effects that relate to the hearing status of siblings, they do provide a clear indication of the effects of the hearing status of parents. Where one or more parents is totally deaf, hearing-impaired children display small but significant advantages in the use of communication modes with manual elements and in academic attainment, reading age, and engagement in the process of education. It is not surprising that the hearing-impaired children of deaf parents should sign better than the hearing-impaired children of hearing parents. The more interesting result is that there are advantages in other domains. Compared with the hearing-impaired children of hearing parents, the hearing-impaired children of deaf parents are likely to be identified earlier leading to earlier provision of appropriate social, linguistic, and educational support. Thus, our data provide indirect evidence of the benefits of early identification.

REFERENCES

Archbold S, Lutman ME, Marshall DH (1995) Categories of auditory performance. *Annals of Otology, Rhinology and Laryngology* 104: 312–14.

Conrad R (1979) *The Deaf Schoolchild*. London. Harper & Row.

Fortnum H, Summerfield Q, Marshall D, Davis A, Bamford J (2001) Prevalence of permanent childhood hearing impairment in the United Kingdom and implications for universal neonatal hearing screening: questionnaire based ascertainment study. *British Medical Journal* 323: 536–9.

Fortnum, HM, Stacey PC, Summerfield AQ (*submitted*) An exploration of demographic bias among participants in a questionnaire survey of hearing-impaired children: implications for comparisons. *International Journal of Pediatric Otolaryngology*.

Kusché CA, Greenberg MT, Garfield TS (1983) Nonverbal intelligence and verbal achievement in deaf adolescents: and examination of heredity and environment. *American Annals of the Deaf* 128: 458–66.

Landgraf JM, Abetz L, Ware JE (1996) *The CHQ User's Manual*. Boston MA: The Health Institute, New English Medical Center.

Meadow KP, Dyssegaard B (1983) Teachers ratings of deaf children: an American-Danish comparison. *American Annals of the Deaf* 12: 900–8.

Meulman JJ, Heiser WJ (1999) *SPSS Categories 10.0*. SPSS Inc., Chicago.

Polat F (2003) Factors affecting psychosocial adjustment of deaf students. *Journal of Deaf Studies and Deaf Education* 8: 325–9.

Powers S (2003) Influences of student and family factors on academic outcomes of mainstream secondary school deaf students. *Journal of Deaf Studies and Deaf Education* 8: 57–8.

Stacey PC, Fortnum HM, Barton GR, Summerfield AQ (2006) Hearing-impaired children in the UK I: Auditory performance, communication skills, educational achievements, quality of life and cochlear implantation. *Ear and Hearing* 27: 161–86.

Stephens D (2005) The impact of hearing impairment in children. In D Stephens, L Jones (eds) *The Impact of Genetic Hearing Impairment*. London: Whurr, pp. 73–105.

Vernon McK, Koh SD (1970) Early manual communication and deaf children's achievement. *American Annals of the Deaf* 115: 527–36.

4 Early Childhood Hearing Impairment and Family History: A Long-Term Perspective

PER-INGE CARLSSON AND BERTH DANERMARK

INTRODUCTION

Hearing impairment is common and affects social participation and quality of life in many different ways (Parving et al., 2001). Genetic hearing impairment has been estimated to account for at least 50% of hearing impairment of early onset (Morton, 1991) the present chapter is based on a cohort study of all people born between 1956 and 1966 with hearing impairment who received audiological rehabilitation at the Department of Audiology at the Central Hospital in Karlstad, Sweden. Several studies describe the situation of children through the years of education (Parving & Christensen, 1993; Dauman et al., 2000) but few studies have considered the long-term outcome and the impact of genetic factors for these individuals.

Most studies dealing with genetic hearing impairment focus on deaf children with or without deaf parents. In the studies by Vernon and Koh (1970) and Conrad (1979) the effects of having a genetic aetiology and of being a child of deaf parents were separated. These authors concluded that it is the fact of having a deaf parent that is important, rather than having a known genetic hearing impairment. Among the few studies dealing with the psychosocial consequences of genetic hearing impairment, Parving et al. (2002) and Huttunen et al. (1999) have focused on education and employment among people with genetic versus non-genetic hearing impairment. Although the genetic hearing-impaired group had poorer hearing in Parving's study, there were no differences in education and postgraduate training between the two study groups. The authors suggest that the lack of difference between the study groups may partially be explained by the higher proportion of subjects provided with hearing aids in the genetic group. Parving also investigated general well-being and found no differences between the two study groups. However, those authors emphasised that

The Effects of Genetic Hearing Impairment in the Family. Edited by D. Stephens and L. Jones.
Copyright © 2006 by John Wiley & Sons, Ltd.

the questionnaire used in the study was insensitive to any psychosocial impact of genetic hearing impairment.

Huttunen et al. (1999) studied late outcome of educational and employment status in a Finnish cohort of people with genetic vs non-genetic hearing impairment. Forty patients participated and 16 (31%) had a genetic aetiology. The cohort as a whole did not achieve educationally as well as their hearing peers. However, subjects with genetic aetiology did not differ from subjects without genetic aetiology in the study. Furthermore, the unemployment rate was more than double in the Finnish cohort compared with the reference population, but the genetic and non-genetic groups did not differ from each other. Huttunen concluded that it is the degree of hearing impairment rather than the aetiology that affects the late outcome.

Today, molecular diagnostics for hereditary hearing disorders is beginning to be available and can be helpful in genetic counselling of hearing-impaired / deaf individuals. However, the majority of people with hearing impairment / deafness do not receive a molecular diagnosis (confirmed mutation/s) or genetic counselling (Arnos et al., 1991). In that context, it is important to bear in mind that having a family history of hearing impairment (FHHI) may influence an individual's life in many respects.

The influence of having a perceived FHHI has been studied by Stephens et al. (2003) in a population study. That study showed an association between having a FHHI and the individual's emotional response to their hearing difficulties. Annoyance experienced as a result of hearing loss, tinnitus or phonophobia was more pronounced in individuals with a FHHI. Thus, those with a FHHI seem to be more affected by hearing problems in general than are those without such a family history.

In the present chapter, we shall discuss how a perceived FHHI affects social and family life, school situation, employment, leisure and audiological rehabilitation in a long-term perspective.

MATERIAL AND DEFINITIONS

The Swedish cohort (born 1956–66) included all individuals with early onset of hearing impairment (diagnosed before the age of 5), affecting one or both ears, who passed through audiological rehabilitation at the Department of Audiology at the Central Hospital in Karlstad, Sweden. The total number of the cohort was 61 people, 56 of whom participated in a first study performed in 1988, including audiometric data, a personal interview and a questionnaire (Bergström, 1991). Fifteen years later, in 2003, a new questionnaire including the same questions as had been asked in the 1988 study was mailed to the subjects. The response rate was 89% (50 out of 56), of whom 30 were females and 20 were males. The respondents did not differ from the non-respondents with regard to gender, the degree of hearing impairment, or presence of a family history.

Audiometric measurements were performed and the results from 1988 and 2003 were compared. Based on the audiometric data, the hearing impairment in the cohort was sensorineural in 47 cases and mixed in 3 cases. Four subjects had a hearing-impaired child but no other hearing-impaired relatives. These four subjects were defined as having no perceived FHHI.

The questionnaire contained 34 questions regarding FHHI, hearing situation, tinnitus, education, working life, family life, leisure and rehabilitation. The question concerning FHHI was worded: *Do any of your relatives have a hearing impairment? If, yes, who?* The subjects were defined as having a FHHI if they answered: *yes.* The questionnaire is shown as Appendix 4.1.

The subjective hearing situation was examined using questions on changes in hearing ability in different situations over the past ten years. Also, the presence of tinnitus and the degree to which tinnitus affected daily life were examined. The mean better ear pure-tone threshold between 0.5 and 4 kHz (M4) was calculated and compared with the audiometric data from 1988. A speech recognition test in quiet was performed. Progression of hearing impairment was defined as a deterioration of >15 dBHL in the mean pure-tone threshold (Stephens, 2001).

The subjects were divided into four groups according to the mean hearing threshold of the better ear. The groups followed standard definitions of hearing impairment and are shown in Table 4.1. The frequencies of subjects in each group are shown in Table 4.2. In 7 of the 50 respondents we were unable to obtain a new audiogram in 2003.

Two types of educational setting were distinguished: (1) integration in an ordinary school with or without extra help of a teacher for hearing-impaired / deaf children and (2) a special school unit for hearing-impaired / deaf children. Three different types of employment status were asked about: (1) stable employment (2) all types of employment (including stable and unstable employment, i.e. all types of contract on a regular basis), and (3) no employment (searching for a job). Also questions about comfort at work, whether any kind of harassment occurred at work and whether the respondents want to leave their work because of their hearing impairment were asked.

Table 4.1 Degree of hearing impairment in the four groups in the Swedish study

Hearing impairment	Degree of hearing impairment
Mild	>20 dB < 40 dB
Moderate	≥40 dB < 70 dB
Severe	≥70 dB < 95 dB
Profound	≥95 dB

Table 4.2 Audiometric results for hearing-impaired individuals with a FHHI, without a FHHI, and in the total cohort

Audiometric results	With a FHHI n = 12	Without a FHHI n = 31	Total cohort n = 43*
Mild	2 (17%)	5 (16%)	7 (16%)
Moderate	6 (50%)	16 (52%)	22 (51%)
Severe	3 (25%)	5 (16%)	8 (19%)
Profound	1 (8%)	5 (16%)	6 (14%)
Progressive	3 (25%)	8 (26%)	11 (25%)

* Audiometric data (2003) are missing from seven individuals

Table 4.3 Hearing-impaired relatives of people in the Swedish cohort

Relatives with hearing impairment	Number
Mother	5
Father	3
Sister	2
Brother	1
Cousin	1
Aunt	1
Father, mother, cousin	1
FHHI (all)	14

Questions on marital status and the number of children who had been born were asked. The number of children they had with a hearing impairment was also investigated. Different activities during leisure time were considered. Audiological rehabilitation was estimated using questions on hearing-aid use, how well the individuals had informed those around them about their hearing impairments and how much audiological rehabilitation they were currently receiving.

Subjects with a FHHI were compared with those without a FHHI regarding the parameters described above and, when available, we also present data for an age-matched population.

For analysing differences between the groups with and without a FHHI Fisher's exact test was used.

RESULTS

Of the participants, 28% (14/50) had a FHHI. Table 4.3 shows which relatives they reported as having a hearing impairment.

Table 4.4 shows the numbers in the different audiometric categories for the groups with a FHHL, groups without a FHHL, and the total cohort. It may be

Table 4.4 Frequencies of different responses for hearing-impaired individuals with a FHHI, without a FHHI, in the total cohort and in an age-matched reference population in Sweden

Questionnaire results	With a FHHI n = 14	Without a FHHI n = 36	Total cohort n = 50	Reference population
Increasing hearing problems	9 (64%)	18 (51%)	27 (55%)*	
Tinnitus	4 (29%)	13 (36%)	17 (34%)	
Hearing aid/s use (>6 hours/day)	9 (64%)	18 (50%)	27 (54%)	
Senior high school	13 (93%)	28 (78%)	41 (82%)	85%
University	5 (36%)[1]	4 (11%)	9 (18%)	32%
Employment (stable)	11 (79%)	22 (61%)	33 (66%)	
Work in noisy environment	3 (25%)	11 (31%)	14 (30%)*	
Want to leave work	4 (33%)[1]	2 (6%)	6 (13%)*	
Married	5 (36%)	8 (22)	13 (26%)	47%
Married/live-in relationships	9 (64%)	23 (64%)	32 (64%)	
Divorced	0	1 (3%)	1 (2%)	12%
Having children	12 (86%)	22 (61%)	34 (68%)	

* Number of responses to the question not equal to 50
[1] $p < 0.05$

noted that fewer people with a FHHI had a profound impairment but if we sum severe and profound impairment the difference disappears.

In Table 4.4, it may be seen that subjects with a FHHI reported increasing subjective hearing problems over the past ten years more often than did subjects without a FHHI, despite the fact that measured progressive hearing loss in the two groups was identical (Table 4.3). The presence of tinnitus did not differ between the two groups. Hearing-aid use was slightly higher among subjects with a FHHI but there was no difference in the total audiological rehabilitation (hearing-aid use, how well the hearing-impaired person had informed those around them about their hearing impairment and how much audiological rehabilitation they were currently receiving) between the two groups.

Subjects with a FHHI went to senior high school and university and had a stable employment more often than did subjects without a FHHI. In the whole cohort, 88% had some kind of contract in the labour market, almost identical to the reference population (89%), and there were no differences between the groups with and without a FHHI. Comfort at work was reported high (94–100%) in both groups, but despite this, 13% in the whole cohort wanted to leave their job because of their hearing problems, and the majority (67%) of these subjects belonged to the group with a FHHI. The total number of subjects who wanted to leave their job was only six, so one cannot draw any firm conclusions from these figures.

Harassment at work was reported by 15% of the subjects; no differences were revealed between the groups with and without a FHHI. Fewer people with a FHHI were working in a noisy environment.

Subjects with a FHHL were more likely to be married than were subjects without a FHHI. However, if we lump together the two groups 'married' and 'live-in relationships', there was no difference. One interesting observation was that subjects with a FHHI were more likely to have children, despite the fact that, in the personal interview in 1988, several of these subjects expressed worries about having a hearing-impaired child. Two subjects in the group with a FHHI had a hearing-impaired child, but this did not differ from the group without a FHHI.

During leisure time, subjects with a FHHI attended courses slightly more often, but there was no difference between the two groups in taking an active part in an association or attending cinemas or theatres.

Overall, statistical analysis showed P-values < 0.05 for two of the questions ('university' and 'wanted to quit work'). Otherwise, the results showed no statistically significant differences between the groups with and without a FHHI for any of the parameters.

DISCUSSION AND CONCLUSIONS

The Swedish cohort study in this chapter showed small overall differences between subjects with and without a FHHI. It must be remembered that, when analysing subgroups in the study group, sample size decreases and differences, or lack of differences, must be interpreted very carefully.

Because this is a long-term follow-up study of a total population in a cohort, some interesting observations can be made. For example, subjects with a FHHI reported increasing subjective hearing problems over the past ten years more often than did subjects without FHHI. This is in accord with an epidemiological study performed by Stephens et al. (2003), which showed that, for those with mild to moderate hearing problems (67.5% in the Swedish cohort), the overall effect of having a FHHI is that such individuals are more affected by any hearing problems than are those without a FHHI. In addition, the best predictor of acceptance of audiological rehabilitation has been found to be the impact of the hearing impairment on the individual (Stephens et al., 1990). Furthermore, subjects with a FHHI used hearing aids more frequently than those without a FHHI in the present Swedish cohort. However, we were unable to find differences between the two groups in the other aspects of rehabilitation.

Another difference noted was that subjects with a FHHI attended high school and university and had a stable employment more often then did subjects without a FHHI. This pattern may be explained by awareness, among individuals in the Swedish cohort with a FHHI, of the vulnerable labour market situation for hearing-impaired people (Danermark et al., 2003). Thus, individuals with a FHHI have striven for a high level of education. In line with this assumption, in the present study, people with a FHHI were less likely to work in noisy environments than those without a FHHI – presumably due to their awareness of how such environments may affect people with hearing problems.

Another interesting observation was that, in the personal interviews conducted in 1988, several of the subjects with a FHHI expressed their worries about having a hearing-impaired child. Despite this, today, subjects in the study with a FHHI were more likely to have had children than subjects without a FHHI. Thus, a FHHI did not seem to play an important role in the decision to have children. In another Swedish study (Carlsson et al., 2004/2005), women with early onset of deafness (profound hearing impairment) had fewer children than did the reference population, so the severity of the impairment may play a more important role in this matter than does having a FHHI.

The overall small differences between the groups with and without a FHHI in the Swedish cohort are in line with the results of the few other studies that have investigated education and employment in connection with genetic vs non-genetic hearing impairment. The Swedish study also included family life, leisure time and audiological rehabilitation, questions that also showed only small differences between the two groups. The majority of studies in the literature that have focused on the psychosocial impact of hearing impairment with genetic and non-genetic aetiologies have been with prelingually deaf children. For mild to moderate hearing impairment (not profound hearing impairment), the few studies that are available have shown no differences between subjects with and without a genetic impairment in terms of psychosocial behaviour. However, there are indications that having a FHHI increases a hearing-impaired person's hearing problems and the general emotional impact of their hearing impairment. We must also remember that not all the effects were negative. For example, a higher level of education was achieved by those with a FHHL in the Swedish cohort. Studies on larger samples, including personal interviews, are required to further reveal the long-term psychosocial outcomes of having a FHHI.

REFERENCES

Arnos KS, Israel J, Cunningham M (1991) Genetic counseling of the deaf. Medical and cultural considerations. *Annals of the New York Academy of Sciences* 630: 212–22.

Bergström B (1991) En uppföljning av hörselskadade ungdomar i Värmland. *Audio Nytt* 4: 18–23.

Carlsson PI, Danermark B, Borg E (2004/2005) Marital status and birthrate of deaf people in two Swedish counties: the impact of social environment in terms of deaf community. *American Annals of the Deaf* 149: 415–20.

Conrad R (1979) *The Deaf Schoolchild*. New York: Harper & Row.

Danermark B, Coniavitis Gellerstedt L (2003) Att höra till: – om hörselskadades psykosociala arbetsmiljö. örebro: örebro Universitet.

Dauman R, Daubech Q, Gavilan I, Colmet L, Delaroche M, Michas N et al. (2000) Long-term outcome of childhood hearing deficiency. *Acta Otolaryngologica* 120: 205–8.

Huttunen K, Sorri M, Väryryen M, Mäki-Torkko E, Lindholm P, Leisti J (1999) Educational outcome and employment of Finns with prelingual genetic vs non-genetic hearing impairment – a 15 years follow up. *European Work Group on Genetics of Hearing Impairment – Info Letter* 6: 36–7.

Morton NE (1991) Genetic epidemiology of hearing impairment. *Annals of the New York Academy of Sciences* 630: 16–31.

Parving A, Christensen B (1993) Training and employment in hearing-impaired subjects at 20–35 years of age. *Scandinavian Audiology* 22: 133–9.

Parving A, Christensen B, Stephens SDG (2002) Genetic hearing impairment and pyschosocial consequences. *Journal of Audiological Medicine* 11: 161–9.

Parving A, Parving I, Erlendsson A, Christensen B (2001) Some experiences with hearing disability/handicap and quality of life measures. *Audiology* 40: 208–14.

Stephens D (2001) Audiological terms. In A Martini, M Mazzoli, A Read, D Stephens (eds) *Definitions and Guidelines in Genetic Hearing Impairment*. London: Whurr, pp. 9–14.

Stephens D, Lewis P, Davis A (2003) The influence of a perceived family history of hearing difficulties in an epidemiological study of hearing problems. *Audiological Medicine* 1: 228–31.

Stephens SD, Meredith R, Callaghan DE, Hogan S, Rayment A (1990) Early intervention and rehabilitation: factors influencing outcome. *Acta Otolaryngologica* Suppl. 476: 221–5.

Vernon M, Koh S (1970) Effects of manual communication on deaf children's educational achievment, linguistic competence, oral skills, and psychological development. *American Annals of the Deaf* 115: 527–36.

APPENDIX 4.1

QUESTIONNAIRE

Family history of hearing impairment

Do any of your relatives have a hearing impairment? [ ] yes [ ] no

If, yes, who? ....

Hearing situation

Do you feel that your hearing impairment has increased during the last 10 years?

[ ] yes [ ] no

How do you feel your total overall hearing level is today compared with 10 years ago?

[ ] much worse
[ ] worse
[ ] equal
[ ] better

Describe your overall hearing level today compared with 10 years ago

....

Tinnitus

Do you have tinnitus? (Any kind of sounds in your ear/s) [ ] yes [ ] no

If yes, describe how your tinnitus affects your daily life..

....

Education

Senior high school [ ] yes [ ] no

Integration in an ordinary school [ ]

Special school unit [ ]

Programme..

University [ ] yes [ ] no
Town..

Programme..

Any other type of education after senior high school

....

Are you studying now?

....

Working life

What kind of work do you do at present?..

– employment status [ ] stable [ ] unstable [ ] any type of employment

[ ] no employment

Previous work

– employment status [ ] stable [ ] unstable

Have you left any job because of your hearing problems [ ] yes [ ] no

Do you use hearing aids at work? [ ] yes [ ] no

If yes: [ ] only on certain occasions
           [ ] daily, less than 2 hours
           [ ] daily, 2 to 6 hours
           [ ] daily, more than 6 hours

Do you use other kinds of technical support at work? [ ] yes [ ] no

If yes, describe the technical support..

Have you informed your co-workers / manager about your hearing impairment?

– co-workers   [ ] yes [ ] no
– manager   [ ] yes [ ] no

How much does your hearing impairment affect you negatively at work?

[ ] very much [ ] much [ ] not much [ ] not at all

How would you describe your contact with your co-workers?

[ ] very good [ ] good [ ] bad [ ] very bad

Do you feel comfortable at work?

[ ] yes [ ] no

Do you want to leave work because of your hearing impairment?

[ ] yes [ ] no

Do you work in a noisy environment?

[ ] yes [ ] no

If yes, [ ] always [ ] often [ ] seldom [ ] never

Have you experienced harassment at work?

[ ] yes [ ] no

Family life

Single [ ]

Live-in relationship [ ]

Married [ ]

Divorced [ ]

If you are married or live in a live-in relationship:

Does your partner have a hearing impairment? [ ] yes [ ] no

Do you have children? [ ] yes, number. . . . [ ] no

Have you adopted a child/children? [ ] yes [ ] no

Do any of your children have a hearing impairment? [ ] yes, number . . . [ ] no

Leisure

Are you a member of a club or association? [ ] yes [ ] no

If yes, describe the association and your role in the association

....

Have you left an association because of your hearing impairment?

[ ] yes [ ] no

How often do you

	more than 4 times/year	1–2 times/year	not at all
(a) Go the cinema	[ ]	[ ]	[ ]
(b) Go to the theatre	[ ]	[ ]	[ ]
(c) Go dancing	[ ]	[ ]	[ ]
(d) Visit church	[ ]	[ ]	[ ]
(e) Attend courses	[ ]	[ ]	[ ]

During leisure time, do you spend more time with hearing-impaired friends than with normally hearing friends?

[ ] yes [ ] no

Do you use hearing aids during your leisure time? [ ] yes [ ] no

If yes: [ ] only at certain occasions
          [ ] daily, less than 2 hours
          [ ] daily, 2 to 6 hours
          [ ] daily, more than 6 hours

Do you use other types of technical support during your leisure time?

[ ] yes [ ] no

If yes, describe the technical support...

Audiological rehabilitation

Describe the audiological rehabilitation you are receiving today

....

Do you think that the audiological rehabilitation you are receiving today is enough?

[ ] yes [ ] no

If no, what are you missing?

....

5 Effects on the Working Life of a History of Hearing Problems in the Family of Origin

LOTTA CONIAVITIS GELLERSTEDT AND BERTH DANERMARK

INTRODUCTION AND EARLIER RESEARCH

It seems that questions concerning the impact of genetic hearing impairment have gradually developed into an interest in questions related to the occurrence of a history of hearing difficulties in the family. One reason for this is that we seldom know the specific genetic hearing impairment, as genetic testing, for various reasons, is rarely carried out. Hearing problems in one's family, on the contrary, could constitute part of a lived or mediated experience and consequently are often known. Moreover, they could, in different ways, have an impact on a person's dispositions, attitudes, coping and perhaps even his or her choices.

Studies reported by Carlsson and Danermark (this volume, Chapter 4) indicate that various comparisons between people with and without a genetic hearing impairment do not reveal any major differences and also that having a family history of hearing impairment (FHHI) seems to be of greater importance to people than having a genetic hearing impairment (see also Kramer et al., this volume, Chapter 6)

Acceptance of audiological rehabilitation has been related to the emotional impact of hearing impairment according to British studies. The impairment itself and activity limitations did not explain all of the emotional impact, however. In a study investigating whether a FHHI influenced the impact that hearing loss had on the individual, Stephens et al. (2003) found that the greater the impact, the more likely there was to be a FHHI.

In a cohort study of 50 people with early onset of hearing impairment, no significant differences in terms of hearing situation, tinnitus, education, working life, family life, leisure and rehabilitation were found between those who had a history of hearing difficulties in their family and those who did not. However, some general observations could be made. People with a FHHI seemed to be more affected by hearing problems than those without (which is in accord with the study by Stephens et al., 2003). They seemed to be more frequent users of hearing aids and to be somewhat better-off in terms of education and work. A question related to the latter observations is whether people with experiences of family hearing difficulties and with a hearing loss themselves since early childhood take measures in terms of, for example, education to be well equipped when entering the labour market (Carlsson & Danermark, this volume, Chapter 4).

It is hardly surprising that people with a history of hearing loss in their families of origin are affected by these circumstances in various ways. A person's psychobiography is moulded through her/his experiences, cultural influences, group affinities etc. during the course of life and contributes to her/his attitudes and predispositions (Layder, 1997). Undoubtedly, such experiences could lead people to make certain decisions regarding education, type of work etc. However, the existence of a history of hearing impairment in the family is only one of many factors having an impact on such decisions. Presumably such an impact would be greater in those with early onset of hearing problems as compared to those with later onset or no hearing impairment. But, as well as affecting important choices in life, having the experience of hearing problems in one's family could possibly influence the way people are affected by and cope with their own hearing impairment, as is indicated in the studies by Stephens et al. (2003) and Carlsson and Danermark (this volume, Chapter 4). More research into the field of the -family history of hearing impairment and the implications for audiological rehabilitation would then be useful.

AIM AND PURPOSE

The aim and purpose of this chapter is to compare some aspects of people in employment who are hearing-impaired between those with or without familial history of hearing problems. The study was conducted in Sweden.

MATERIALS AND METHOD

The *source* of empirical data in this study is (a) *a short questionnaire* sent to people with a hearing loss (patients at audiological clinics) who had three years earlier answered (b) *a comprehensive questionnaire* on working life conditions and health. In some cases (c) *national statistics* were also used.

In the original sample of 781 patients aged 20–64 years, 539 responded (70%). Of these, 94 were excluded because they had, for various reasons, not been working for the last three years, mainly due to early retirement, but also to long-term sick leave and unemployment. In conclusion, the first data collection (carried out in the late 2001) left us with a sample of 445 respondents in the labour force with hearing impairment. The original sample was randomly drawn from all patients visiting audiological clinics over the previous 24 months in the Örebro and Värmland counties of Sweden. Comparison of non-respondents with respondents did not show any differences with regard to sex, age or diagnosis. Furthermore, we have no indications that using a sample from the selected counties would be associated with any systematic bias. Details of the theoretical and empirical considerations, data collection, empirical results and analysis etc. in relation to the original sample may be found in Danermark and Coniavitis Gellerstedt (2003, 2004a,b) and in Coniavitis Gellerstedt and Danermark (2004).

Respondents were re-contacted 3 years later and asked about their current situation and any changes since 2001 in relation to work, and to answer three questions about the presence of hearing problems in the family.

This second questionnaire was sent to 434 people (11 had died or emigrated since 2001 or could not be reached by mail) of whom 376 (87%) responded. The empirical data presented in this article are based on answers from these 376 respondents to the short questionnaire of 2004 and to the comprehensive questionnaire of 2001.

Some basic characteristics of the 2004 sample are shown in Table 5.1

Non-respondents were somewhat younger and there seemed to be a sex-related pattern regarding diagnosis and severity of hearing loss: sensorineural hearing loss was more common among female than male respondents but among non-respondents the pattern was the reverse. More severe hearing losses were also more common among female than male respondents and this pattern was even more accentuated among non-respondents.

Table 5.1 Basic characteristics of sample

	Men	Women	Total
2004 sample	268	166	434
Number of questionnaires sent out	(62%)	(38%)	(100%)
Respondents	226	150	376
Non respondents	42	16	58
Response rate	84%	90%	87%
Mean age 2004			
Respondents	57	55	56
Non-respondents	56	52	55
Sensorineural hearing loss			
Respondents	71%	82%	75%
Non-respondents	76%	50%	69%
Mean pure tone average (PTA)			
Respondents	25	37	30
Non-respondents	24	43	29
Marked hearing loss (PTA ≥ 56)			
Respondents	5%	13%	8%
Non-respondents	0%	23%	5%

OPERATIONALISATION AND PREVALENCE OF FAMILY HISTORY

Respondents were asked whether anyone in their family has (or had) hearing problems and, if this was the case, they were also asked to fill in a table indicating the relative(s) in question and the corresponding age of onset. The *relatives* pre-printed in the table were mother, father, sister, brother, grandparents: mother's mother, mother's father, father's mother, father's father (this detailed way is the common way of designating grandparents in the Swedish language), daughter, son and 'other family member, who?' *Age of onset*: The question '*Since what age has this relative had problems with hearing?*' was to be answered by filling in the table with the following intervals given: His/her whole life; Since childhood/adolescence; Since he/she was aged 20–44; Since he/she was aged 45–64; After 64 years of age; Age of onset unknown to the respondent.

Obviously information gathered in this way picks up a wide range of occurrences of hearing loss in the family. Indeed, 60% of the respondents indicated that one or more members of their family has (or had) problems with hearing loss, while 36% have no family member with hearing loss and 4% answer that they do not know (for further details, see Table 5.2).

For the purpose of this article *Family History of Hearing Impairment* (*FHHI*) is defined as onset of hearing problems before the age of 45 in the respondent's mother and/or father and/or onset before the age of 20 in the respondent's brother and/or sister (FHHI, family of origin, see below). This would presumably mirror an occurrence of hearing impairment in the respondent's family of origin during her/his childhood/adolescence. Coding of family history according to the following criteria has been made:

1. *FHHI, family of origin* (*first-degree relatives*): Occurrence of family history in family of origin (mother and/or father with onset before the age of 45 and/or sibling before the age of 20)

Table 5.2 Occurrence of family history, sex and age

	2004 respondents	Without family history* (3)	With family history (2)	FHHI, family of origin (1)
Women	**100% (n = 150)**	28%	72%	15%
<50 years	100% (n = 32)	38%	62%	19%
>50 years	100% (n = 118)	25%	75%	14%
Men	**100% (n = 226)**	48%	52%	10%
<50 years	100% (n = 37)	51%	49%	24%
>50 years	100% (n = 189)	48%	52%	7%
Both sexes	**100% (n = 376)**	40%	60%	12%
<50 years	100% (n = 69)	45%	55%	22%
>50 years	100% (n = 307)	39%	61%	10%

* Including those with a family history not known to respondent

2. *With family history of hearing impairment*: People coded as 1 (above) or occurrence of family history in family of origin with onset at later age than in 1 above and/or any other relative (including their own child and spouse) with onset at any time in life

3. *Without family history of hearing impairment*: No family history (134 respondents) or no family history known (17 respondents)

Table 5.2 shows that the occurrence of a family history among our respondents (people in the labour force who are patients at audiological clinics) was 12% when defined as occurrence of hearing problems in the respondent's family of origin during the respondent's childhood/adolescence (mother and/or father with onset before the age of 45 and/or sibling with onset before the age of 20).[1] Occurrence of a family history more generally among any relative (including own children and spouse) and with onset at any time in life was 60% among our respondents.

Table 5.2 also indicates that occurrence of a family history of hearing problems seems to be overall more frequently reported by women in our sample ($\chi^2 = 11.0$, 1 df, p = 0.001). Moreover, we can observe that middle-aged people (and in particular women) report a history of hearing problems in their family more frequently than younger people following the broad definition ('With family history' in Table 5.2). This is, perhaps, not surprising as the onset of age-related hearing impairment might be a more frequent topic of conversation among ageing relatives. Finally, however, we also observe that reports of a history of hearing problems in family of origin ('FHHI, family of origin' in Table 5.2) appears to be more frequent among younger than among older respondents (22% as compared to 10% – NS). At least two circumstances could bring about this (possible) pattern. One is that the prevalence of hearing difficulties in the population (in Sweden) is increasing, at least among women and young people (Statistics Sweden, 2003: 46; Swedish Government Official Reports, 2001: 56, p. 50) and, thus the number of people experiencing hearing problems in family of origin also increases. A further possible explanation is that people with a history of hearing problems in their family of origin may have left the labour market (due to early retirement, for instance) to a larger extent in the older age-group as compared to the younger one. We shall return to this later.

The prevalence of a history of hearing problems in the family in our study differs from other reports due to differences in populations and differences in operationalisation. Stephens et al. (2003) estimate for instance that 11% in a total population (of people with and without hearing impairment) have a family history of hearing impairment. Family history is then defined by a 'Yes' answer to the following question: 'Did any of your parents, children, brothers or sisters have great difficulty in hearing before the age of 55 years?' In their

---

[1] Occurrence rises to 30–35% among women and 26% among men (if we include occurrence of hearing problem in any of the parents with onset before the age of 65).

study of 50 people with hearing impairment with onset before the age of 5 years, Carlsson and Danermark (this volume, Chapter 4) found that 28% of them had a family history of hearing impairment. A French study was carried out via a website ('France Acouphènes') where people could answer the following question: 'Do or did other members of your family (brothers, sisters, parents, grandparents etc.) have problems with their hearing?' 122 out of 300 (41%) reported having a family history of hearing problems and/or tinnitus (this volume, Chapter 12).

RESULTS

INTRODUCTION

The question to be investigated is whether there are significant differences between people in the labour force with hearing impairment who (a) have and (b) have not experienced hearing problems in their family of origin (parents, siblings) during their childhood/adolescence. The initial assumption is that having a FHHI in family of origin matters and has an impact on the experienced consequences of hearing impairment, coping and even choices in life.

In the subsequent presentation results are systematically given for the total group of respondents, for those without family history ((3) in Table 5.2) and for those with a FHHI in family of origin ((1) in Table 5.2). The rationale for presenting results also for the entire group of 2004 respondents is to give a point of reference to an ordinary group of audiological patients in the labour force.

Furthermore, results are presented separately for men and women. This makes comparisons with Carlsson and Danermark (this volume, Chapter 4) difficult, but is considered necessary because of – among other things – the gender-related patterns of hearing loss mentioned above (Table 5.1) and the gender-segregated labour market in Sweden.

After a short presentation of work changes for our respondents in the previous three years, information about respondents' hearing losses are given and then the question of experienced consequences and coping is addressed. Finally we turn to indicators of important choices in life.

RECENT CHANGES IN RELATION TO THE LABOUR MARKET

Only people (20–64 years of age) in the labour force were asked to answer the first (2001) questionnaire. Three years later (2004) 17% of the men and 14% of the women had reached the age of 65[2] and had retired. Among the respondents of working age about 80% were still working in 2004 while remaining 20% were not, due to early retirement,[3] long-term sick leave, unem-

---

[2] 65 years of age is the standard age of retirement in Sweden.
[3] 86% of those in 2004 who had taken early retirement reported that hearing impairment played some or a major part for their early retirement.

Table 5.3 Percentages (%) with childhood onset of hearing impairment

	2004 respondents	Without family history	FHHI, family of origin
Women	14 (n = 134)	22 (n = 36)	18 (n = 22)
Men	8 (n = 207)	9 (n = 100)	29 (n = 21)
Overall	10 (n = 341)	12 (n = 136)	23 (n = 43)

n designates number of respondents in the corresponding category

ployment etc. Percentages are roughly the same for men and for women with a FHHI in family of origin and men and women without family history.

HEARING LOSS

Onset of hearing impairment

About every tenth respondent had childhood onset (onset since birth or before the age of 8 years) of hearing impairment. Childhood onset is more common among female than among male respondents. We recall that only respondents in the labour force are included.

For instance: out of 36 women without a family history in our sample, 22% have childhood onset and of 22 women with FHHI in family of origin 18% have childhood onset (Table 5.3).

Comparing the three groups (women, men and both sexes respectively) without family history with the corresponding group having a FHHI in family of origin, no significant differences were found (between the women, between the men and between both sexes, respectively).[4]

Severity of hearing loss

In Table 5.1 we saw that women on average had more severe hearing losses than men in terms of mean pure tone average (PTA).

However, both men and women in our sample with a FHHI in their family of origin seem to have more severe hearing losses than those men and women without (Table 5.4). However, differences were significant only when calculated for the total group.

Tinnitus

About half of the respondents had tinnitus. Tinnitus seems to be somewhat more frequent among male respondents (Table 5.5).

---

[4] All tests of significance in the following are between 'Without family history' and 'FHHI, family of origin'.

Table 5.4 Mean pure tone averages

	2004 respondents	Without family history	FHHI, family of origin
Women	37	38	43
Men	25	23	30
Overall	30	27	37

Women: ns, Men: ns, Overall: rho = −0.154; p = 0.015

Table 5.5 Percentages with tinnitus

	2004 respondents	Without family history	FHHI, family of origin
Women	44 (n = 148)	34 (n = 41)	48 (n = 23)
Men	51 (n = 223)	57 (n = 109)	23 (n = 22)
Overall	48 (n = 371)	51 (n = 150)	36 (n = 45)

Women: ns, Men: χ^2 = 8.31; 1 df; p = 0.004

Men with a FHHI in family of origin, however, more rarely have tinnitus than men without a family history while the opposite is possibly the case for women.

Conclusions on hearing loss

There are no differences between those without a family history of hearing problems and those with FHHI in family of origin in terms of onset from birth or early childhood. People with a FHHI in family of origin, however, seem to have more severe hearing impairments as compared to those without any family history of hearing impairment and men with a FHHI in family of origin more rarely have tinnitus than men without a family history.

HEALTH, WELL-BEING AND COPING

Health and well-being

On the basis of several questions about health and well-being two simple indices were constructed. No significant differences were observed between respondents with hearing impairment without a family history and people with hearing impairment with FHHI in family of origin (Figure 5.1). Neither sex nor age had an impact on this image of similarity.

Consequences

According to Stephens et al. (2003) and Carlsson and Danermark (this volume, Chapter 4), people with a family history of hearing problems seem to

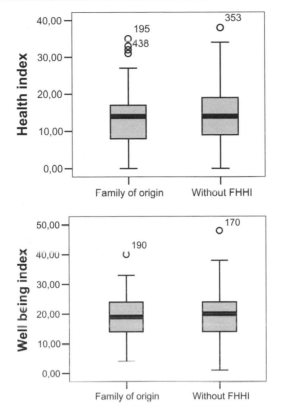

Figure 5.1 Health index and well-being index by family history.

be more affected by their own hearing impairment than those without a family history. In our study, information about consequences of hearing impairment *in the work environment* was requested. There were no significant differences between respondents without a family history and respondents with a FHHI in family of origin: about a quarter of respondents indicated 'big consequences'.

Use of hearing aid at work

Respondents were asked whether they had a hearing aid or not and if they had, they were asked if they use their hearing aid at work. In Table 5.6, 'Yes'-answers to this question are calculated as percentage of total sample (that is, including those who do not have a hearing aid). About half of the respondents use hearing aids at work with women being the more frequent users.

Both women and men with a FHHI in their family of origin seem to use hearing aids at work more frequently than those without. Differences are not

Table 5.6 Percentages using hearing aid at work

	2004 respondents	Without family history	FHHI, family of origin
Women	63 (n = 150)	55 (n = 42)	74 (n = 23)
Men	40 (n = 226)	35 (n = 109)	54 (n = 22)
Overall	49 (n = 376)	40 (n = 151)	64 (n = 45)

No difference was statistically significant

statistically significant, but a similar pattern was found also by Carlsson and Danermark (this volume, Chapter 4). We recall that there are indications that people with a FHHI in their family of origin have more severe hearing impairments than respondents without a family history (Table 5.4). When comparing the use of a hearing aid among respondents (both sexes) with mild hearing impairment ('Not significant' and 'Slight' according to M4) the difference between those without a family history and those with a FHHI in family of origin disappears.

Conclusions on health, well-being and coping

No differences in reported health, well-being, consequences at work and (when controlling for severity of hearing loss) use of hearing aids were found.

CHOICES

We will now turn to two circumstances that could be indicators of long-term decisions and choices in life – occupation and work environment in terms of exposure to noise. In the section we shall also make use of national statistics.

Occupation

In Table 5.7 an account of occupational belonging (aggregated level) is given for, on the one hand, our respondents with hearing impairment and, on the other hand, the total working population in Sweden.[5] Of course, comparisons are blurred by the very small numbers and the age of respondents with hearing impairment as well as by possible coding errors.

The main picture (Table 5.7) is that there seems to be no major difference between the occupational structure of men and women (patients at audiological clinics) with hearing impairment and the population at large when examining occupation on this level.

[5] According to the publication *The Work Environment 2003*, based on the comprehensive samples (about 14,000) of the employed population according to Swedish Labour Force Surveys during the fourth quarter of 2003 and published by the Swedish Work Environment Authority and Statistics Sweden.

Table 5.7 Occupational structure

Occupation SSYK code number	National statistics (16–64 years of age) 2003	2004 respondents	Without family history	FHHI, family of origin
1. Legislators, senior officials and managers	3	2*	0	5*
2 + 3**	41	36	23	38
4 + 5 + 6 + 7 + 8***	50	54	72	48
9. Unskilled occupations	6	8	5	9
Total women	**100%**	**100%** (n = 140)	**100%** (n = 39)	**100%** (n = 21)
1. Legislators, senior officials and managers	7	10*	9*	19*
2 + 3**	36	35	29	43
4 + 5 + 6 + 7 + 8***	52	51	57	33
9. Unskilled occupations	3	4	5	5
Total men	**100%**	**100%** (n = 208)	**100%** (n = 97)	**100%** (n = 21)

* Including non-specified 'foremen' etc.
** Code 2 and 3 (professionals and technicians and associate professionals) require the equivalent of university-level education
*** Code 4–8 (clerks, service workers and shop sales workers, skilled agricultural and fishery workers, craft and related trades workers, plant and machine operators and assemblers) require the equivalent of secondary education
Women: $\chi^2 = 8.64$; 3 df; p = 0.034: Men: ns

However, the hypothesis that people with a family history of hearing impairment tend to have relatively high education (e.g. Carlsson and Danermark, this volume) is supported in our sample, at least as far as women are concerned, as a significantly larger proportion of women with a FHHI in family of origin have occupations requiring university education as compared to women without a family history. The same tendency, although not statistically significant, was observed among men in the sample. It should again be noted, though, that a selective mechanism could be operating here if people leave the labour market through early retirement more often when having a hearing impairment and in addition having an occupation not requiring high education, possibly associated with a difficult work environment.

Exposure to noise at work

According to national statistics on exposure to noise at work,[6] the percentage of men in this situation has been fairly stable during the 1990s while there has

[6] Swedish Work Environment Authority & Statistics Sweden 2001 and 2003. Exposure to high level of noise = you are not able to talk in a normal voice during at least a quarter of the working time.

Table 5.8 Percentages exposed to noise at work

	2004 respondents	Without family history	FHHI, family of origin
Women	45 (n = 144)	35 (n = 40)	52 (n = 23)
Men	61 (n = 211)	69 (n = 105)	50 (n = 22)
Overall	55 (n = 355)	59 (n = 145)	51 (n = 45)

No difference was statistically significant

been an increase of about 5% among women aged 30–49 years. In 2001, 29% of economically active men and 16% of women aged 16–64 years were exposed to noise at work. Furthermore, exposure to noise seems to decrease with age. National statistics also indicate which occupations are associated with a noisy work environment.

In our sample of people (on average much older than the national sample) with hearing impairment, levels of exposure to noise are much higher: 61% of the men and 45% of the women report that they work in a noisy environment (Table 5.8). The higher levels are perhaps not surprising considering, firstly, the comparatively more general question in our questionnaire[7] and, secondly, the occurrence of noise-induced hearing impairment as a consequence of noisy work environments among people (possibly among men in particular) in our sample of patients from audiological clinics. The question arises whether people are trapped in certain occupations and workplaces and cannot and/or do not want to change to a less noisy environment.

There does not seem to be a difference between those without a family history and those with a FHHI in their family of origin as far as noise in the workplace is concerned. About half of our respondents find themselves in noisy working surroundings.

Conclusions on choices

Women (and possibly also men) with a FHHI in their family of origin seem more likely to work in graduate professions than those without a family history but there does not seem to be a difference between the groups working in a noisy environment.

SUMMARY AND DISCUSSION

The question to be investigated was whether there are significant differences between people in the labour force with hearing impairment that (a) have and

[7] 'Do you work in an environment of noise or intrusive sounds?'

(b) have not experienced hearing problems in their family of origin (parents, siblings) during their childhood/adolescence. The initial assumption was that having a FHHI in family of origin matters and has an impact on the consequences of hearing impairment, coping and even choices in life.

To sum up the results of our comparison between those in employment who have a FHHI in their family of origin and those who do not have a family history of hearing problems at all, we find few statistically significant differences. People with a FHHI in family of origin do seem to have more severe hearing impairments as compared to those without any family history but there are no differences between the two groups in terms of onset from birth or early childhood. However, men with a FHHI in family of origin less frequently have tinnitus as compared to men without a family history. No differences in reported health, well-being, consequences at work and (when controlling for severity of hearing loss) use of hearing aid could be observed between those with a FHHI in family of origin and those without family history. Furthermore, there does not seem to be a difference between these groups in terms of exposure to noisy work settings. However, women (and possibly also men) with a FHHI in their family of origin seem more likely to work in graduate professions than those without a family history.

Can we conclude, then, that having a FHHI in family of origin does not matter? The present results would rather indicate that respondents with a FHHI in family of origin have a way of coping with their own hearing impairment so that health, well-being and consequences of impairment at work is similar to those of people without a family history of hearing problems, even though the hearing impairment of the former is generally more severe.

A supplementary conclusion could be that women, and possibly also men, with a FHHI in their family of origin seem to have prepared themselves educationally for the demands of the labour market and have developed comparatively successful ways of coping with their hearing problems. However, it could also be that precisely the individuals with a FHHI in their family of origin who have invested in higher education, are still in the labour market while others with a FHHI in their family of origin have retired.

As we have information only about people with hearing impairment who were in the labour force in 2001 we could not know whether people with hearing impairments outside the labour force constitute a group similar to our respondents in terms of FHHI in family of origin and without family history or if there is, for example, a larger proportion of people with FHHI in their family of origin outside the labour force. We could, as pointed out earlier, not exclude the possibility of a selective mechanism generating the patterns observed in our study.

Certainly, further investigation into the impact of having a FHHI would require more data and larger samples than were available for the present study. However, qualitative research methods in investigating a strategically chosen sample of women and men with hearing impairment, in order to understand the various processes leading to the impact of having or not having a history of hearing problems in the family (or in their close circle), would be a priority. Such research could then provide an input for further quantitative studies into family history and its audiological implications.

REFERENCES

Coniavitis Gellerstedt L, Danermark B (2004) Hearing impairment, working life conditions, and gender. *Scandinavian Journal of Disability Research* 6: 225–45.

Danermark B, Coniavitis Gellerstedt L (2003) *Att höra till – om hörselskadades psykosociala arbetsmiljö* (Belonging – On psychosocial working conditions of people with hearing impairment). Örebro: Örebro University.

Danermark B, Coniavitis Gellerstedt L (2004a) Psychosocial work environment, hearing impairment and health. *International Journal of Audiology* 43: 383–9.

Danermark B, Coniavitis Gellerstedt L (2004b) Social justice: Redistribution and recognition – a non-reductionist perspective on disability. *Disability & Society* 19: 339–53.

Layder D (1997) *Modern Social Theory: Key Debates and New Directions.* London: UCL Press.

Statistics Sweden (2003) *Funktionshindrade 1988–1999* (Disabled 1988–1999). Levnadsförhållanden. Rapport 97. Stockholm: Statistics Sweden.

Stephens D, Lewis P, Davis A (2003) The influence of perceived family history of hearing difficulties in an epidemiological study of hearing problems *Audiological Medicine* 1: 228–31.

Swedish Government Official Report SOU 2001: 56 *Funktionshinder och välfärd* (Impairment and Welfare).

Swedish Work Environment Authority & Statistics Sweden (2001, 2003) *Arbetsmiljön 2001 resp 2003* (*The Work Environment 2001* and *2003* respectively).

II Prospective Studies – Late Onset Hearing Impairment

6 Effects of a Family History on Late Onset Hearing Impairment: Results of an Open-Ended Questionnaire

SOPHIA E. KRAMER, ADRIANA A. ZEKVELD AND DAFYDD STEPHENS

'Having a family history of hearing loss made me determined not to ignore the problem. It made me aware of the danger of social isolation.'

INTRODUCTION

In the field of audiology, the role of having a family history of hearing loss and particularly its psychosocial impact on adults having hearing loss themselves, is still a relatively unexplored area of research. While extensive literature is available on the adverse psychosocial effects of hearing loss in general (Danermark, 2005; Kramer, 2005; Stephens, 2005), almost no information exists on the specific impact of having a family history. This is in contrast with the rapidly growing number of studies in genomic medicine in this area (Martini et al., 1996; Toriello et al., 2004).

So far, very few studies have addressed the effect of a family history of hearing loss in adults. One example is the investigation reported by Stephens et al. (2003). In that study the presence of a family history as a factor which could influence the emotional impact was explored in a household survey including more than 34,000 subjects. It was found that the greater the impact of hearing loss, the more likely there was to be a family history of hearing problems. However, a major limitation of that study is that the questions were designed for general purposes, rather than to examine the specific effects of having a family history of hearing impairment.

Preliminary results of a study on the effects of having a family history of otosclerosis are described by Lemkens (2005). Among nine participants, the impact of having a family history was perceived as mainly positive, since it had helped them to be prepared for any potential difficulties. Also, the family history provided them the opportunity to share their problems with other family members. Anxiety about their children's future was a negative consequence. The very few studies on the psychosocial consequences of genetically caused deafblindness (Usher syndrome) are described by Möller (2005).

In order to address the deficit in our knowledge on the effects of having a family history of non-syndromal late onset hearing impairment, we decided to conduct a qualitative study using an open-ended questionnaire asking people about the impact of having a family history of hearing loss. This questionnaire was administered both in Cardiff (Wales) and in Amsterdam (the Netherlands). Examining the Welsh data, we were primarily interested in determining whether having a family history of hearing loss is mainly a positive, a negative or a neutral experience. The data were analysed accordingly and the results of that study have been reported in detail by Stephens and Kramer (2005). Examining the Dutch data, we were primarily interested in the identification of themes representing various groups of attitudes towards having a family history of hearing loss. The present chapter focuses on the Dutch results and considers them in relation to the findings obtained in Wales.

RESEARCH STUDY

METHOD

To explore the area of family history of hearing loss, an open-ended questionnaire was designed. Open-ended questions can be administered as a substitute of a personal interview or to complement such an interview. While responses to open-ended questions may be difficult to interpret and while the process of coding may be time consuming, open-ended questions give the respondents a great freedom of expression. Using this method of data collection, the respondents are allowed to share any information that is regarded as essential to them. Also, an open-ended procedure implies no bias due to a limited response range. Early in the research process, an open-ended approach or an interview is indispensable to determine the possible range of responses. Such information is required prior to considering the development of a structured questionnaire with a set of closed questions (Frary, 1991).

To collect data on the impact of having a family history of hearing loss, we first verified whether the respondent had or had previously had a relative with hearing problems. If yes, the respondent was invited to proceed and to report as many effects of the family history as he or she could think of. Figure 6.1 shows the open-ended questionnaire. For the Dutch population, the questionnaire was translated into Dutch (Figure 6.1, lower panel).

You have mentioned that <u>other</u> members of your family have or have previously had hearing problems.

Does your family history of hearing loss have any effect on your <u>reaction</u> to <u>your own</u> hearing problems? (please tick the answer that applies most to you)

☐ YES ☐ NO

If YES, please list any ways this knowledge has affected you. Write down as many effects as you can think of:

....
....
....

Op dit moment vindt er een onderzoek plaats naar gehoorverlies dat erfelijk bepaald is. Het onderzoek is onder andere gericht op de psychosociale gevolgen van erfelijk gehoorverlies. Daar is nog weinig of niets over bekend.

Heeft <u>u zelf</u> hoorproblemen en hebben uw ouders, broers, zusters en/of kinderen die ook? Dan is de volgende vraag voor u bedoeld. We hopen dat zoveel mogelijk lezers met erfelijk bepaald gehoorverlies bereid zijn de onderstaande vraag te beantwoorden. Die is als volgt:

Op welke manier heeft het feit dat gehoorverlies in uw familie voorkomt (erfelijk is), <u>uw</u> reactie op uw <u>eigen</u> gehoorverlies beïnvloed? Schrijf zoveel mogelijk reacties op.

....
....
....

Figure 6.1 The open-ended questionnaire used in the present study. The upper panel shows the English version. The lower panel shows the Dutch translation. The formats of the questionnaires are slightly different, since the English version was handed out in the clinic, while the Dutch version was posted on the website.

In Cardiff, the open-ended questionnaire was administered to those consecutive patients seen in the Audiological rehabilitation clinics of the Welsh Hearing Institute from whom the clinician had elicited a family history of hearing problems. In the Netherlands, the Dutch version of the questionnaire was posted on the website of the Dutch Society of Hard-of-Hearing people.

Table 6.1 Characteristics of the respondents participating in the present study

	N	Effect Yes/No	Gender M/F	Age Min	Age Median	Age Max
Cardiff	100	57/43	34/66	31	67	92
Amsterdam	42	41/1	18/24	19	56	90

CONTENT ANALYSIS

Data were processed according to the qualitative content analysis as described by Graneheim and Lundman (2004). Examples of studies on different topics in which such a qualitative content analysis was applied are those of Shields and King (2001) and Barroso (1997). Creating categories is the core feature of qualitative content analysis. A category is a group of content that shares a commonality. The qualitative content analysis classifies and compares groups of responses. The initial unit of analysis (meaning unit) comprises the particular statement of the respondent. The procedure entails a progressive classification of the responses from 'meaning units' to 'condensed meaning units' then to 'sub-themes' and finally 'themes'. Examples of that process are given in Table 6.2, which shows representative meaning units, condensed meaning units, sub-themes and finally the themes formed in the present study. The qualitative analyses in this study were conducted independently by two researchers. Evaluation of these processes was done by a third person. A process of reflection and discussion resulted in agreement on the final set of themes identified.

PARTICIPANTS

As mentioned in the introduction, data were collected both in Cardiff (Wales) and in Amsterdam (the Netherlands). In Cardiff, a total of 100 patients participated and were included in the study. In the Netherlands, a total 41 adults replied and returned their reactions either by email or by regular post. Details of both the Welsh and the Dutch participants are shown in Table 6.1.

In Cardiff about 40% of the respondents reported that their family history had no effect on their reaction to their own hearing difficulties, while in the Netherlands only one person reported that it had no such effect.

RESULTS

AMSTERDAM DATA

Reports from the participants in Amsterdam yielded a total of 90 meaning units. Qualitative analysis of the responses resulted in the identification of six themes:

'expectation/anticipation', 'acceptance of hearing loss', 'help-seeking', 'sharing knowledge', 'offspring/worry about future' and 'role modelling'. Examples of meaning units in each of those categories are given in Table 6.2. The particular statements of the respondents towards their family history could be positive, negative or neutral. Within most of the themes, positive, negative and neutral attitudes were observed. However, the majority of the statements within the theme 'sharing knowledge' were positive, while the majority of the responses within the theme 'expectation/anticipation' were neutral. A striking example of a negative reaction was given in the category 'acceptance of hearing loss'. While most of the participants reported that having a family history of hearing loss had helped them to accept the problem, one or two individuals reported that the inherited impairment prevented them from blaming anyone or any incident, making it impossible for them to accept the loss.

Responses within the category 'help-seeking' referred to both the time of help-seeking and to the familiarity with help-seeking. An example of the latter sub-theme is '*My broad experience with hearing loss in the family gave me confidence as to where to get the best help and which questions to ask*'. Within the theme 'offspring/worry about future' some respondents reported serious concerns about their children's future. Others, however, mentioned that having a family history of hearing loss did not prevent them from having children and that the lives of those with a hearing impairment should be regarded as of full value.

Observation of the attitudes within the category 'role modelling' clarified that a positive attitude towards the presence of their own hearing loss may stem from both positive and negative role models.

As it is relevant to know whether the identification of a theme is based on a few meaning units only or on a substantial number of statements, the number of meaning units in each theme was counted and the results are presented in Table 6.3. The theme with the largest reported statements (N = 23) was 'sharing knowledge'. The remaining themes had comparable numbers of meaning units.

CARDIFF DATA

In Cardiff, the primary aim of the study was to explore whether having a family history of hearing loss is a positive, a negative or a neutral phenomenon (Stephens & Kramer, 2005). Therefore, condensed meaning units (in total 150) were grouped into a positive, a negative, a neutral or a general theme. In total, 30% of the meaning units were what might be termed 'general effects', not obviously related to the family history, but related to the hearing loss in general. An example of such a general effect is '*I feel I miss out a lot, I don't enter into conversation*'. Of the remaining 70% of the meaning units, 57% were positive, 19% negative and 24% neutral. Table 6.4 shows the distribution of the positive, negative and neutral responses of both the Cardiff data and the Amsterdam data. The most common positive impact concerned realising the

Table 6.2 Example of the content analysis entailing a progressive classification of the responses from 'meaning units' to 'condensed meaning units' then to 'sub-themes' and finally 'themes'. For each identified theme, two examples are given

Meaning unit	Condensed meaning unit	Sub-theme	Theme
'I had no inhibitions about wearing hearing aids after having observed the benefit my aunt gained and difficulties my mother's denial continue to cause . . .'	Observed benefit of hearing aids. Observed difficulties of denial within the family	Observed effects of hearing aid use. Observed negative effects of denial to use hearing aids.	Role-modelling
'My father always refused to admit that he was hearing-impaired, which had adverse effects . . .'	Observed negative effects of father's denial of hearing loss	Observed negative effects of denial	
'Both my father and grandfather had serious hearing problems, so becoming hearing-impaired myself was no surprise for me. I was expecting it.'	Expectation of hearing loss, since it was observed among family members	Expecting getting a hearing loss	Expectation/ Anticipation
'When I was about twelve years of age, I realised that I had a chance of becoming hearing-impaired.'	Realisation of having a family history of hearing loss	Realising having a chance of becoming hearing-impaired	
'My attitude towards hearing loss was not negative, since I'd seen it in the family and grew up with it.'	No negative attitude towards hearing loss due to family history	No negative attitude	Acceptance

Quote		Sub-theme	Theme
'Having family members with hearing loss helped me to accept my own hearing problems.'	Family history helped to accept own hearing loss	Family history helps acceptance	
'Having a family history of hearing loss made me determined to seek help sooner.'	I was determined to seek help sooner	Seeking help sooner	Help-seeking
'I started to use hearing aids in an early stage.'	I started to use hearing aids in an early stage	Hearing aids in an early stage	
'Having a family history of hearing loss made me stronger, since I could share important issues with my close relatives.'	Sharing information with my relatives made me stronger	Sharing information with relatives	Sharing knowledge
'Whenever I have problems with my hearing loss, I ask family members how they dealt with such difficulties.'	In case of problems, I ask my family members	Asking family members for solutions	
'Our children are still normally hearing, but I am worried about their future.'	I am worried about the future of my children's hearing	Worried about future	
'I feel guilty about the fact that I have carried over the hearing impairment to my children.'	I feel guilty about carrying over the hearing loss	Feelings of guilt	Offspring/worry about future

Table 6.3 The total number of reported meaning units per theme and the distribution of positive, negative and neutral responses. The table shows the results of the Amsterdam data

Theme	Total number of meaning units within each theme	Distribution of the number of positive, negative and neutral meaning units		
		Positive	Negative	Neutral
Role modelling	13	7	2	4
Expectation/anticipation	10	0	1	9
Acceptance	15	4	8	3
Help-seeking	11	7	3	1
Sharing knowledge	23	12	4	7
Offspring/worry about future	18	2	9	7

Table 6.4 Proportion of positive, negative and neutral attitudes towards the family history of hearing loss in Cardiff and in Amsterdam

Effects	Example	Cardiff data	Amsterdam data
Positive	Realising importance of hearing aids/early help seeking	57%	36%
Negative	Anxious about future/offspring	19%	30%
Neutral	Not realising hearing problems were hereditary or indifferent attitude towards a family history	24%	34%

importance of hearing aids and early help-seeking. Common negative effects were concern for the future of themselves and their children. Neutral impacts were reported ignorance, denial of a family history or an indifferent attitude towards having a family history.

DISCUSSION

The results of this study give an impression of the themes playing a role in the family history of hearing loss and its effect on those having hearing loss themselves. The identification of six themes, each with a comparable number of statements, emphasises the diversity of the effects that the concept of family history may be associated with. It is not only the diversity, but also the content of the themes that underlines the potential value of the family history both in research activities and in clinical care. The present findings highlight, further explain and substantiate the role of the family history of hearing loss, alongside with the advances in genomic medicine within this area. In particular they highlight its role in feelings of guilt, in feelings of preparedness, in the provision of sources in advice and, particularly, in providing role models. Such role models may have either positive or negative impacts on the hearing-impaired individual.

Before discussing the findings of this study, it must be noted that the themes identified are not necessarily mutually exclusive. A condensed meaning unit may sometimes fit into more than one theme and overlap between themes should not be ignored. Also, ambiguity in the meaning of words may induce weakness in reliability and validity of the results. However, within the process of reflection and discussion among the three researchers, the context of the particular statement (sentences preceding and following the particular statement) was taken into account as well. It helped to identify the underlying meaning of a reported statement in cases of doubt and helped take forward the classification of the responses from 'meaning units' to 'condensed meaning units' and finally into 'themes'.

An interesting result of this study is the distribution of positive, negative and neutral attitudes towards the family history of hearing loss.

The Cardiff data show that the majority of the responses (57%) fell into the positive category, while the minority of the reactions (19%) were negative. This pattern was also observed in the Amsterdam data, even though the differences in proportion between the categories were not as large as in the Cardiff data. This could be due to the self-selection bias in the Dutch sample, all having chosen to join the Society for Hard-of-Hearing people, perhaps because of lack of acceptance of their hearing impairment. In the Cardiff sample, 40% denied any effect of their family history. It could well be these were the people who did not experience positive effects, but felt a desire to please the researchers. Thus they did not wish to express any negative effects.

The Amsterdam data give a clarification as to how the positive, negative and neutral attitudes are divided over the various themes. The results show that most by far of the attitudes within the themes 'role modelling', 'help-seeking' and 'sharing knowledge' were positive, while the responses within the theme 'anticipation/expectation' were mainly neutral.

Predominantly negative reactions were found within the theme 'offspring/worry about future'. Comparable findings were reported by Lemkens (2005). Such an identification as to which themes are observed as being mainly positive, negative or neutral may yield relevant information for clinicians working with people who have a family history of hearing loss and for those involved in counselling. Such information is essential when the utility and the structural implementation of a family history tool in clinical practice is discussed.

Regarding the results, it must be considered that the samples in the present study are not representative of the general population of people with hearing impairment. There is no information about non-respondents within this context. It may well be that only those having specific experiences or having explicit attitudes towards their family history decided to respond, while those who were unaware of their family history did not feel the need to participate.

Similarly, it may well be that only those having predominantly positive feelings towards their family history decided to respond, while those having mainly negative feelings did not want to be confronted with the effects again by writing them down.

Further systematic studies to explore the impact of having a family history of hearing loss are required. An inquiry using a structured questionnaire and exploring awareness of family history is currently in preparation.

Nevertheless, the present study provides relevant information to those who wish to further explore the family history of hearing loss either clinically or for research purposes.

REFERENCES

Barroso J (1997) Social support and long-term survivors of AIDS. *Western Journal of Nursing Research* 19: 554–82.

Danermark B (2005) A review of the psychosocial effects of hearing impairment in the working age population. In D Stephens, L Jones (eds) *The Impact of Genetic Hearing Impairment*. London: Whurr, pp. 106–36.

Frary RB (1991) A brief guide to questionnaire development. Blacksburg, Virginia: Office of Measurement and Research Services, Virginia Polytechnic Institute and State University.

Graneheim UH, Lundman B (2004) Qualitative content analysis in nursing research: concepts, procedures and measures to achieve trustworthiness. *Nurse Education Today* 24: 105–12.

Kramer SE (2005) The psychosocial impact of hearing loss among elderly people: a review. In D Stephens, L Jones (eds) *The Impact of Genetic Hearing Impairment*. London: Whurr, pp. 137–64.

Lemkens N (2005) The effects of otosclerosis. In D Stephens, L Jones (eds) *The Impact of Genetic Hearing Impairment*. London: Whurr, pp. 195–200.

Martini A, Read A, Stephens D (eds) (1996) *Genetics and Hearing Impairment*. London: Whurr.

Möller K (2005) The impact of combined vision and hearing impairment of deafblindness. In D Stephens, L Jones (eds) *The Impact of Genetic Hearing Impairment*. London: Whurr, pp. 165–94.

Shields L, King SJ (2001) Qualitative analysis of the care of children in hospital in four countries – Part 1. *International Pediatric Nursing* 16: 137–45.

Stephens D (2005) The impact of hearing impairment in children. In D Stephens, L Jones (eds) *The Impact of Genetic Hearing Impairment*. London: Whurr, pp. 73–105.

Stephens D, Kramer SE (2005) The impact of having a family history of hearing problems on those with hearing difficulties themselves: an exploratory study. *International Journal of Audiology* 44: 206–12.

Stephens D, Lewis P, Davis A (2003) The influence of a perceived family history of hearing difficulties in an epidemiological study of hearing problems. *Audiological Medicine* 1, 228–31.

Toriello HV, Reardon W, Gorlin RJ (eds) (2004) *Hereditary Hearing Loss and Its Syndromes*. Oxford University Press, New York.

7 Factors in the Effects of a Family History on Late Onset Hearing Impairment

**DAFYDD STEPHENS, SOPHIA E. KRAMER
AND ANGELES ESPESO**

INTRODUCTION

Until recently there has been little investigation of the influence of having a family history of hearing problems on adults with hearing difficulties themselves (e.g. Stephens et al., 2003; Danermark, 2005; Kramer, 2005). Within the present series of studies we have attempted to probe patients' views as to the effects which they had experienced.

In an open-ended questionnaire administered to individuals who reported a family history of hearing problems, we were able to identify a number of effects, positive, negative and neutral on the individual's reaction to their own hearing loss (Stephens and Kramer, 2005; Kramer et al., this volume, Chapter 6). Within those studies, we were unable to determine which of these effects related to each other and which were commonly experienced within the general population with late onset hearing impairment.

From the open-ended study we took 20 of the most commonly reported effects, positive, negative and neutral and composed a questionnaire in a closed-set format. Each item represents a statement and the respondents were asked whether each statement was 'definitely true', 'probably true', 'probably not true' or 'definitely not true' for them. The questionnaire was administered to 192 individuals who had a hearing impairment and who reported a family history of such an impairment. We examined the relationship between questions, their factorial basis and how they related to demographic factors. (Kramer et al., *submitted*).

In that study, five orthogonal factors which accounted for 58.1% of the total variance were identified. These factors were:

1. awareness of family history – positive effects (21.8% of variance)
2. awareness of family history – negative effects (10.2%)
3. effects of hearing loss in general (9.3%)

The Effects of Genetic Hearing Impairment in the Family. Edited by D. Stephens and L. Jones.
Copyright © 2006 by John Wiley & Sons, Ltd.

4. importance of hearing loss *per se* (9.0%) and
5. distinctiveness of individual hearing (7.9%).

We examined the demographic determinants of these, and only factor 2 appeared to be related to the particular population under study among the three groups which we had used as a source for these data.

The three different populations from which these data were derived were:

1. a population seen in an audiological rehabilitation clinic
2. a population aged 55–65 years who were subjects or potential subjects of a genetic study and
3. those who responded to a website questionnaire.

Within the present chapter we shall examine in more detail differences and similarities between these three subject populations.

METHOD

QUESTIONNAIRE

This comprised 20 statements made by patients in response to our earlier open-ended questionnaire in which they were asked to list any effects of their family history of hearing impairment on their reaction to their own hearing impairment (Stephens & Kramer, 2005; Kramer et al., this volume, Chapter 6). The questions were selected on the basis of the number of times the statement was made together with obtaining a balance between positive, negative and neutral comments.

Each individual within the present investigation was asked to indicate whether each of the 20 statements selected was 'Definitely true', 'Probably true', 'Probably not true' and 'Definitely not true' for them. The English questionnaire is shown as Appendix 7.1.

SUBJECTS

Participants in this study comprised 192 individuals, 87 males and 105 females, derived from the three populations as mentioned above. The first population comprised a consecutive series of 98 patients reporting a family history of hearing loss seen in the Audiological Rehabilitation Clinics of the Welsh Hearing Institute in Cardiff. Thirty-eight were male and 59 were female, and their mean age was 63 years (SD 17.2, range 17–92 years). Their mean better ear hearing level across both ears (500, 1000, 2000 and 4000 Hz) was 44.3 dBHL (SD 20.8 dB) and their mean worse ear hearing level 53.9 dBHL (SD 26.0 dB).

The second group comprised 58 subjects seen as part of a genetic and aetiological study on age-related hearing impairment also at the Welsh Hearing Institute. All were aged between 55 and 65 years (mean 60.0 years SD 3.5

years, range 54–65 years) and did not have any marked asymmetry in their hearing loss. Thirty-three were male, 25 female and their mean better ear hearing level was 37.3 dBHL (SD 17.5 dB) and their mean worse ear hearing level 44.8 dBHL (SD 19.6 dB). All had sensorineural hearing impairment.

The third group comprised 36 subjects who responded to a question '*If you yourself as well as any other members of your family (parents, brother and sisters, children) have hearing problems, please let us know of any ways that having other people in your family with hearing problems has affected **your** reaction to your **own** hearing problems*' placed on the GENDEAF website (www.gendeaf.org) and on the website of the Dutch Society of Hard-of-Hearing People (Nederlandse Vereniging voor Slechthorenden, NVVS). The responses to this open questionnaire are discussed elsewhere (this volume, Chapter 6). Those responding were also emailed the same closed-set questionnaire used for the Cardiff subjects. A Dutch translation was sent to those responding from the Netherlands. Fifteen of the 36 respondents were male and 21 female. Their mean age was 54.5 years (SD 12.5 years, range 21–75 years).

As the responses within the Dutch group were obtained via a website, we did not have audiometric information on this group. We therefore used a surrogate measure derived from the National Study of Hearing (Davis, 1995) which asked 'Do you have difficulty following TV programmes at a volume others find acceptable without any aid to your hearing?' We had previously used this in a population study on the effects of a family history on hearing impairment (Stephens et al, 2003; this volume, Chapter 1). In a separate study (this volume, Chapter 13) on the influence of a family history on tinnitus complaint behaviour, the relationship between these response categories and the mean hearing level was defined (N = 102). The results of this are shown in Table 7.1. The TV measures correlated at a level of Tau = 0.59 with their worse ear hearing level, averaged across 500 Hz, 1, 2 and 4 kHz.

Of the 34 respondents to the question, 6 reported no problem, 5 a slight problem and 23 a moderate problem. If we take Table 7.1 as a representative basis for the conversion, it suggests that the Better Ear Hearing Level for this group is approximately 40.8 dBHL and the worse ear 54.6 dBHL.

Table 7.1 Relationship between TV measure and better and worse ear hearing levels. The mean hearing levels averaged across the octave frequencies 500 Hz to 4000 Hz are shown

TV	Better ear hearing level		Worse ear hearing level	
	Mean	sd	Mean	sd
No Problem	12.9	10.7	20.4	20.9
Slight Problem	20.0	10.0	26.6	12.8
Moderate Problem	28.5	10.3	35.5	11.8
Severe Problem	48.9	19.7	66.1	25.3

RESULTS

DEMOGRAPHIC COMPARISON OF GROUPS

There was no significant difference in the gender balance across the three groups ($\chi^2 = 4.8$, 2 df, P = 0.09). However, an analysis of the age showed a significant difference between the groups (f = 4.7, p = 0.01). Individual group comparisons showed no difference between groups 1 and 2 but both groups were significantly older than group 3 (1 vs 3; t = 3.0, p = 0.004; 2 vs 3, t = 2.5, p = 0.09).

A comparison of the hearing levels of groups 1 and 2 showed significant differences with worse hearing in group 1 for both Better Ear Hearing Level (6.9 dB, t = 2.1; p = 0.004) and for Worse Ear Hearing Level (9.0 dB; t = 2.3; p = 0.025). It is impossible to be sure whether the 'Internet' group differed from the other two groups, although the simple conversion data in Table 7.1 suggest they might have hearing levels somewhere between groups 1 and 2.

Data for the age band of onset of the hearing problems were available for groups 2 and 3, with few data available for group 1. Results were grouped on the basis of presence of hearing problems from birth, from birth to 15 years, 15–40 years and 40–65 years. These are shown in Table 7.2, in which it may be seen that the subjects from group 2 were more likely to indicate a later onset of their hearing loss ($\chi^2 = 28.4$; 3 df; p < 0.001) than those in group 3.

QUESTIONS

The affirmative responses to all the questions are shown in Table 7.3. For simplicity, the responses to 'Definitely true' and to 'Probably true' have been amalgamated. It may be seen from this that with the sole exception of question 12 (Having a family history has influenced major life decisions (e.g. choice of career) for me) all questions indicated an effect of having a family history. The results for question 12 are considered in more detail below and are picked up in the discussion.

When we analysed the questions in terms of the factors identified by Kramer et al. (submitted) we found notable differences between affirmative responses to the different categories. These are shown in Table 7.4, which indicates the

Table 7.2 The reported age of onset of hearing loss reported by subjects in groups 2 and 3 (numbers and percentage per age band)

	Age of onset			
Group	Birth	<15 years	15–40 years	40–65 years
Group 2	1 (2%)	3 (5%)	9 (15%)	45 (78%)
Group 3	6 (18%)	4 (12%)	11 (33%)	12 (36%)

Table 7.3 Positive responses for the questions used

Question no.	Summary wording	Category (from Kramer et al., submitted)	% agree
1	Aware of social isolation	Awareness of FH – Positive	63.5
2	I didn't think it important enough to ask	Importance HL/Help-seeking	30.7
3	Determined not to ignore problem	Awareness of FH – Positive	73.2
4	Didn't realise hearing problems hereditary	(Classified)	63.0
5	More aware of other people's HL	Awareness of FH – Positive	83.2
6	More fatalistic	Effects HL in general	52.4
7	More open about my problems	Awareness of FH – Positive	78.5
8	Long diagnosis to no effect	Importance HL/Help-seeking	40.7
9	More empathy for others I meet	Awareness of FH – Positive	79.7
10	Concern about children's hearing	Awareness of FH – Negative	65.0
11	Not worried about using HA	(Hearing aid)	85.2
12	Influenced career decisions	Distinctiveness of individual hearing status	17.5
13	Encourage others too proud	Awareness of FH – Positive	83.3
14	Prospects of HL depressing	Effects HL in general	70.8
15	Not seeking own problems	Awareness of FH – Negative	45.0
16	Expected problems	Awareness of FH – Negative	54.5
17	Comfort that family coped	Awareness of FH – Positive	64.7
18	Worried about enjoying music	Effects HL in general	69.5
19	Early help seeking	Awareness of FH – Positive	55.3
20	Thought everyone the same	Distinctiveness of individual hearing status	23.4

Table 7.4 Mean % of subjects agreeing with statements in the different factors from Kramer et al. (submitted)

Awareness of family history – Positive	72.7
Awareness of family history – Negative	54.8
Effects of HL in general	64.2
Importance HL and help seeking	35.7
Distinctiveness of individual hearing status	20.5

highest proportion of agreements with factor 1 (Awareness of family history – positive effects) and a smaller agreement with negative effects and non-specific effects.

Of the 20 questions across all subjects 1.3% were not completed by group 1, 0.2% by group 2 and 1.1% by group 3. In most cases no more than 4 subjects out of 192 across the three groups failed to complete the questions, except for question 10 which 9 (8 from group 1) failed to complete. This is not surprising bearing in mind its wording '*It worries me that my children may develop hearing problems in the future'* and that many participants may not have had children.

Next we examined the distribution of the responses by subject group to each question using chi square tests. No significant differences were found for 12 of the 20 questions (1, 5, 6, 7, 10, 11, 13, 15, 16, 17, 18, 19). The questions showing significant differences are discussed below.

Responses to specific questions

Question 2

'Because of my family history, I didn't think my hearing loss important enough to do anything about my own hearing loss' differed significantly across groups ($\chi^2 = 23.6$; 6 df; p = 0.001). Groups 1 and 2 did not differ, but both differed significantly from group 3 (1 vs 3, $\chi^2 = 19.4$, p < 0.001; 2 vs 3, $\chi^2 = 15.7$, p = 0.001). While 37.8% and 36.2% of groups 1 and 2 respectively agreed with the statement, only 2.8% of group 3 did, with 80.6% definitely disagreeing.

Question 3

'Having a family history of hearing loss made me determined not to ignore the problem' showed a smaller difference ($\chi^2 = 13.2$; p = 0.041) with groups 1 and 2 and 1 and 3 not differing from each other significantly, but group 2 differing from group 3 in which 88.9% agreed with the statement compared with 67.2% in group 2 (2 vs 3; $\chi^2 = 10.3$; p = 0.02).

Question 4

'I didn't realise hearing problems were hereditary' was agreed with by 11.1% of group 3 compared with 45.9% and 37.9% of groups 1 and 2. Again there was no significant difference between groups 1 and 2 but both differed significantly from group 3 (1 vs 3, $\chi^2 = 14.4$, p = 0.03; 2 vs 3, $\chi^2 = 8.0$, p = 0.045).

Question 8

'My hearing problems were a long time being diagnosed so had no effect on me' was stated as true by 46.9% and 46.6% of groups 1 and 2 but by only 14.3% of group 3 ($\chi^2 = 14.3$; p = 0.027). The differences between group 3 and both groups 1 and 2 were significant (1 vs 3, $\chi^2 = 13.1$, p < 0.05; 2 vs 3, $\chi^2 = 10.1$, p < 0.02).

Question 9

'My experience of a history of hearing loss in the family gave me empathy with people who would possibly find it irritating if I continually asked for repetition or rephrasing' showed a slightly different pattern of results with most from group 3 agreeing with the statement, less from group 1 with group 2 occupy-

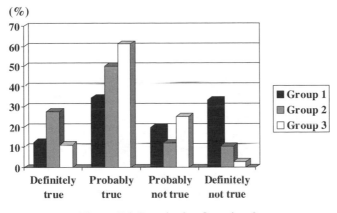

Figure 7.1 Results for Question 9.

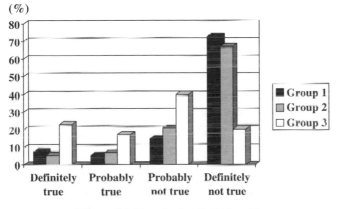

Figure 7.2 Results for Question 12.

ing an intermediate position. The overall difference between groups was significant (χ^2 = 22.7; p = 0.001), but the only difference between groups to be significant was between groups 1 and 3 (χ^2 = 19.1; p < 0.001). These results are shown in Figure 7.1.

Question 12

'Having a family history of hearing loss has influenced major life decisions (e.g. choice of career etc.) for me' reverted to the pattern of results found with Questions 2, 3, 4 and 8 with a significant difference between group 3 and both groups 1 and 2 (1 vs 3, χ^2 = 29.3, p < 0.001; 2 vs 3, χ^2 = 20.3, p < 0.001), but no significant difference between groups 1 and 2. The results are shown in Figure 7.2 which indicates fewer subjects in group 3 disagreeing with the statement.

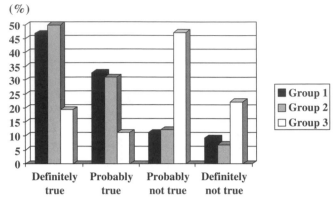

Figure 7.3 Results for Question 14.

Question 14

'The likelihood of decreasing hearing with age is a depressing prospect' again follows the pattern of groups 1 and 2 not differing from each other, but both differing significantly from group 3 (1 vs 3, $\chi^2 = 29.4$; $p < 0.001$; 2 vs 3, $\chi^2 = 24.0$, $p < 0.001$). Thus the large majority (80%) of both groups 1 and 2 consider the statement to be true whereas two-thirds of group 3 consider it not to be true for them (Figure 7.3).

Question 20

'Until I came to clinic I thought everyone could hear the same as me' shows a similar pattern, but the overall differences are less marked ($\chi^2 = 15.5$; $p < 0.02$). The main difference is that fewer subjects in group 3 (27.8%) state that it is definitely not true for them, than in groups 1 and 2 (56.1% and 65.5% respectively). The differences between 1 and 3 overall showed a χ^2 value of 8.9 ($p < 0.05$) and, between 2 and 3, $\chi^2 = 14.3$; $p = 0.003$).

FACTOR ANALYSES

We might question the overall factor analysis performed across all subjects for all questions given the differences in pattern of response between groups for 8 of the questions. It seemed reasonable therefore to repeat the factor analysis on the 12 questions, which do not differ significantly between groups. For this analysis we followed Kramer et al. (submitted) in excluding questions 4 and 11 which did not relate significantly to any of the other questions when we performed a correlation matrix. This identified three factors from those questions, which explained 56.4% of the total variance. These are shown in Table 7.5.

Table 7.5 Factor analysis on the twelve questions which did not differ across groups

Factor	% variance	Questions loading significantly	Description
1	22.9	1, 5, 6, 7, 13	Awareness of family history – positive effects
2	18.1	16, 17, 20	Uncertainty
3	15.4	10, 15, 18	Awareness of family history – negative effects

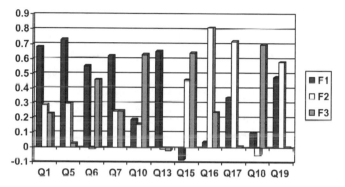

Figure 7.4 Loadings from the individual questions on the three factors shown in Table 7.5.

This highlights the key factors of Positive Effects and Negative Effects of a Family History and of Uncertainty. The loading of the specific questions on the three factors is shown in Figure 7.4.

As respondents from group 1 and from group 2 did not differ significantly in terms of their responses to any of the individual questions, we also performed a factor analysis on the response to the 18 related questions with the subjects from these two groups combined (n = 156).

This resulted in four factors, two of which are the same as those shown in Table 7.3, with five of the six questions loading on the other two factors having been excluded from the previous analysis. The different factors are shown in Table 7.6, and account for 54.5% of the total variance.

These factors appear to reflect the main elements of the responses emerging consistently in all the clinic subjects.

There were too few subjects who responded to the questionnaire via the website for us to perform a factor analysis. We consequently performed a correlation matrix using the Kendall Tau non-parametric correlation test. This showed only one cluster of significant correlations (p < 0.01). This was broadly similar to factor 1 in Table 7.6, with significant correlations between questions

Table 7.6 Factor analysis on all 18 questions based on the responses from subjects in Groups 1 and 2

Factor	% variance	Questions loading significantly	Descriptor factor	Equivalent in Table 7.5
1	25.0	1, 3, 5, 6, 7, 9, 16, 17, 19	Awareness of FH – positive effects	1
2	12.0	10, 14, 15, 18	Awareness of FH – negative effects	3
3	10.2	2, 8, 16	Passiveness	–
4	7.4	12, 13, 20	Broad outlook	–

1, 3, 5, 7, 17, 18. The last (18) was not found in the other groups and was '*I am worried that my enjoyment of music will be impaired*'.

RELATIONSHIP TO DEMOGRAPHIC FACTORS

From the amalgamated data from groups 1 and 2, we calculated the relationship between the individual factors (Table 7.6) and the demographic factors gender, age, age of onset of hearing loss, awareness of family history and hearing levels. There was no notable relationship with age, gender or age of onset.

Hearing level, both in the better ear and in the worse ear, was related negatively to factors 2 (tau = -0.016; p = 0.009, tau = -0.18, p = 0.003) and 4 (tau = -0.16, p = 0.009; tau = 0.15, p = 0.014). Thus those with worse hearing were more concerned about aspects of their family history of hearing loss, and more likely to report that they were rather fatalistic about the consequences of their family history. Awareness of family history related to factor 1 (tau = -0.15; p = 0.017) and to factor 3 (tau = 0.17; p = 0.01). This indicates that those aware of their family history report themselves as seeing the positive aspects of such. They also tend to be less passive in their response to it.

In addition we related the cluster identified from the correlation matrix on group 3 (equivalent to factor 1) to the demographic variables and again found a significant relationship only to awareness of their family history (tau = 0.51; p = 0.001).

DISCUSSION

This chapter is broadly an extension of the analyses reported elsewhere by Kramer et al. (*submitted*) for the overall study population.

The responses obtained from the individual questions suggest that the large majority of respondents are affected by their family history in one way or another. They suggest that the majority of the responses are in a positive direction and that this occurs even though almost two-thirds of the respondents indicated that they did not realise that hearing problems were hereditary. Such a response does not preclude them having family members whom they took as role models without realising that they suffered from the same condition. Often they might attribute a parent's hearing impairment to noise exposure, infection or trauma rather than to a genetic disorder.

It does indicate that there was no real difference in the responses given between two different clinical populations in Cardiff, but that there were a number of important differences found in the Dutch respondents to questions placed on a website. The differences found between these groups generally indicate that the Dutch Website Group indicate more definite effects of the family history (Questions 2, 3, 8, 12, 14) compared with the clinical samples, although the response to Question 12 could be related to their younger age. Indeed there was a significant correlation between the response to this question and the subject's age (tau = 0.13; p = 0.023), even though the correlation was not large.

It is interesting that the self-selected Dutch respondents showed more positive effects of a family history and that the 'Knowledge of family history' questions indicated that 89% of the Dutch population were aware of the hereditary effect compared with 46% and 38% of the two Cardiff populations.

The general factorial structure found for the two groups of Cardiff subjects is broadly similar to the pattern for the whole group with 'Awareness of FH – positive effects' and 'Awareness of FH – negative effects' being the two most important factors. In addition the relationships with demographic variables mirrored the overall results, positive effects being related to awareness of the family history and negative effects to hearing level. The relationship found between factor 3 (passiveness) and family history awareness is interesting in that those with awareness were generally less passive. This is broadly similar to the result found with factor 1, although interestingly factors 1 and 3 showed no significant relationship to each other.

The results of this study and the identification of a similar factor structure in the separate samples again confirm that awareness of family history may be considered as a potential tool to promote psychosocial well-being among those with hearing loss having psychosocial difficulties resulting from their hearing impairment.

To facilitate this, role modelling activities should be promoted. These should include the role of awareness of family history in counselling programmes. However, it is important to be aware of the fact that those with greater loss may experience just negative effects of a family history.

The findings in this chapter seem to emphasise the fact that increasing awareness may be relevant for some groups of people with hearing loss, while for others (those with severe hearing impairment) it may even have adverse effects.

Thus, distinction of different groups constitutes an important contribution to our current knowledge within this respect.

REFERENCES

Davis A (1995) *Hearing in Adults*. London: Whurr.

Danermark B (2005) A review of the psychosocial effects of hearing impairment in the working age population. In D Stephens, L Jones (eds) *The Impact of Genetic Hearing Impairment*. London: Whurr, pp. 106–36.

Kramer SE (2005) The psychosocial impact of hearing loss among elderly people. A review. In D Stephens, L Jones (eds) *The Impact of Genetic Hearing Impairment*. London: Whurr, pp. 137–64.

Kramer SE, Stephens D, Espeso A (2006) The impact of having a family history of hearing problems on those with hearing difficulties themselves: a structured questionnaire (*submitted*).

Stephens D, Kramer SE (2005) The impact of having a family history of hearing problems on those with hearing difficulties themselves: an exploratory study. *International Journal of Audiology* 44: 206–12.

Stephens D, Lewis P, Davis A (2003) The influence of a perceived family history of hearing difficulties in an epidemiological study of hearing problems. *Audiological Medicine* 1: 228–31.

APPENDIX 7.1

Name: Date:

Hospital No.:

The following are statements made by other people with hearing loss in their families. Please indicate whether they are true or not in your case.

	Definitely True	Probably True	Probably Not True	Definitely Not True
1. It made me aware of the danger of social isolation	☐	☐	☐	☐
2. Because of my family history, I didn't think it important enough to do anything about my own hearing loss for a while	☐	☐	☐	☐
3. It made me determined not to ignore the problem	☐	☐	☐	☐
4. I didn't realise hearing problems were hereditary	☐	☐	☐	☐
5. It made me more aware of other people with hearing problems	☐	☐	☐	☐
6. It made me more fatalistic about my hearing problems	☐	☐	☐	☐
7. It made me realise the need to be open about problems so others can help	☐	☐	☐	☐

	Definitely True	Probably True	Probably Not True	Definitely Not True
8. My hearing problems were a long time being diagnosed so had no effect on me	☐	☐	☐	☐
9. It gave me empathy with people who would possibly find it irritating if I continually asked for repetition or rephrasing	☐	☐	☐	☐
10. It worries me that my children may develop hearing problems in the future	☐	☐	☐	☐
11. I am not worried about using a HA as I know how much of a problem it is for others without one.	☐	☐	☐	☐
12. It has influenced major life decision (e.g. career) for me	☐	☐	☐	☐
13. I try to encourage others who are too proud to seek help	☐	☐	☐	☐
14. The likelihood of decreasing hearing with age is a depressing prospect	☐	☐	☐	☐
15. Had I not known of my relatives' deafness, I think I would continually be casting round for the cause of my own problems	☐	☐	☐	☐
16. I expected problems in later life because of the family history	☐	☐	☐	☐
17. I had some comfort from the fact they had coped in more difficult circumstances	☐	☐	☐	☐
18. I am worried that my enjoyment of music will be impaired	☐	☐	☐	☐
19. It made me aware of the problem and prompted me to seek help sooner.	☐	☐	☐	☐
20. Until I came to clinic I thought everyone could hear the same as me	☐	☐	☐	☐

8 The Impact that a Family History of Late Onset Hearing Impairment Has on Those with the Condition Themselves

SARAH COULSON

INTRODUCTION

Late onset hearing impairment is considered to be the development of hearing loss after language has been learnt. Hearing impairment has an impact not only on the person diagnosed but also their family and friends. Having a relative with the same condition may have an impact on how the person deals with their own hearing loss.

Stephens and Kramer (2005) explored the impact family history has on those with hearing loss themselves. In this study patients with a family history of hearing loss from an audiological clinic were asked whether their family history had had an impact of their reaction to their hearing loss. Fifty-seven per cent reported an impact and these impacts were divided into positive, negative and neutral categories. Positive impacts were reported to be: realisation of the importance of hearing aids, early help-seeking, the understanding of others and the understanding of problems experienced. Negative impacts included: anxiety for the future, worries about the effect on offspring and being more conscious of problems. Neutral impacts included non-realisation of a family history, denial of family history or impact and awareness of family history.

Stephens & Kramer (2005) is one of very few papers that has specifically researched the impact family history has on those with late onset hearing impairment. It highlights the complex nature of feelings and issues surrounding this particular group of individuals, and provides an important insight into how family history impacts on those also affected with the condition, a major question in this study.

The present study focuses on the experience of adults with late onset hearing impairment who have had relatives who had the same condition. This

The Effects of Genetic Hearing Impairment in the Family. Edited by D. Stephens and L. Jones.
Copyright © 2006 by John Wiley & Sons, Ltd.

qualitative study is based on the data obtained from ten individuals and one couple in a semi-structured interview. The accounts given by the subjects were analysed in depth using a theme-orientated discourse analysis approach and themes were drawn out from the data. Experiences with the affected relative and coping mechanisms were explored in depth.

The results show that people's experiences of relatives with hearing impairment differ between those that had a broad knowledge of their relative and those who did not. Those that did have varied memories of their relative/s spoke widely of relational issues rather than transactional ones. This study shows the complexities underpinning the mechanisms used by someone with hearing loss when they have had experience of a relative/s with the same condition.

METHOD

This study uses a qualitative approach in both the data collection and analysis. As many previous studies have been quantitative, there is a need for more of an in-depth understanding of the complex nature of hearing impairment with family history.

Each patient was interviewed for 45–60 minutes using a semi-structured interview. A semi-structured interview was used because it allows the participants to answer the questions freely, describing experiences that they are comfortable discussing, thus providing a greater depth of understanding of the issues important to the participants. The sample consisted of individuals who had been seen in the Welsh Hearing Institute, University Hospital of Wales, Cardiff, for their hearing loss and had at least one relative who also had hearing impairment later in life. The sample was taken from successive clinic lists. The sample varied in age with varying experiences of their affected family member.

DATA ANALYSIS

The data were analysed using theme-orientated discourse analysis identifying themes in the interview transcripts. This analysis was used as it allows the exploration of the verbal interactions between interviewer and interviewee. These verbal interactions or language allows us to communicate and fulfil everyday tasks and is central to this analysis. To allow the researcher to fully familiarise herself with the data, the tapes were transcribed in a readable paper format. These transcripts were read and re-read allowing the researcher to identify themes. The transcripts were then split into two groups, those individuals who had extensive experience and memory of their affected relative/s, and those who did not. Further categorising and analysis of the Family Knowledge group was performed to analyse and understand the impact this family knowledge had on the participant and their coping mechanisms.

RESULTS

Two distinct groups emerged from the data, the Family Knowledge Group and the Non Family Knowledge Group. The Family Knowledge Group (four individuals) are those where the participant describes a broad knowledge and memories of their affected relative's hearing loss and life and that this family member/s has played a part in the participants' life. Thus, the Non Family Knowledge Group (seven individuals) are those where the participant does not have many memories or knowledge of their relative with hearing loss. In these cases the family member may not have lived with them, with memories being limited, or the participant did not talk about their family member in relation to their hearing loss.

FAMILY KNOWLEDGE GROUP

Relational and transactional issues in and out of the family sphere

The data in the Family Knowledge Group showed clear differences of coping strategies in and out of the family environment. There was also a split between experiences described as relational and those described as transactional. By splitting the data into these four categories the researcher was able to obtain a more in-depth appreciation of the data and analyse them further. The following sections examine these four categories in greater depth, beginning with explanations of the four distinct entities of family sphere, non-family sphere, transactional and relational. These entities will then be combined to form four categories, providing an examination of the relational and transactional issues in and out of the family sphere.

Transactional/Relational

The data were split into transactional and relational data. Transactional data were the discussion of everyday mundane tasks often involving non-human contact, such as the television or the cooker timer. Relational is rather more complex, this was categorised as the discussion of relational networks, roles, self (including loss of face), sharedness and character. These relational/transactional extracts either involved the family sphere or were outside the family sphere. The extracts below describe these transactional and relational experiences.

Extract 1 (Transactional)

S: *Do you remember your grandmother having any similar problems? (Similar problems such as not hearing mumbling or people asking if you have your hearing aid in)*

I: *. . . thinking about it, my grandmother's natural style was to talk, and I would be the one listening. So she could just rabbit along; it would only be an issue*

*if I tried to speak and then it would be, a bit louder, look a little bit lost. She
never got at me for it she was just frustrated at the quality of the hearing aid.
Frustration.* (C7)

In this extract the respondent is describing his grandmother's style of talking
so that she did not include others in the conversation. This is a transactional
response as it shows an everyday coping mechanism for her deafness.
However, it can be seen that the respondent then ends the transactional
response with descriptions of his grandmother's frustration at the quality of
her hearing aid. This could be understood as a relational response, therefore
many transactional responses are often ended with a relational explanation
and relational/transactional descriptions are often closely interlinked.

Extract 2 (Relational)

S: *Are there any bad effects of knowing that you have a family history, had any
bad effect on how you view your hearing loss or anything? Anything positive or negative or in between?*

I: *. . . well no, it comes back to the question of the positive aspects in a way.
Um, remember my mother and more of my grandmother I have the sense
that hearing loss was part of the quirky nature of who they were. Um, I just
imagine I will be a sort of quirky person like that.* (C7)

In this extract the respondent is describing his mother and grandmother's
quirky personality and that is how he sees himself being in the future. This is
a relational description of the character of the family members, character
playing a part in the respondents' way of dealing and coming to terms with
his future and his hearing loss.

Family Sphere / Outside Family Sphere

Participants usually discussed matters that are either things that involved the
family or those that did not. Therefore a split was made between data that
involved the family or spouse and those that did not. Descriptions of other
affected family members in their own entity were put into the 'outside family
sphere' group as they were taken to be a separate person. The following
extracts provide examples of what is meant by 'family sphere' and 'outside
family sphere'.

Extract 3 (Family Sphere)

S: *So what did you do differently, instead of shouting at her?*

I: *I was very much around her, the youngest child. I had her attention, I would
not say to her, so that she would know, I would have her full attention then.
I knew that we didn't need to shout* (giggle) (C1)

This extract is a respondent describing how she used to communicate with her mother so that she could hear, thus is something that was inside the family sphere.

Extract 4 (Outside Family Sphere)

S: *... you mentioned that your father had the television very loud, do you find that you turn the TV up louder?*

I: *I put the 888 thing, I put the words up, and I can read so rapidly. But the other thing in that sense to hearing, I actually take in information from the written word.* (C9)

This extract is a respondent describing her use of teletext so that she does not have to have the television up too loud, she finds that she can read quickly so that she understands the conversation on the television. This is an example of a coping mechanism outside the family sphere; it does not include other family members.

Having described the four entities of family sphere, non-family sphere, transactional and relational separately, we will now examine these entities included in four categories, allowing a greater understanding of the data. These categories are:

1. Family Sphere – Transactional
2. Family Sphere – Relational
3. Outside Family Sphere – Transactional
4. Outside Family Sphere – Relational

Family Sphere – Transactional

This category included everyday tasks that were described that involved the family, for example, how family members communicate with the hard-of-hearing member.

The extracts below illustrate the data analysed, allowing for further analysis and conclusions. Further extracts can be seen in Coulson (2004).

Extract 5

S: *It may not be too bad not to hear him sometimes ... So looking back at your mother and her hearing loss, how does that knowledge, that your mum had hearing loss, affect how you feel about yours?*

I: *... I know as a child I felt very protective, people were impatient with her ... I used to rush home on a Friday when she did the shopping ... I used to catch up with her and go to the same shops every week ... and they knew my mother and every week I used to have to say you will have to speak up my mother can't hear you. And the next week we would be back to square*

*one again, I used to get so frustrated about it; it helped me deal (with) people
to be more considerate with me.* (C1)

In this extract the respondent is describing her memory of rushing home from
school to help her mother do the weekly shopping. She describes the difficulties her mother had in communicating with the shopkeepers, and the feelings
of frustration she had with the shopkeepers at their inconsideration for her
mother's hearing loss and her need to protect her mother from their ridicule.
This very transactional process, going to do the shopping, has a very relational
aspect, the feelings of frustration – a protection by the daughter.

From this category it can be clearly seen that the participant is describing
coping and communication mechanisms used by them when they were
younger, in order to communicate with their hard-of-hearing relative. It also
includes communication tactics used by their family members with them, the
participant. These tactics and ways of coping have been learnt either from the
past, from when they were a child, or from now with their spouse. They have
been learnt and adapted to allow the participant and their family to cope with
everyday communication problems. This has appeared in many other cases,
extracts including:

Extract 6

I: *As long as she was looking at you she was alright. It was partly lip-reading
and partly hearing. But you dare not walk behind her, she would not hear
behind you. Again, she was not profoundly deaf in the prof's definition but
she was certainly very hard of hearing.* (C9)

This extract describes another coping strategy used by a family to communicate with a hard-of-hearing relative. They used positioning so that their relative could see their face and lips so that she could understand what they were
saying. By walking behind her they knew that she could not hear the conversation so they learnt how to stand or sit so that they were positioned in the
best way in order to communicate. Lip-reading, as described by Hallberg and
Carlsson (1991) is a non-verbal communication strategy which is part of the
'controlling the social scene', which is an active strategy used by the hearing-
impaired to control the situation so that they can communicate. This is in contrast to the Non Family Knowledge Group where coping strategies were far
less active and controlling of the social scene.

Communication problems between family members and particularly
spouses have been widely researched (Stephens et al., 1995; Piercy, 2002).
Communication plays a large part in relationships; if we cannot communicate
with our spouse and other family members, then frustration and blame result
(Hétu et al., 1993).

Further extracts in this category include family members telling the respondent that they are getting deaf.

Extract 7

I: *Medical background, knowing there was a system of helping me, that is what encouraged me, knowledge, family encouraging me. And also the teasing 'you're getting deaf now' and that kind of thing, so I was encouraged by the family.* (C9)

Family members telling their relative that they are deaf and cannot hear properly or are not being fully involved in the family is something that Glass (1985) described in his research. He also described the monopolisation of conversations so that they do not give other people the opportunity to speak, and thus no opportunity to misunderstand. This can be seen in extract 3.

Family Sphere – Relational

This category includes extracts that involve the interaction of family members that involve a relational aspect as described in the relational category. This category is extremely complex and a further analysis of this group can be seen in a later section. The following extracts show examples of experiences of relational issues in the family sphere.

Extract 8

S: *I suppose, basically knowing that you have a family history – has that had any effect on how you feel about your hearing loss? For example do you find it reassuring that someone else in your family had the same problems, or do you find it (a) frightening sort of effect?*

I: *Sort of silly thing, this is why I was talking about the Munchausen's . . . It was (a) sort of silly feeling that I wanted to follow in their footsteps . . . you know that would show that I was in their lives . . . And so I don't know whether that is quite a profound thing because they died and (I) sort of followed them in a way.* (C7)

This respondent is describing his desire to follow in his mother's and grandmother's footsteps, in the way of having hearing impairment. To him, having hearing loss has brought him closer to them. However, before he was diagnosed as having hearing loss he thought he had a form of Munchausen's because he thought that he had made up the symptoms of hearing loss so that he can follow in his relatives' footsteps.

Extract 9

S: *Do you notice any of that in your brother or your parents and their hearing loss? (loss of confidence)*

I: *The family was the centre of her world, we would make allowances for it, so I don't think it bothered her in the slightest. And quite frankly as a family, were not the types of people that made a fuss about life. We are able to take things in our stride, which unfortunately other people are not. So you're lucky in that sense.* (C9)

This category of the data includes a complex web of coping and communication mechanisms, included in which are descriptions of the affected relatives' personality. The family ethos and personality of the affected member shape the coping mechanisms used by the family members and are remembered, learnt and are put into place when the participant is older and uses them to cope with their own hearing loss.

Outside Family Sphere – Transactional

This category covers the descriptions of everyday tasks that do not involve family members. The following extract provides an example of transactional experiences outside the family sphere.

Extract 10

S: *. . . are there any negative aspects of your mother's hearing loss that you feel yourself or your mother had? When you go into the shops and people didn't understand.*

I: *Yes that is I suppose. Even now when I shop at Sainsbury's, so if you are paying by card they always ask you do you want cash back do you want to save your vouchers. So I never wait to be asked, I don't want cash back thank you and I am saving my vouchers. Often I am packing and they are saying it to me and I used to miss it, excuse me, if I know a question is coming I will answer it before they have a chance to ask me. I find that a great help sometimes.* (C1)

This respondent describes using a pre-learnt script when doing the shopping. Interestingly this is the same respondent from which extract 5 was taken. In extract 5 she described the weekly shopping she did with her mother.

When communicating with strangers, each person has a clear role, the cashier and the customer in a shopping situation, to give an example. If we do not fulfil our role satisfactorily then the boundaries between those roles has been changed. In this extract, if the customer, the respondent in this case, does not hear the cashier ask the routine questions and the cashier has to repeat themselves or make themselves heard so that the customer can hear, then the professional relationship between them has changed. The customer has lost face as they have not fulfilled their role to the usual standard and their disability has become apparent to the cashier. This showing of their hearing loss has meant that they have lost their social standing and this is something that they try to prevent at all costs. Thus by learning scripts and other coping mechanisms their face can be maintained and their disability hidden and they can live a life of normality. A large amount of our verbal interactions with people, especially strangers, is spent saving face. It is argued that this is done by using 'politeness strategies' in order to establish roles, especially when managing uncertainties in social settings (Brown & Levinson, 1987). This respondent (extracts 5 and 10) describes protecting her mother from the ridicule of the shopkeepers. Loss of face was important to her, when she was a child and now as an adult. As a child she was trying to protect her mother's embarrassment by asking the shopkeepers to speak up as her mother could not hear. By doing this for her mother, she learnt coping mechanisms that helped her mother cope and were in-built and stored for her to use when she herself developed hearing loss. In one respect she was one step ahead of those who had not had this learning exposure as a child.

This is also an example of how a transactional event can have a relational aspect where the description of an everyday or mundane task ends with a relational, emotional description or comment. This is in contrast to the Non Family Knowledge Group where transactional comments rarely ended with a relational aspect.

These extracts involve the use of coping mechanisms in order to achieve everyday tasks such as listening to the radio or doing the shopping. Some coping mechanisms are straightforward practical actions, such as turning the television or radio up so that it can be heard, or how they position themselves within a group. However, some involve the use of a learnt, prepared script, so that none of the conversation is misunderstood or ignored. By learning this script in the everyday sense of shopping, the participant will avoid the embarrassment of missing out on the interaction between them and the cashier, thus the prevention of loss of face. The notion of face is an important one, seen throughout the cases, and is one that seems to be of great importance in the public sphere.

Outside Family Sphere – Relational

This category includes extracts where the participant describes experiences that involved an emotional aspect, not involving the family. The following extract describes relational issues experienced outside the family sphere.

Extract 11

I: *So now it's getting pretty bad, as I am completely misunderstanding one or, but if I am with my friends I am always saying what did she say, I'm hanging in there – it's stressful really.* (C1)

This respondent is describing the decline of her hearing; as a result she is misunderstanding words. With her friends she is asking what the other people in the conversation say, and feels that she is not totally involved in the conversation. She describes feelings of 'hanging in there' resulting in feelings of stress.

This category is the description of events where communication has been difficult resulting in a relational aspect including loss of face and embarrassment. In this extract the respondent describes feelings of stress and embarrassment at the inability to converse with both friends. Hallberg and Carlsson (1991) show categories describing examples of restriction in social interactions. Within this are two categories, 'Frustration and aggression' and 'Frustration of the need of self-assertion'. In extract 11 the respondent's description of her meeting with friends falls under both categories with their examples under the frustration and aggression category, 'the hearing person is irritated at the environment' and under the frustration of the need of self-assertion category, 'being left out' being shown in this extract. Those authors described situations of hearing-impaired people being unable to follow group conversations which causes frustration not only with their surroundings and the people they are conversing with, but also with themselves.

In extract 11, the respondent is describing feelings of 'hanging in there' and the stress this caused. This indicates that she is trying desperately to be part of the conversation but is not quite able to understand the full conversation. By 'hanging on' she has a desire to be involved but still has not been able to develop a satisfactory coping mechanism that allows her to join in group conversations. She wants to be conversing normally and not have this obstacle in her way. Normality is the key to all coping mechanisms used by this group. Perhaps loss of face and self-esteem is at risk if she asks for repetition or clarity of the conversation. Perhaps she does not want to be a hindrance in the social group, and they are intimidating.

The need to minimise the effect of hearing loss and the coping strategies that develop in order to maintain their social identity, has been discussed by Goffman (1990). Goffman argued that, in order to minimise the obtrusiveness of their stigma, people can learn the essence of a social interaction. By learning set interactions, for example at a dinner party, a person with hearing loss can keep their 'secret' and hide their disability.

This shows that even with the exposure to learning opportunities at an early age, and with personal experience, hearing loss still results in difficulties in communication that are hard to overcome.

Feelings of being left out and embarrassment are feelings of inferiority, as described by Hallberg and Carlsson (1991). Coping mechanisms are developed and learnt by those who are hearing-impaired in order to control situations to the best of their ability so that they manage everyday life. By managing and coping with everyday life they can try to avoid embarrassment and loss of face. However, some situations they cannot control, as when the situation may involve other people who cannot be controlled, such as that in extract 11. The breakdown of these communication coping strategies leads to embarrassment and stress and ultimately feelings of inferiority, which leads to the realisation of their disability. Interestingly, the respondents' coping mechanisms usually are ways that do not allow strangers to see their disability. However it is possible that sometimes it is felt that it is safe to put those defences down, and show their disability. A way of showing their disability would be the use of a hearing aid. Goffman (1990) argues that by wearing a 'stigma symbol' the person would be disclosing their disability. This disclosure would change their social identity and have a variety of consequences on their social interactions.

This category also includes thoughts of hearing loss and other disabilities and how other people's situations are more difficult than their own. Examples of this can be seen in the next subsection under 'Other-Experiential'.

Conclusion

Looking at transactional aspects of communication and coping mechanisms for the family sphere and outside family sphere groups, we can see some differences. In the outside family group the coping mechanisms used are generally pre-learnt and prepared scripts when dealing with people outside the family, for example, doing the shopping and dealing with customers at work. However, in the family sphere group, coping strategies used in order to communicate are more direct, such as asking for things to be said, facing them or presenting their good ear, or even just isolating themselves from conversation. When communicating with strangers there is a fear that their self-esteem, face and social standing are at risk if they are perceived to be disabled or needing more assistance or not able to fulfil their job requirements. At home, with the family, this is not so much an issue and the hearing loss can be apparent and has more of a disease association.

Relational aspects in and out of the family sphere are also described differently. Within the family sphere, coping mechanisms revolve around heroic descriptions of their affected family member, their personality and ethos, providing a way for them to cope with everyday difficulties of hearing loss. Participants' relatives are described as exceptional, not a grumbler, calm and quiet. With family sayings including, 'if you can manage, then do', 'we take things in our stride' and 'there is no such thing as can't until you have tried'. These all provide a framework of coping that the next generation of family members with hearing loss have used as a way to cope with the difficulties of hearing loss. Situations within the family are also described that could be far worse than their own, such as not having other family members with hearing loss or not having family ethos/sayings allowing them to cope.

Relational aspects described outside the family sphere are generally difficulties in communication with friends and people that the participant knew. These are descriptions of embarrassment, stress, feelings of stupidity, which come when coping strategies used for communication break down. They also, interestingly, describe situations that would be far worse than their own, such as having a terminal illness. These are possibly ways of convincing themselves that hearing impairment is not as bad as it could be and that it isn't anything that causes too much difficulty in their life.

A MORE DETAILED EXAMINATION OF
RELATIONAL STRATEGIES

Further analysis has been undertaken of the relational data and four clear distinctions of data have emerged. I shall begin by looking at the familial category of data, where the participant describes how they believe that hearing impairment is passed down through the generations. I shall next provide an in-depth examination of the relational aspects and experiences described within the family. I continue with an analysis of how experiences of hearing impairment provide learning experiences and how this affects coping. Finally I examine how individuals describe situations worse than their own and how this may be a way of coming to terms with their condition.

Familial

This group includes data where the participant has described an understanding that hearing impairment can be passed down the family. The following extracts describe how the participants believe that their hearing impairment can be passed on.

Extract 12

I: *My daughter is 44 now in September, I think she is going to be like me, (son) has good hearing, but she is going to follow me, she has to go get her ears syringed quite frequently. So I would imagine she is going to have the same problems as me. She is exactly like I was at that age.* (C10)

This respondent is describing the similarities between her and her daughter in terms of hearing loss. She believes that, because she is following the same pattern of ear syringing, she is likely to develop hearing loss later in life. This shows that this respondent believes that hearing loss can be passed down through generations and is something that is just accepted.

Extract 13

I: *Right – I had the sense that with my grandmother it was a more dramatic thing, I had the sense that my mother was taking after my grandmother.* (C7)

This respondent also believes that hearing loss is passed down through the family (genetic).

This understanding of where their hearing loss has come from may, in some way, help them to come to terms with the condition and not to dwell on what may have caused it. This is in contrast to the Non Family Knowledge Group where some respondents wondered what may have caused their loss and wanted reassurance that they had not caused the condition through neglect or something they had done wrong. Extracts from the Non Family Knowledge Group include:

Extract 14

I: *In my mind it was separate, I always wondered what it was, I could hear some things but not others.* (C5)

This respondent has just described what she thought her mother and father's hearing loss was caused by, and in this extract she is saying that hers is separate, but she always wondered what caused hers. She then continued, a few turns later, to state that, if her ear infections as a child had been treated differently then she may not have hearing loss as an adult.

Extract 15

I: *Oh gosh, have I been doing that I would hate something to happen to me and it to be my own fault. Cause I try to take all the right precautions . . .* (C3)

This respondent is describing how he would hate it if he did something to cause something to be medically wrong with him. He speaks a lot about how he looks after himself and eats the right food, and is justifying to himself that he has not caused the hearing loss.

Both these extracts show that those in the Non Family Knowledge Group and those generally that have not had exposure to close relatives with hearing loss have less chance to come to terms with their hearing loss and battle for an explanation of its cause.

Family-Relational

These descriptions are the relational aspects of the family sphere including roles, face, embarrassment and characterisation of affected relatives.

I have discussed the notion of face and embarrassment of miscommunication in the previous section. However, there is another aspect of the family-relational category – characterisation of affected relatives. This is the way that respondents have described their relative's personality in a heroic sense. Examples of these descriptions can be seen below:

Extract 16

I: *No she didn't, but she was an exceptional person, she was lovely she would let everyone get on with it.* (C1)

This respondent was asked '*Did you find your mother getting irritated?*' Her response described the idyllic personality of her mother.

Extract 17

I: *She was a very . . . a lady that didn't go around rushing about into to things she took things in her stride, she never . . . She was a very calm person, I don't know whether that was anything to do with the deafness but I felt it help her deal with the deafness it might have been her way . . . she was a calm lady didn't get over agitated, coped with crisis very well.* (C1)

This respondent again describes their mother as taking things in her stride and coping very well in a crisis and with her hearing loss.

Extract 18

I: *No, reassuring because she was such a calm person, I think that is why I was bothered that I was going deaf but I wasn't panicky.* (C1)

The respondent describes their mother as a calm lady and they found this reassuring with their own hearing loss.

These positive descriptions of family members' personalities show that the respondents thought highly of their relative and the way that their personality allowed them to cope well with their hearing loss. It is unclear whether the family member's personality shaped the way that they coped or that their personality developed and changed into a form that allowed them to cope with their hearing loss. Either way the respondents may have learnt from their positive outlook and personality as a good way of coping and as something they aspire to themselves.

Family-Experiential

Included in this group are descriptions of experiences where the participant has been provided with a learning opportunity from their affected relative. Examples include:

Extract 19

I: *Yes, yes there is no such thing as can't until you have tried. One of my mother's little sayings, so I never thought, I always felt push on.* (C1)

This respondent is recalling one of her mother's sayings which she uses as one of her own personal beliefs, thus has learnt a coping ethos from her mother.

Extract 20

I: *I think, Aren't I fortunate that I have something that I can wear, whereas my dad had to just have put up with it? I would have loved him to have access to something like this.* (C10)

This respondent is comparing their hearing aid with one her father had, hers being a lot better, and she feels fortunate that she does not have to put up with the difficulties that her father had.

By growing up with a relative with hearing loss, these participants have been provided with opportunities to learn from their relatives' experiences in coping with their hearing loss. Having these opportunities has allowed the participants to be prepared and learn how to cope with their hearing loss in various situations of everyday life. Those with hearing loss who have not had this opportunity to learn from other family members may not cope as well with their own hearing loss. This contrast in coping can be seen in the Non Family Knowledge Group. The group that had not had continuous or broad exposure to a family member with hearing loss do not have the same ability to cope with everyday communication tasks as those that have had the broad exposure and knowledge of affected family members. This can be seen in extracts 27 and 28, where coping mechanisms used are shutting off because they cannot hear in church and opening their purse for the cashier to take the correct money. These contrast with the advanced developed coping mechanisms used by the Family Knowledge Group of learning scripts, positioning themselves and using technical help, such as hearing aids. Due to this successful use of evolved coping mechanisms, the Family Knowledge Group appear to be more comfortable and adapted to their hearing loss and the disadvantages it brings.

People with hearing loss do not solely learn coping mechanisms from other family members with the condition, but also from their own everyday lives and experiences. These personal experiences, however, only provide limited opportunities to learn coping mechanisms as they are often accidental opportunities that are not reliable. However, the family experience provides a continuous, reliable and systematic exposure to learning opportunities. Therefore such individuals are in a better starting position than those that have not had the learning exposure earlier in life.

Participants' personal sphere of learning and coping produces ways of dealing with and putting into perspective their situation of being hearing-impaired. Examples include:

Extract 21

I: *Yes. I don't think my hearing loss has been severe enough to for me to think it to be a handicap as such. It is a gradual thing and you just adapt to it. It is only when you get a hearing aid that you notice how much you were missing.* (C10)

This respondent describes their reaction to hearing impairment and it not being considered to be a handicap; it is something they have adapted to. Having a hearing aid has made them appreciate how much they were missing.

Extract 22

I: *No, none at all. None whatsoever, it was just that I accepted it thinking that it was an age-related thing, but always in that fashion, I'm not a worrying kind of person.* (C9)

This respondent describes that they were not worried about their hearing loss; it was just accepted as something they got when they were older.

By having this exposure to other relatives with hearing loss, the participants may also be in a better position to appreciate and come to terms with their own disability. If they have seen a relative take the disability in their stride, then the condition itself is nothing to fear and is not to be thought of as a disability or disadvantage. This is where someone with an understanding of and exposure to a family member with hearing loss can use those learning opportunities and apply them to their own personal learning opportunities, combining to produce a large pool of coping mechanisms. Family ethos and beliefs can play a large role in coping and provide a level of normality and belief of how one should cope and behave in the public and private spheres. In this way hearing loss is not thought of as something to worry about or dwell on or to be considered as a disadvantage or disability. This is again in contrast to those in the Non Family Knowledge Group as they do not appear to have these family beliefs or coping strategies that allow them to be positive and forward about their hearing loss. They, as a group, generally dwell on their disabilities and speak of blame towards others and their communication abilities that do not allow them to join in conversations or social activities. There seems to be less of an ability to cope with the outside world and those around them; and they do not appear to be able to adapt to their environment and learn new communication strategies in order to cope with everyday tasks.

Other-Experiential

Participants often describe their situation, of being hearing-impaired, of being much better than other situations, such as being visually impaired and being seriously or terminally ill. Examples from the transcripts include:

Extract 23

I: *Yes and because of the background working with some seriously ill people it makes you realise how lucky you are. We accept that. Too many people complain without that much to complain about.* (C9)

This respondent has a large family of medical professionals and describes an awareness of serious medical conditions. She believes that there are far worse conditions than hearing loss and it makes her realise how fortunate she is that she only has hearing loss and not anything worse. She also states that people complain about things when they really do not have anything to complain about, so be grateful for what you have.

Extract 24

I: *It didn't worry me it didn't frighten me . . . growing up it is like somebody born without sight is the same as hearing it can't be easier . . . it is something you haven't known.* (C1)

This respondent is describing hearing loss as something they are not frightened of and compare it to somebody born without sight.

These comparisons to other disabilities or diseases are similar to Hallberg and Carlsson's (1991) findings and their 'minimising the disability' category, within their group of strategies used for managing their hearing impairment.

The Non-Family Knowledge Group do not make any of these other experiential claims of comparing their condition to that of others which they perceive to be worse than their own. It is suggested that those that do not have a broad knowledge of or exposure to other family members with hearing loss have not been able to come to terms with their loss, and perceive it to be a disability that hinders them in everyday life.

Conclusions from Family Knowledge Group

The Familial category showed that the majority of those respondents with a broad knowledge of their family member/s with hearing loss, made a genetic link for the cause of their own hearing loss. This was shown to be in contrast with the Non Family Knowledge Group, where the respondents pondered and worried over the cause of their hearing loss. It is argued that the Family Knowledge Group are more able to come to terms with their own hearing loss as they have a personal understanding and belief for the cause, they feel that it was passed on from their parents. For some, this knowledge that their hearing loss has come down the generations from their grandparent to parent is of some reassurance.

The Family-Relational category showed how notions of face, embarrassment and characterisation of affected relatives shaped how our respondents coped with their own hearing loss. The notion of face, is an important aspect to protect and, by using sophisticated coping mechanisms, the self-esteem and confidence of the hearing-impaired person can be maintained. Within the family, however, this notion of face becomes less important as there is less at stake, as your family will not make judgements upon you based on your hearing ability. Characterisation of the affected relative/s is a large theme throughout the transcripts and is the positive, idyllic-like descriptions of family members with hearing loss. These personalities left a mark on our respondents and provided them with a benchmark of how to cope with and adapt to their hearing loss. It is perhaps a way of saying, 'If X didn't grumble, then I shouldn't either'.

The Family-Experiential category looked at the ways in which family members with hearing loss have provided our respondents with learning opportunities which have allowed them to successfully adapt to and cope with their own hearing loss. Included in this is the role of family ethos and beliefs and the learning of coping strategies from the respondent's personal sphere.

The Other-Experiential category describes how respondents describe other situations that would be worse than their own. It is argued that this shows their adjustment to hearing loss and their appreciation of what they have. It is possible that this outlook on life has been influenced by their family members' beliefs and understanding.

I have discussed the impact family knowledge has had in terms of Familial, Family-Relational, Family-Experiential and Other-Experiential categories. It can be seen that, by having an experience of other family members with hearing loss and their coping mechanisms, there is greater exposure to learning experiences. This exposure allows those with hearing loss to be more understanding of the cause of disease, to have a more positive outlook, to develop more successful coping mechanisms and to be more able to come to terms with their disability.

NON FAMILY KNOWLEDGE GROUP

Examination of responses by participants with little family experience and/or exposure

The Family Knowledge Group is analysed and discussed in greater depth in the previous subsection, as this group is where the author's main interests lie.

The remainder of this chapter is a summary of the findings from the Non Family Knowledge Group. There are several clear similarities between the responses from these cases, mainly revolving around transactional actions.

Transactional responses

The majority of the cases in the Non Family Knowledge Group predominantly describe their family member/s with hearing loss in a very transactional, factual way, with no relational or emotional descriptions of personality or coping mechanisms. The interview is mostly based on factual stories of diagnosis of their hearing loss and stories often irrelevant to the question asked. In some ways it appeared that the participant was avoiding talking in depth about their memories of their relative and their hearing loss. This avoidance could be that their memories of their family member were not good ones or perhaps that they simply did not remember anything about their relatives' hearing loss. Of those who did describe their family members with hearing loss, the descriptions were often not positive. The vast majority of descriptions in and out of the family sphere were transactional, with few or no relational descriptions. Examples of these transactional descriptions include:

Extract 25

I: *My father had some slight trouble, you know. I can remember my mother having a hearing aid but not the reasons, you know. But my father was always off and on with everything, but my mother, my father not having a hearing aid, I can remember that. I can remember him saying yes, and we used to say it was the war and things like that, you know.* (C5)

In this case the respondent is describing their memories of their mother's and father's hearing loss. There are no personal or emotional responses included, it is factual and to the point.

Extract 26

I: *Well, my mum, just had a hearing aid put in and everything was fine. There was one auntie, X who died long before my mother died. I mean she had to write everything down and hold it up. Really, with hearing aids and everything. You would write it down and she would write it back, this is going back late 50s mid to late 60s.* (C2)

This respondent is describing his mother's and aunt's hearing loss and the coping mechanisms they used. Like the previous extract this is factual story-telling with no personal details of personality or emotional impact of the hearing loss.

As these extracts show, their family member and their hearing loss is described in a very factual, transactional way with no emotional aspect.

Coping and communication

Another interesting similarity of the cases emerged when coping and communication mechanisms were considered in depth. Examples of some extracts are included below:

Extract 27

I: *If there is a lot of people, say I go to the church service and I don't put it in, I cannot get all the words. So I just sit there and just shut off. It doesn't worry me, I just don't bother trying to listen.* (C4)

This respondent describes her attendance at church, for which she doesn't wear her hearing aid and consequently cannot understand the whole of the service, and therefore switches off.

Extract 28

I: *Yes, yes. Except when they ask for money, I get the pounds and tens out and I got a load of loose change here. The change goes in my purse, I lift it out and throw it onto the counter and take what you want.* (C6)

When shopping, this lady cannot hear how much money the cashier needs so she just opens her purse and asks the cashier to take the right money from her purse.

These extracts describe coping mechanisms for everyday tasks, such as doing the shopping or going to church. The first extract shows the participant not bothering to listen at church, and not having developed any form of coping mechanism to help her hear better in church. She is still attending church so is not 'avoiding the social scene' as described by Hallberg and Carlsson (1991). However, her behaviour is included in their description of 'Maintaining social interactions'. This is a way of coping with an everyday task by maintaining the task (going to church) and trying to make the best of it and not 'become a bother'. By doing this she has become tolerant of the environment around her and the public's lack of understanding of hearing loss. Hallberg and Carlsson (1991) continued to describe the cost involved in preserving such social interactions. 'More things have to be regarded as not so important, and restricted involvement in conversations have to be tolerated.' From this we can see that this respondent perseveres with her attendance at church at the cost of not being fully involved with the service. This lack of any proactive coping mechanism for their hearing loss leaves them becoming less involved with their environment around them. Further findings are that many of the participants described themselves as avoiding certain situations where they found communication difficult. This lack of coping may be linked with their lack of exposure to learning opportunities with family members with the same condition.

Extract 28 also shows the lack of any proactive coping strategy for an everyday task such as doing the shopping. This informant does not use any strategy which may allow her to hear better, but asks the cashier to help themselves to the correct amount of money. By doing this the informant has shown their disability and has taken a disabled role. S/he is not frightened to lose face or social standing or show their hearing loss in public. This is in distinct contrast to the Family Knowledge Group, which was discussed in more detail earlier.

Further similarities are the denial of their own hearing loss and the blaming of communication difficulties on others. An example taken from extracts is given below:

Extract 29

I: *These sound engineers don't drop it when the dialogue comes on.* (C11)

This respondent describes his anger at the television producers not reducing the music when the dialogue comes on, something which he feels very strongly about.

Blaming others, such as TV presenters and friends and family, for the respondents' inability to hear a conversation is a way of covering up their lack of coping mechanisms to overcome such difficulties. This again shows the inability or desire to form ways of dealing with or overcoming their hearing loss in order to allow them to achieve everyday tasks.

OVERALL CONCLUSIONS

This group of individuals have shown that, by not having a broad knowledge of their family member/s with the same condition, they generally have limited coping mechanisms. The coping mechanisms they use to overcome communication difficulties tend to be avoidance techniques, blame, denial, and shutting off. Mechanisms also used in the public sphere are open gestures of asking for help, such as opening their purse and asking the cashier to take the correct money in order to pay for something. By doing this the respondent has shown the cashier that they are disabled and need their help, and have lost face in doing so. It is suggested that by not having been exposed to learning opportunities for coping with hearing loss, that they have to learn from their own experiences. These experiences may be limited and their may be more at risk for the respondent in terms of embarrassment and loss of face.

The respondents talk widely of routine, factual and transactional issues, even when describing their family member with the same condition. There are few or no relational issues discussed, in and out of the family sphere. They also, as a group, tend to take the disabled role, of needing help and assistance, which may be an indication that they see themselves as hearing-impaired rather than someone who is hard of hearing.

The research has identified clear differences between those who have a broad exposure to and experience of a family member/s with hearing loss and those who do not. Those who have had a wide exposure to and experience of a family member with hearing loss have had a large opportunity to learn coping mechanisms from their relative/s. These opportunities have enabled them to adapt more easily and successfully to their own hearing loss, and have made them more positive about their disability than those that have not had this exposure. Although coping mechanisms can be learnt on a personal sphere, these are often a more risky enterprise in terms of face and confidence, thus are limited and often off-putting to the individual.

Another difference between the two knowledge groups is in the discussion of transactional and relational issues. The Family Knowledge Group speak predominantly of relational issues, inside and out of the family. Transactional issues are discussed, however, but they often are ended with a relational comment. In contrast to this the Non Family Knowledge Group speak predominantly of transactional issues and factual descriptions about their hearing loss. They often discuss and describe family members less positively than the knowledge group.

Individuals in the Family Knowledge Group with late onset hearing impairment have different coping mechanisms depending on the environment they happen to be in. Outside the family sphere, communicating with strangers in shops or at work, coping mechanisms are tailored so that the hearing-impaired does not get embarrassed or lose self-esteem or face. Inside the family sphere communication and coping strategies can be far more relaxed.

Relational aspects also differ between inside and outside the family sphere. Inside the family, beliefs and family ethos play a large part in shaping coping mechanisms, whereas outside the family sphere descriptions are limited to communication breakdown with friends, leading to loss of face and confidence.

I argue that by having a broad and varied experience of a family member with hearing loss the hearing-impaired individual has more ability to cope with their hearing loss both outside and in the family sphere. These experiences shape the way they think, cope and view their disability, providing an excellent framework to build on through their own personal experiences and lives.

REFERENCES

Brown P, Levinson S (1987) *Politeness: Some Universals in Language Usage.* Cambridge: Cambridge University Press.

Coulson S (2004) The impact family history of late onset hearing impairment has on those with the condition themselves. MSc Dissertation. Cardiff University.

Glass LE (1985) Psychosocial aspects of hearing loss in adulthood. In H Orlans (ed), *Adjustment to Hearing Loss.* San Diego, CA: College-Hill, pp. 167–78.

Goffman E (1990) *Stigma: Notes on the Management of Spoiled Identity.* Harmondsworth: Penguin.

Hallberg LMR, Carlsson SG (1991) A qualitative study of strategies for managing hearing impairment. *British Journal of Audiology* 25: 201–11.

Hétu R, Getty L, Jones L (1993). The impact of acquired hearing loss on the intimate relationship: implaications for rehabilitation. *Audiology* 32: 363–81.

Piercy S, Piercy F (2002) Couple dynamics and attributions when one partner has an aquired hearing loss: implications for couple therapy. *Journal of Marital and Family Therapy* 28: 315–26.

Stephens D, France L, Lormore K (1995) Effects of hearing impairment on the patient's family and friends. *Acta Otolaryngologica* 115: 165–7.

Stephens D, Kramer SK (2005) The impact of having a family history of hearing problems on those with hearing difficulties themselves: an exploratory study. *International Journal of Audiology* 44: 206–12.

9 Influence of a Family History of Hearing Impairment on Participation Restriction, Activity Limitation, Anxiety and Depression

ANGELES ESPESO AND DAFYDD STEPHENS

INTRODUCTION

Elsewhere in this book various authors have explored the impact of a family history of hearing problems on a range of aspects of the psychological impact of hearing impairment. There is, however, conflicting evidence from different studies and, within the present investigation, we have examined the impact of a family history in a carefully controlled and defined population. We consider the impact on Activity Limitation, Participation Restriction and Psychological Well-being.

Stephens et al. (2003) found, in a population study, that the possibility of having a family history of hearing difficulties was greater in those who reported hearing problems (19.7%) than in those without such a difficulty (8.9%).

In a follow-up with further analyses from that study they found that this applied equally in elderly respondents (>60 years old) in whom 68% of males and 52% of females with a family history reported hearing problems as compared with 45% of males and 28% of females without such a family history. In addition, in both studies, they found that those with hearing difficulties were more likely to report participation restrictions (Stephens et al., this volume, Chapter 1).

In contrast to the population study, which indicated that in those with a family history of hearing problems their hearing loss had a greater impact, Stephens and Kramer (2005) found a different pattern of results in a clinic population. They took only subjects who had a FHHL and asked them to list any impact that their family history had on them. These subjects reported three times as many positive effects as negative effects.

The Effects of Genetic Hearing Impairment in the Family. Edited by D. Stephens and L. Jones.

We have sought, within the present study, to determine whether an individual with a family history of hearing impairment differs in terms of Activity Limitation, Participation Restriction and Psychological Well-being from those without such a family history.

METHOD

In order to carry out this study we obtained ethical approval from Cardiff & Vale NHS Trust Research and Development Office and the Bro Taf Local Research Ethical Committee.

A group of 109 patients, seen as part of a genetic and aetiological study on age-related hearing impairment at the Welsh Hearing Institute (WHI) in Cardiff, gave informed consent to take part in this study. Within that study we recruited patients passing through the WHI clinics who were born between 1938 and 1949 and who had a symmetrical acquired non-syndromal sensorineural hearing loss.

The patients interested in taking part in the study were divided into two groups: a first group *with* a family history of hearing impairment and a second group *without* a family history of hearing impairment. A patient will be considered to be part of the first group if one or both parents were/are affected by any kind of hearing loss.

The 109 patients presented with different levels of sensorineural hearing loss. Exclusion criteria for participation in the study were having a hearing impairment due to a conductive hearing loss caused by a previous otitis media, middle ear effusion or an ear operation, having Menière's disease or a vestibular Schwannoma.

All patients were between 55 and 66 years of age (mean = 61.4 years; SD = 3.5).

All individuals underwent a pure tone air and bone conduction audiometry and otoadmittance testing so that the main audiometric criterion of having a sensorineural hearing loss would be confirmed objectively.

Both groups were given two well established questionnaires, the Quantitative Denver Scale (Alpiner et al., 1971) and the Hospital Anxiety and Depression Scale (HAD) (Zigmond & Snaith, 1983; Snaith, 2003), to be returned by post.

The Denver Scale of Communication Function consists of 34 questions divided into two main groups: Questions 1 to 23 test the participation restriction of the patient in different situations of his/her life. Questions 24 to 34 probe the activity limitations of the patient. The first 23 questions can be subdivided into different groups: Questions 1–6 test the patient's *attitude towards peers*; Questions 7–15 determine any *social problems* caused by the patient's hearing impairment; finally Questions 16–23 look into the impact on *communication skills/difficulties* of the hearing-impaired patient. In all parts, each

In a scale of 0–10, how much does your hearing problem affect your life?

(please circle as appropriate)

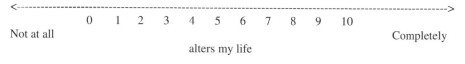

Figure 9.1 Visual analogue scale.

question is answered ticking only one of the following statements: *1. Definitely agree; 2. Slightly agree; 3. Irrelevant; 4. Slightly disagree; 5. Definitely disagree.*

At the end of the questionnaire we inserted an overall assessment of the impact of having a hearing loss on the patient's life in general by using a visual analogue scale (VAS) as shown in Figure 9.1. Even though there has been controversy on the use of VAS (Steiner & Norman, 1995; Kerr & Stephens, 2000), we considered this test to be a useful method of measurement in the context of this study.

The second questionnaire, the Hospital Anxiety and Depression Scale or HAD Scale consists of 14 closed-set questions and was designed to help any physician to determine how the patient feels about his/her medical condition/s (Zigmond & Snaith, 1983; Snaith, 2003). Questions 1, 3, 5, 7, 9, 11 and 13 assess the patients' anxiety (max score 21 points) and questions 2, 4, 6, 8, 10, 12 and 14 assess the patients' depressive feelings (max score 21 points). Scores on each scale can be interpreted in ranges: normal (0–7), mild (8–10), moderate (11–14) and severe (15–21). In this particular study it is used to assess the patient's current anxiety and depressive symptomatology in relation to their hearing impairment and determine if their response has been affected by the presence of a history of hearing loss in their family.

All patients were instructed not to take too long over their replies as their immediate reaction will be more accurate.

RESULTS

GENDER AND AGE

109 patients agreed to take part in this study; 51 patients had no family history of hearing impairment (FHHI): 26 male and 25 female. Of those with a FHHI (58 individuals) 32 were males and 26 females. The gender breakdown did not differ significantly between groups ($\chi^2 = 0.19$; NS).

The age range of these patients was between 55 and 66 years old with a total mean of 61.3 years of age. The mean age of the males was 61.2 and that of the

Table 9.1 Independent samples t-test: Age – FHHI

	FHHI	N	Mean	Std. Deviation	t	p
Age	no FHHI	51	62.0	3.30	1.76	0.08
	with FHHI	58	60.8	3.51		

females was 61.6 years. There was no significant difference between the age of the patients in the two FHHI groups (t = 1.77; p = 0.08) (Table 9.1).

DENVER SCALE RESULTS

One hundred and eight participants answered the 34 questions that form the Denver Scale of Communication Function. When comparing the means of the total score of the Denver Scale for the two FHHI groups, no significant difference was found (t = –0.78; p = 0.44).

We also examined the answers of both groups after dividing the questions into the two main domains of *Participation Restriction* and *Activity Limitation*. This again showed no significant difference between the two FHHI groups for either the Participation Restriction (t = –0.83; p = 0.41) or the Activity Limitation questions (t = –0.34; p = 0.73).

The statistical analysis of the three Participation Restriction subscales likewise showed no significant differences between the two FHHI groups.

Examining the answers obtained from the two FHHI groups on the individual questions using the non-parametric Mann–Whitney U-test, we found that Questions 10, 23 and 31 showed a significant difference between the groups:

- Question 10: '*I tend to be negative about life in general because of my hearing problem*' is a participation restriction question studying the attitude of the patient towards their peers. Those *with a FHHI* present a more positive attitude about their life despite their hearing impairment (Z = –2.00; p = 0.04).
- Question 23: '*I do not like to admit I have a hearing problem.*' This is a participation restriction question studying the communication attitude of the patient. Those *with a FHHI* are more likely to disagree with the statement that they do not like to admit to having a hearing impairment (Z = –2.15; p = 0.03).
- Question 31: '*In church I have much difficulty hearing the sermon.*' This is an activity limitation question studying specific difficult listening situations. Those *with a FHHI* disagree more with the statement (Z = –1.98; p = 0.05).

VISUAL ANALOGUE SCALE (VAS)

Three male patients and one female patient did not complete the VAS.

The mean answer on the visual analogue scale in the group *without a FHHI* was 5.5 (SD = 2.8), while in the group *with a FHHI* it was 5.4 (SD = 2.6) (t = 0.16; p = 0.87).

HAD SCALE

One subject did not answer any of the HAD Scale questions.

Comparison of the mean scores of the HAD questions both for the individual questions and for the agglomerated scores (Anxiety and Depression) showed no significant difference between the two groups of FHHI (Anxiety t = −1.07, p = 0.28; Depression t = −0.47, p = 0.64).

The HAD scores on each scale can be interpreted in ranges: normal (0–7), mild (8–10), moderate (11–14) and severe (15–21). On analysing the ranges in each FHHI group it was found that 60.8% of patients *without a FHHI* were within the normal range for the anxiety questions and 84% were within the normal range for the depression questions. In the group of patients *with a FHHI* 47% presented a 'Normal' range in the anxiety questions and 80% present 'Normal' ranges in the depression questions. When looking at the severe range of the anxiety questions and the depression questions there were no differences between the FHHI groups.

In general, when comparing the FHHI groups in terms of their anxiety bands, there was no significant difference between those with or without FHHI ($\chi^2 = 0.43$, NS). The same outcome was found when compared on their depression bands ($\chi^2 = 0.9$, NS).

OTHER ANALYSES

The mean Better ear threshold (500 Hz–4 KHz) was 38.3 dB (SD 16.3 dB) and the mean Worse ear threshold (500 Hz–4 KHz) was 47 dB (SD 19.5 dB). On analysing the two FHHI groups separately, those without a FHHI presented a mean Better ear threshold of 40 dB (SD 15 dB) and a mean Worse ear threshold of 50 dB (SD 19 dB). In the group with a FHHI the mean Better ear threshold was 37 dB (SD 17.5 dB) and the Worse ear threshold was 44.3 dB (SD 20 dB). None of the differences between the two FHHI groups was not significant (Better ear (t = 0.96; p = 0.34) and Worse ear (t = 1.52; p = 0.13)).

A Kendall non-parametric correlation matrix was calculated in both FHHI groups. It included the following variables: gender, age, better ear and worse ear hearing levels, Denver Scale questions, divided into main groups (PR and AL) as well as its subgroups (attitude towards peers, social problems and communication), and the HAD scales of anxiety and depression. The correlation matrices showed that (Table 9.2):

1. The Better ear hearing level in the group *without FHHI* correlated significantly with Participation Restriction score ($\tau = -0.23$; p = 0.02), the

Table 9.2 Correlations of hearing levels to FHHI groups and Participation Restriction/Activity Limitation

QUESTIONS (Denver Scale)	BETTER EAR				WORSE EAR			
	Without FHHI		With FHHI		Without FHHI		With FHHI	
	Kendall's tau-b Correlation coefficient (τ)	p value (p)	Kendall's tau-b Correlation coefficient (τ)	p value (p)	Kendall's tau-b Correlation coefficient (τ)	p value (p)	Kendall's tau-b Correlation coefficient (τ)	p value (p)
Activity Limitation	−0.28	0.006	−0.341	0.000	−0.24	0.02	−0.24	0.011
Participation Restriction	−0.23	0.02	−0.11	0.246	−0.2	0.054	−0.106	0.257
Attitude towards peers	−0.16	0.112	−0.157	0.097	−0.12	0.23	−0.106	0.262
Social problems	−0.24	0.015	−0.125	0.185	−0.17	0.08	−0.169	0.073
Communication	−0.22	0.03	−0.046	0.624	−0.21	0.03	−0.052	0.58

Activity Limitation score ($\tau = -0.28$; $p = 0.006$), Social problems ($\tau = -0.242$; $p - 0.015$) and Communication ($\tau = -0.22$; $p = 0.028$). However, the Better ear in the group *with FHHI* correlated significantly only with the Activity Limitation score ($\tau = -0.341$; $p = 0.000$).

2. Likewise, the Worse ear hearing level in the group *without a FHHI* correlated significantly with Participation Restriction Communication score ($\tau = -0.213$; $p = 0.033$) as well as the Activity Limitation score ($\tau = -0.239$; $p - 0.018$). Again, the Worse ear in the group *with FHHI* correlated significantly only with the Activity Limitation score ($\tau = -0.341$; $p = 0.000$).

Discussion

Within the present project we investigated whether an individual with a family history of hearing impairment (FHHI) might differ in their activity limitations, participation restrictions and psychological well-being from those not presenting such a family history. We had found no difference in the gender breakdown between the groups nor the mean age between the groups *without a FHHI* and *with a FHHI*.

We were unable to demonstrate any significant differences in Activity Limitation, Participation Restriction or Psychological Well-being.

We did, however, found that those *with a FHHI* had a more positive attitude towards their life despite their hearing impairment (Denver Question 10). Furthermore, those *without a FHHI* did not like to admit having a hearing impairment. Similarly, Stephens and Kramer (2005) also found that, among their sample of patients, those aware of their family history of hearing loss seem to be more positive about hearing problems than those without. However, it is possible but unlikely that these findings could have happened by chance, as both effects might be anticipated in those with a FHHI having more insight into their problems.

This study has shown that among those patients *with a FHHI* who complain of having more difficulties in specific listening situations, such as listening to the television or the radio unless the volume is turned up loud, someone calling from another room, using the phone, etc., will have a higher depression score on the Hospital Anxiety and Depression Scale. These findings differ from those observed by Saglier et al. (2005), who found in a population of 171 patients that the presence or absence of a FHHL did not affect the psychological state of those with hearing difficulties themselves.

It was interesting to note that, while in those with no FHHI there was a significant correlation between impairment and both Activity Limitation and Participation Restriction, in those with a FHHI, the significant correlation disappeared. Elsewhere, Noble (1998) and others have found a smaller relationship between impairment and 'Handicap' than between impairment and 'Disability'. These results suggest that the presence of a FHHI may explain part of this difference.

Kramer et al. (*submitted*) found that 63% of patients with a family history of hearing loss did not realise that their hearing problems were hereditary.

Among the group of patients with a FHHI in our study (58 subjects) who were asked to complete the family history questionnaire 22 were aware of their family history and 36 were not. We examined the relationship between their response to question 4 ('*I didn't realise hearing problems were heredi-tary*') and the questions in the Denver Scale. We found a significant rela-tionship (t = −1.93; p = 0.003) to Question 6 ('*People sometimes avoid me because of my hearing problems*'). It seems that those subjects aware of their family background of hearing loss are able to integrate into social life with a more active approach (Kerr & Stephens, 2000). It is important to understand that people with hearing impairment, particularly the elderly, sometimes find severe difficulties in following discussion and conversations and then feel excluded from certain intellectual activities (Noble, 1998; Kramer, 2005).

There was no significant relationship between knowledge of family history and overall HAD scores of Anxiety and Depression, but a significant rela-tionship with HAD Questions 4 ('*I can laugh and see the funny side of things*') (Z = −3.244; p = 0.001) and 13 ('*I get sudden feelings of panic*') (Z = −2.7; p = 0.007). In these we found that those aware of their family history of HL present with more symptoms.

REFERENCES

Alpiner JG, Chevrette W, Glascol E, Metz M, Olsen B (1971) The Denver Scale of Communication Function (University of Denver, Denver).

Danermark B (2004) A review of the psychological effects of hearing impairment in the working age population. In D Stephens, L Jones (eds) *The Impact of Genetic Hearing Impairment.* London: Whurr, pp. 106–36.

Kerr P, Stephens D (2000) Understanding the nature and function of positive experi-ences in living with auditory disablement. *Scandinavian Journal of Disability Research* 2: 21–38.

Kramer S (2005) The psychosocial impact of hearing loss among elderly people: a review. In D Stephens, L Jones (eds) *The Impact of Genetic Hearing Impairment.* London: Whurr, pp. 137–64.

Noble W (1998) *Self-assessment of Hearing and Related Functions.* London: Whurr.

Snaith RP (2003) The Hospital Anxiety and Depression Scale. *Health and Quality of Life Outcomes* 1: 29.

Steiner D, Norman G (1995) *Health Measurement Scales.* Oxford: Oxford Medical Publications.

Stephens D, Kramer S (2005) The impact of having a family history of hearing prob-lems on those with hearing difficulties themselves: an exploratory study. *International Journal of Audiology* 44: 206–12.

Stephens D, Lewis P, Davis A (2003) The influence of a perceived family history of hearing difficulties in an epidemiological study of hearing problems. *Audiological Medicine* 1: 228–31.

Weir NF, Stephens SDG (1976) Personality measures in ENT outpatients. *Journal of Laryngology and Otology* 90: 553–60.

Zigmond AS, Snaith RP (1983) The Hospital Anxiety and Depression Scale. *Acta Psychiatrica Sandinavica* 67: 361–70.

10 Does a Family History of Hearing Impairment Affect Help-Seeking Behaviour and Attitudes to Rehabilitation?

CLAIRE WILSON AND DAFYDD STEPHENS

INTRODUCTION

Hearing impairment affects 19% of the 51–60 year age group and 60% of the over 70 year age group (Davis, 1989). Help-seeking for hearing impairment involves several steps. The patient first has to be aware of his impairment and a need for rehabilitation, and (in the UK health system) also seek referral through his general practitioner. However, many patients are dissatisfied with the results after hearing aid fitting. Attempting to reduce this dissatisfaction requires examination of the influences and attitudes affecting referral. The majority of older individuals are not self-motivated but have been persuaded to attend for a hearing aid by a relative (O'Mahoney et al., 1996). Wilson and Stephens (2003) found that whether or not the patient was self-motivated did not affect the outcome of auditory rehabilitation. However, like other authors (Brooks, 1989; Gatehouse, 1994), they found individuals with a more positive attitude toward hearing aids were both more satisfied with their hearing aids and used them more.

Do individuals with a family history of hearing impairment have a more positive attitude, or exhibit earlier help-seeking behaviour, than those with no family history? The studies described here aim to further explore the effect of attitude toward hearing aids and the help-seeking behaviour in those with a family history of hearing impairment.

The null hypothesis of the two pilot studies described is:

Having a family member with a hearing impairment does not affect the individual's attitude to auditory rehabilitation.

The Effects of Genetic Hearing Impairment in the Family. Edited by D. Stephens and L. Jones.
Copyright © 2006 by John Wiley & Sons, Ltd.

METHOD

In both studies family history refers to parents or siblings, i.e. first-degree relatives, with a hearing impairment sufficient to require hearing aid use, or cause difficulties in communicating.

STUDY 1

A questionnaire was administered to consecutive new patients (not previous hearing aid users) seen at the Welsh Hearing Institute audiological rehabilitation clinic over a 6-month period. Patients were asked questions about the duration of hearing difficulties, 'How long ago was your hearing perfect?' They were also asked whom they perceived to be the motivating person (self/others) behind the referral as described by Wilson and Stephens (2003). The individual's attitude towards a hearing aid was graded by the clinician from −3 to +3 on a visual analogue scale, with −2 to −3 representing individuals who appeared to have a negative attitude, −1 to +1 a neutral attitude and +2 to +3 representing a positive attitude. All patients at a follow-up visit 3 months after the hearing aid fitting were asked to grade their satisfaction with their hearing aid on a visual analogue scale ranging from total dissatisfaction (0) to complete satisfaction (10). The clinician noted the site (e.g. being worn, in a box) and the type of hearing aid, whether it was fitted correctly, the patient's manipulative skills and the patient's reported use of the aid. The mean level of hearing for 500 Hz, 1 kHz, 2 kHz and 4 kHz for the better and worse hearing ear was also noted. During the consultation, information regarding a family history of hearing impairment was noted. The authors then re-analysed the results in order to determine whether or not having a family history of hearing impairment affected the attitude of the subjects, as well as any of the various outcome measures (i.e. site of hearing aid at review appointment (worn correctly, incorrectly or not worn), satisfaction with, reported use and manipulation skills of hearing aid) reported in the earlier study.

STUDY 2

A questionnaire was administered to consecutive patients seen at a Welsh Hearing Institute audiological rehabilitation clinic, over a 6-month period. Patients were asked if there was a family history of hearing impairment and, if so, who was affected. They were also asked about the duration of their hearing problems 'How long ago was your hearing perfect?' and the motivating factor for referral (self/other). As in Study 1, their attitude toward a hearing aid was graded by the clinician from −3 to +3 on a visual analogue scale, with −2 to −3 representing individuals who appeared to have a negative attitude −1 to +1 neutral attitude and +2 to +3 representing a positive attitude.

The mean level of hearing for 500 Hz, 1 kHz, 2 kHz and 4 kHz for the better and worse hearing ear was also noted.

In both studies the same clinician (DS) extracted and collected the data. All correlations and statistical analyses of the data were performed using chi-square, Kendall's tau and t tests.

RESULTS

STUDY 1

Fifty-eight sets of notes could be retrieved from the 140 individuals in the initial study. The demographics of those with and without a family history of hearing impairment are shown in Table 10.1.

In these analyses, like Wilson and Stephens (2003), self-referred individuals were found to have a more positive attitude toward hearing aids (p = 0.063).

As shown in Table 10.2, a significant relationship was found between the longest reported duration of hearing problems and family history of hearing impairment (p = 0.024), i.e. those with a family history had been aware of their hearing problems for a longer period of time. There was also a significant relationship between maternal hearing impairment and the duration of reported hearing problems prior to consultation (p = 0.037), suggesting that those with

Table 10.1 The demographics of those with and without a family history in study 1

	Family history	No family history
Male	14	15
Female	17	12
Mean age	69 years	71 years
Better hearing level	42 dBHL	43 dBHL

Table 10.2 Relationships between demographic variables and family history in study 1

	Family history of hearing impairment	Paternal hearing impairment	Maternal hearing impairment	Parental hearing impairment
Attitude	NS	p = 0.034	NS	NS
Self-reported duration of hearing problems	NS	NS	p = 0.037	NS
Longest reported duration of hearing problems	p = 0.024	NS	NS	NS
Self-referral	NS	NS	NS	p = 0.040

Table 10.3 The relationship between family history and outcome measures

	Family history of hearing impairment	Paternal hearing impairment	Maternal hearing impairment	Parental hearing impairment
Site of hearing aid	NS	NS	NS	NS
Manipulation	NS	NS	NS	NS
Satisfaction	NS	NS	NS	NS
Use	NS	NS	NS	NS

Table 10.4 Demographics of those with and without a family history in study 2

	Family history	No family history
Male	15	17
Female	12	18
Average age	64 years	71 years
Better hearing level	37 dBHL	40 dBHL

a family history of hearing impairment actually delay seeking hearing aid referral or that they were more sensitised to its onset.

A significant relationship was also found between attitudes towards a hearing aid and paternal hearing impairment ($p = 0.034$), i.e. if the father had a hearing impairment there was less motivation to use a hearing aid.

A further significant relationship was noted between parental hearing impairment and self-referral ($p = 0.040$). Indicating that those with a family history are more likely to attend voluntarily rather than as a result of pressure from those around them.

From Table 10.3 it can be seen that no significant relationships can be found between outcome measures recorded in study 1, i.e. site of hearing aid at review appointment (worn correctly, incorrectly or not worn), satisfaction, reported use, manipulation skills and any of the family history variables.

STUDY 2

Sixty-two questionnaires were completed. The demographics of those with and without a family history are shown in Table 10.4.

As in study 1, self-referred individuals were found to have a more positive attitude toward a hearing aid ($p = 0.024$). As can be seen from Table 10.5, there was no significant relationship with family history and duration of hearing impairment or attitude to hearing impairment.

Comparison of Tables 10.1 and 10.4 show that those with a family history in study 2 were younger and had better 'better ear hearing' than those subjects seen in study 1.

Table 10.5 Relationship between demographic variables in study 2

	Family history of hearing impairment	Paternal hearing impairment	Maternal hearing impairment	Parental hearing impairment
Attitude	NS	NS	NS	NS
Self-reported duration of hearing problems	NS	NS	NS	NS
Longest reported duration of hearing problems'	NS	NS	NS	NS
Self-referral	NS	NS	NS	NS

There was also a significantly greater 'longest reported duration of hearing problems' in study 2 than in study 1 (t = 2.65; p = 0.009).

DISCUSSION

In both studies, those who were self-referred were more likely to have a positive attitude towards use of their hearing aid.

Significant relationships to a family history were found in study 1, i.e. a family history and longer reported duration of hearing problems (p = 0.024). Increased duration of hearing problems with a maternal hearing impairment (p = 0.037), and a more negative attitude towards a hearing aid with paternal hearing impairment (p = 0.034). The only 'positive' relationship with a family history was that those individuals with one or both parents affected were more likely to have sought help of their own accord, rather than as a result of pressure from those around them. In study 2 no significant relationships where found. No relationship to family history was found when outcome variables measured in study 1 were examined.

In both studies numbers were small. In study 1 the family history data were collected retrospectively from available notes. In many cases notes were not available (due to microfilming of the notes and deaths). Data collection in study 2 was prospective, collected by the same individual (DS). From Tables 10.1 and 10.4 it can be seen that the individuals in study 2 were younger and had more sensitive hearing levels. During the interval between the end of the first study and the start of the second study digital hearing aids were introduced into the department. The positive media coverage regarding digital hearing aids may have resulted in increased referral numbers; this may have been responsible for the longer duration of hearing problems in study 2 compared with study 1 (p = 0.009), possibly by encouraging those reluctant to seek help with analogue hearing aids. Whether and how this may have influenced the family history relationships found in the first study is not immediately apparent.

The significant relationships found in study 1 appeared to show that those with a family history are less likely to access hearing rehabilitation services earlier than those without a family history, or at least to have perceived an earlier onset of their problems. However, the relationship found between parental hearing impairment and self-referral indicates that those with a family history are more likely to attend of their own volition rather than as a result of external pressure.

No such relationships were found in study 2. The results of study 1 may suggest weak evidence of an effect on help-seeking behaviour in those with a family history, therefore rejecting our null hypothesis that a family history of hearing impairment does not affect the individual's attitude to auditory rehabilitation.

In addition, in a separate unpublished study, we found no relationship between family history and hearing aid outcome measures. Analysis of changes in patient complaint as assessed using the client-orientated scale of improvement – COSI (Dillon et al., 1997) found that neither the reduction in complaints nor the magnitude of the residual complaint was influenced by whether or not the individual had a family history (Stephens, personal communication).

The results of this study are in contrast to work by Jacobsen et al. (2004) who looked at attitudes to the development of prostate cancer in those with a family history. They found that those with a family history considered themselves more vulnerable to developing prostate cancer and were more likely to undergo screening than those without a family history. They suggested that heightened concern about developing the disease is an important motivating factor. In keeping with theories of protective health care, a meta-analysis of breast cancer screening behaviour reported women with a family history were more likely to have been screened (McCaul et al., 1996).

Theories of health belief models form a major framework for understanding acceptance of health and health behaviour (Janz & Becker, 1984). The four dimensions of the health belief model are, perceived susceptibility, perceived severity, perceived benefits and perceived barriers. By applying the health belief model one can attempt to understand the results of our pilot studies.

1. Perceived susceptibility: many individuals may not feel that they are at increased risk of having a hearing impairment when they have an affected family member. The aetiology of the hearing impairment may be considered due to noise, ear infections or operations rather than to genetic factors. Sill et al. (1994) found 62% of later onset hearing loss reported one or two parent(s) with some form of hearing loss compared to 49% of early onset (≤ 20 years of age) regardless of reported cause for hearing impairment. Although results from this American study (4039 returned questionnaires), failed to show that fully recessive or dominant models explained the early

or later onset hearing loss, it highlights the importance of genetic factors in adult onset hearing impairment. A genetic effect on the inheritance of later onset of hearing loss was also found by Gates et al. (1999) in their twin study.

2. Perceived severity: hearing impairment affects quality of life but is not perceived as life threatening requiring early treatment.

3 & 4. Perceived benefits and barriers. Society's attitude towards individuals with a hearing impairment may affect their willingness to accept a hearing aid, i.e. the hearing aid 'effect'. Past experience of a relative having positive or negative experiences with a hearing aid may also affect referral patterns. Van den Brink et al. (1996) found that the revised health belief model including the person's subjective norm, i.e. his belief that the people who are important to him think he should, or should not, perform the health-related behaviour, provided valuable insight into attitude factors in help-seeking for hearing impairment.

In conclusion, we found weak evidence that having a family history of hearing impairment actually makes one less likely to access hearing rehabilitation services, i.e. delaying their help-seeking behaviour. Further studies examining attitude to susceptibility and aetiology of hearing impairment in families may be useful.

REFERENCES

Brooks DN (1989) The effect of attitude on benefit obtained from hearing aids. *British Journal of Audiology* 23: 3–11.

Davis AC (1989) The prevalence of hearing impairment and reported hearing disability among adults in Great Britain. *International Journal of Epidemiology* 18: 911–17.

Dillon H, James A, Ginis J (1997) Client orientated scale of improvement (COSI) and its relationship to several other measures of benefit and satisfaction provided by hearing aids. *Journal of the American Academy of Audiology* 8: 27–43.

Gatehouse S (1994) Components and determinants of hearing aid benefit. *Ear and Hearing* 15: 30–49.

Gates GA, Couropmitree NN, Myers RH (1999) Genetic associations in age related hearing thresholds. *Archives of Otolaryngology and Head and Neck Surgery* 125: 654–9.

Jacobsen PB, Lamonde LA, Honour M, Kash K, Hudson PB, Pow-Sang J (2004) Relation of family history of prostate cancer to perceived vulnerability and screening behaviour. *Psycho-Oncology* 13: 80–5.

Janz NK, Becker MN (1984) The health belief model: a decade later. *Health Education Quarterly* 11: 1–47.

McCaul KD, Branstetter AD, Schroeder DM (1996) *Health Psychology* 15: 423–9.

O'Mahoney CF, Stephens D, Cadge BA (1996) Who prompts patients to consult about hearing loss? *British Journal of Audiology* 30: 153–8.

Sill AM, Stick MJ, Prenger VL, Phillips SL, Boughman JA, Arnos KS (1994) Genetic epidemiological study of hearing loss in an adult population. *American Journal of Medical Genetics* 54: 149–53.

Van den Brink RHS, Wit HP, Kempen GIJM, van Heuvelen MJG (1996) Attitude and help seeking for hearing impairment. *British Journal of Audiology* 30: 313–24.

Wilson C, Stephens D (2003) Reasons for referral and attitudes toward hearing aids: do they affect outcome? *Clinical Otolaryngology* 28: 81–4.

11 The Impact of a Family History of Hearing Impairment on Rehabilitative Intervention: A One-Year Follow-Up

CHRISTOPHE SAGLIER, FERNANDO PEREZ-DIAZ,
LIONEL COLLET AND ROLAND JOUVENT

INTRODUCTION

Hearing loss affects 3 million people over the age of 55 years in France, and is a serious handicap for those who suffer from it. Alongside noise trauma, age is an important factor in the onset of hearing disorders (Syka, 2002). Such age-linked hearing loss, or 'presbyacusis' (Sheldon, 1948; Abrams, 1978; Herbst & Humphrey, 1981; Jones et al., 1984; Gates et al., 1990) is found in 33–60% of elderly subjects. The French pollster IPSOS, in its 2001 Hearing Day survey, estimated almost 62% of over 70s to have some sort of hearing deficit.

There have been several studies of the psychological aspects of hearing loss. Kalayam et al. (1991) found associated psychiatric disturbance in half of their patients with hearing disorders. These figures are in agreement with those of Eastwood et al. (1985) and Mahapatra (1974). Several studies further indicated a link between deafness and the emergence of paranoid or schizophrenic disturbance (Kay et al., 1964; Cooper, 1976) – although other studies have since invalidated these results (Altshuler & Sarlin, 1963; Stephens, 1980; Moore, 1981; Kalayam et al., 1991; Prajer & Jeste, 1993). Indeed, according to Kenneth & Altshuler (1971), schizophrenic disturbance appears no more frequently in deaf than in hearing subjects – although these authors did find increased impulsiveness and aggression in the deaf.

We conducted an initial study in 2004 (Saglier et al.) that enabled us to define the 'presbyacusic' population. The results revealed no major psychiatric pathology in hearing-impaired subjects but did, however, reveal some quite marked differences from control subjects. Firstly, hearing-impaired subjects experienced greater cognitive difficulty than controls, as also found by Uhlmann et al. (1986), Davis et al. (1991) and Kalayam et al. (1995).

The Effects of Genetic Hearing Impairment in the Family. Edited by D. Stephens and L. Jones.
Copyright © 2006 by John Wiley & Sons, Ltd.

It further emerged that hearing-impaired subjects experienced less social pleasure than controls: i.e. they may, to a slight but significantly greater degree, be presenting with social anhedonia, or a diminished capacity to feel pleasure in being in relationship with other people. Denmark (1969) and later Mulrow et al. (1990a) have already shown hearing loss to entail severe communication disorders resulting in social and emotional isolation for the sufferer. According to Mulrow et al. (1990b), hearing-impaired subjects cease to find social satisfaction and feel a lack of self-esteem. This social isolation can lead to severe emotional disturbance such as depression or pathological anxiety.

Although there have been several reports of non-negligible depressive and anxiety states in hearing-impaired populations (Herbst & Humphrey, 1981; Jones et al., 1984; Mulrow et al., 1990a, b; Kalayam et al., 1995; Cacciatore et al., 1999), we found no tendency to emotional disturbance in hearing-impaired subjects. On the other hand, we did notice that the greatest disturbance in hearing-impaired subjects were less psychological than psychosensory, with massive sensory hyperaesthesia and hyperacusis (auditory hyper-sensitivity). Hearing loss seemed to cause not only unpleasant if not unbearable auditory sensations, but also increased visuo-vestibular and gustatory sensitivity.

Since the primary treatment for hearing disorders consists in wearing a hearing aid, it seemed logical to study the effect a hearing aid might have on the associated psychological and psychosensory disturbances.

Hearing aids have been reported to improve communication and socialisation (Mulrow et al., 1990b), depressive disorders (Appollonio et al., 1996; Cacciatore et al., 1999), and cognitive disorder after 6 weeks of rehabilitation, with Ojéda et al. (2004) further reporting improvement in episodic memory processes.

We found that the improvement induced by the hearing aid mainly concerned hyperaesthetic and hyperacusic psychosensory disturbances. Even so, hyperaesthesia and hyperacusis scores remained significantly higher than in normally hearing subjects even after the hearing aid had provided some improvement. Thus, despite a positive hearing-aid effect over 6 months, hearing-aid-fitted subjects did not show total remission of their psychosensory symptoms.

Stephens et al. (2003) further demonstrated a correlation between the emotional reactions associated with hearing loss and the type of hearing loss concerned. Thus, disability-induced emotional reactions were particularly associated with familial hearing loss – i.e. hearing-loss in a context of family history of deafness – with emotional change occurring secondary to the onset of hearing loss. This is all the more important as the emotional impact of hearing loss would seem to be the major factor in the acceptance of a hearing aid (Stephens et al., 1991).

It is thus important to know what psychological impact hearing loss may have when it occurs in subjects with a family history of hearing impairment, and how this affects their emotional development secondary to hearing-aid fitting.

METHOD

SUBJECTS

One hundred and seventy-seven hearing-impaired subjects, presenting for hearing-aid fitting in a dedicated centre, were included (76 male, 101 female; mean age: 70 years 3 months, SD = 11.9 years) for assessment before (T_0), at 6 months after (T_6) and at 12 months (T_{12}) after fitting.

QUESTIONNAIRES

Subjects were assessed by means of self-administered psychopathology questionnaires relating to the following areas:

- *Depression:* Geriatric depression scale (GDS) (Brink et al., 1982)
- *Cognitive disorder:* Self assessment scale for cognitive difficulties in daily life (CDS) (MacNair & Kahn, 1983)
- *Anxiety:* State-trait anxiety inventory (STAI) (Spielberger, 1983)
- *Social isolation:* Social anhedonia scale (SAS) (Eckblad et al., 1985)
- *Sensory complaints:* Sensory hyperaesthesia scale (Jouvent et al., 2000, unpublished); auditory sensitivity or hyperacusis scale (Khalfa et al., 2002)

We further interviewed the 117 subjects regarding any family history of hearing impairment, asking the following question: 'Are there members of your family (brothers, sisters, parents, grandparents, etc.) who suffer or have suffered from deafness?'

RESULTS

CHARACTERISTICS OF THE STUDY POPULATION

Familial deafness

Of the 171 subjects who answered the question regarding familial deafness, 88 reported no family history, while 83 knew of the presence of hearing loss within their family; i.e. 48.35% of the hearing-impaired subjects in our sample had a family history of hearing impairment. These findings are in agreement with those of Karlsson et al. (1997) and Gates et al. (1999).

The prevalence of a family history of hearing impairment in 'presbyacusic' subjects is thus high, with almost half of them knowing a close relative affected by hearing loss.

Use of hearing aids

Of the 171 subjects, 149 'Fitted' hearing-impaired subjects (77 male, 72 female; mean age: 69 years 10 months) were reassessed at 6 (T_6) and 12 months (T_{12}) after hearing-aid fitting. 20 other hearing-impaired subjects gave up the use of their hearing aid during the first 6 months of rehabilitation – i.e. before T_6. These 'Withdrawals' (16 male, 4 female; mean age: 68 years 11 months) were also reassessed at 6 and 12 months. Two subjects were excluded from the analysis, having given up and later resumed the use of their hearing aids.

At T_0, the 149 'Fitted' hearing-impaired subjects were also asked: 'How long have you had hearing problems?'

'Fitted' hearing-impaired subjects with a family history: age and gender

There was no significant gender difference ($\chi^2 = 0.52$; $p = 0.47$) between the group reporting a family history and the other hearing-impaired subjects.

The educational level did not differ between the two groups ($\chi^2 = 7.21$; $p = 0.13$).

The degree of hearing loss was similar in the two groups (right ear: $t = 0.11$; $p = 0.91$; left ear: $t = -0.43$; $p = 0.66$).

Prior to fitting, hearing-impaired subjects without a family history of hearing impairment had experienced hearing problems for a similar period of time (mean: 6.76 years; SD: 8.27) as those with (mean: 7.12 years; SD: 8.91) ($t = 0.25$; $p = 0.80$), i.e. the number of years of hearing loss was equivalent between groups.

The mean age of the subjects with family history of hearing impairment was significantly lower (67 years 11 months, vs 71 years 9 months; $\chi^2 = 2.28$; $p = 0.02$).

QUESTIONNAIRE RESULTS

There were no significant differences between the 'with' and 'without family history' groups for GDS, STAI, CDS, SAS or sensory hyperaesthesia scores, whatever the test-time (before, or 6 or 12 months after fitting). Thus the presence or absence of a family history of hearing impairment would not seem to affect hearing-impaired subjects' psychological state: it does not cause psychological alteration, or cognitive or emotional disturbance in hearing-impaired subjects.

On the other hand, the results do describe a tendency for subjects with a family history of deafness to react differently in psychosensory terms. While their hyperacusis scores prior to fitting were scarcely different from those of subjects without a family history of hearing impairment (Figure 11.1), they remained hypersensitive at 6 months' rehabilitation, whereas other hearing-impaired subjects tended to show a fall-off in hyperacusis over the same period ($t = 1.92$; $p = 0.06$).

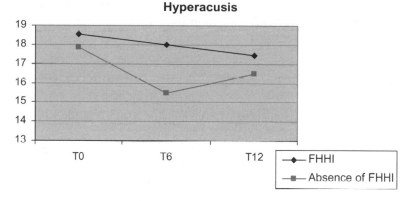

Figure 11.1 Change in hyperacusis scores over 1 year according to presence or absence of family history of hearing impairment.

Thus, at 6 months, hyperacusis scores tend to be lower in subjects 'without' than 'with family history' (t − 1.99; p = 0.05).

Likewise, scores on the emotional component of the hyperacusis scale after 6 months were higher in subjects 'with' than 'without familial history' (t = −2.10; p = 0.04). This emotional component refers to disturbance due to noise occurring in silence, and to the impact of noise on concentration and on stress (Khalfa et al., 2002). A link between family history of hearing impairment and emotional intolerance of high intensity noise was previously highlighted by Stephens et al. (2003).

This divergence, however, would seem to be ephemeral, in as much as scores at 12 months post-rehabilitation were once again broadly similar. Hearing-impaired subjects without a family history of hearing impairment were stable in their hyperacusis scores between 6 and 12 months post-fitting.

Consequently, people presenting with a family history of hearing impairment do not show psychological disorders that are specific or different from those found in other hearing-impaired subjects. They do, however, seem to be less sensitive to the impact of their hearing aid on their hyperacusis.

Withdrawals

The same number (n = 10) of subjects 'with' and 'without family history' stopped using their hearing aids. Family history was thus not a differentiating (minority) trait with respect to withdrawal from rehabilitation, ruling out the otherwise conceivable hypothesis that giving up the hearing aid might depend on whether the hearing impairment had a familial background or not.

Focusing on those subjects who did give up their hearing aid, little difference on the various scales emerged between those with and without family history of hearing impairment. Only the social component of the hyperacusis scale (noise impact on social life) at 6 months post-fitting differed between the two groups (t = −2.13; p = 0.05).

DISCUSSION

The prevalence of family history of hearing impairment is high in hearing-impaired subjects, at nearly 50%.

Furthermore, the hearing-impaired subjects presenting with a family history of hearing impairment in our sample tended to be 'younger' than the others at time of hearing-aid fitting. The interval between the initial perception of hearing loss and hearing-aid fitting, on the other hand, was broadly similar in both groups. It follows that the hearing-impaired subjects presenting with a family history of hearing impairment became aware of an initial perception of hearing loss earlier than the others. These findings are open to a number of interpretations (Figure 11.2).

Firstly, hearing-impaired subjects presenting with a family history of hearing impairment may undergo earlier auditory system deterioration than those without such family history. And yet they wait just as long to begin rehabilitation.

Secondly, hearing-impaired subjects presenting with a family history of hearing impairment may not have been affected earlier, but rather have been alerted by their family history. Having a family model of hearing impairment, they were better informed of the signs and symptoms of hearing loss. Like-wise, they might actually expect to become hearing-impaired. Elderly people

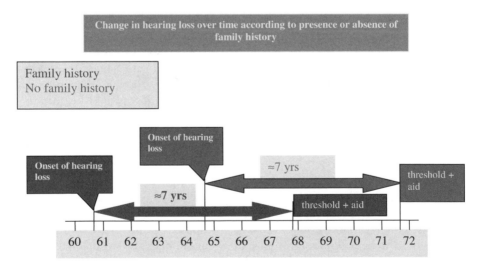

Figure 11.2

interviewed in clubs have indeed claimed to be hard of hearing purely on the grounds that their mother or father became so as they got older and that they themselves consequently were bound to suffer from hearing loss: 'It's in the genes.' Now, these people did not necessarily actually show any hearing loss significant for their age: they just expected it, being prepared by their family background making them more attentive to any hearing problem they might have.

Our results did not find family history of hearing impairment to be a factor in the emergence of psychological problems in hearing-impaired subjects. Many studies have, indeed, reported the emergence of psychological and emotional disturbances in the hearing-impaired (Kay et al., 1961; Mahapatra, 1974; Cooper, 1976; Herbst & Humphrey, 1981; Jones et al., 1984; Eastwood ct al., 1985; Uhlmann ct al., 1986; Mulrow ct al., 1990a,b; Davis et al., 1991; Kalayam et al., 1991, 1995; Cacciatore et al., 1999), but the causes remain vague. Hearing loss appears for a number of reasons (ageing, illness, excessive noise exposure etc.), which suggests that the consequences likewise may be varied and specific to each aetiology. We were unable to relate the family history of hearing impairment to the psychological and psychosensory disturbances described in hearing-impaired subjects in the literature. Studying causative factors of hearing impairment other than family history might help identify the mecha nisms underlying psychological changes.

The reported beneficial effect of the hearing aids on psychological distur bance varies from study to study. Some have found hearing aids to reduce disturbance of mood (Mulrow ct al., 1990b; Cacciatore ct al., 1999), of episodic memory (Ojéda et al., 2004), and of sensory hyperaesthesia and hyperacusis (Saglier et al., 2004).

The present study sought to establish whether the hearing-aid effect on the psychological state of hearing-impaired subjects might vary with the presence or absence of a family history of hearing impairment.

We found that the hearing-impaired subjects reporting a family history of hearing impairment in our sample did not show the beneficial effect of the hearing aid on their hyperacusis experienced by the others during the first 6 months of rehabilitation. We mentioned earlier the hypothesis that familial hearing impairment may be a specific pathology, one feature of which would be earlier onset. This differential pathology might also account for the fact that hearing-impaired subjects without a family history of hearing impairment showed a fall-off in hyperacusis with hearing-aid fitting, whereas hearing-impaired subjects with familial deafness did not. The hearing-aid effect may differ, since it is in fact acting on two distinct pathologies.

We would thus be confronting two quite different pathologies in these two groups. The former, familial group, being aware of auditory disturbance and of hearing aids, have limited expectations regarding any beneficial effect of the hearing aid, having some idea of its field of action and of its possible drawbacks. The latter, non-familial group, for whom the hearing aid represents 'the cure' for hearing impairment, expect and strive to find very positive hearing-aid effects on their auditory symptoms (hyperacusis).

This explanation, however, remains speculative, especially inasmuch as our results point to no more than a tendency towards improvement in hearing-impaired subjects without a family history of hearing impairment. In other words, the scores vary only slightly between the two groups and the various times of assessment. It would therefore be more correct to say that there is no definite hearing-aid effect on the psychology of hearing-impaired subjects according to whether or not they have a family history of hearing impairment.

REFERENCES

Abrams M (1978) *Beyond Three Score Years and Ten: A First Report on a Survey of the Elderly.* Mitcham: Age Concern.

Altshuler KZ, Sarlin MB (1963) Deafness and schizophrenia: a family study. In JD Rainer, KZ Altshuler (eds) *Family and Mental Health Problems in a Deaf Population.* New York: Columbia University.

Appollonio I, Carabellese C, Frattola L, Trabucchi M (1996) Effects of sensory aids on the quality of life and mortality of elderly people: a multivariate analysis. *Age and Ageing* 25: 89–96.

Bargues ML (1992) *Mal entendre au quotidien.* Paris: Odile Jacob.

Brink TL, Yesavage JA, Lum O (1982) Screening tests for geriatric depression. *Clinical Gerontologist* 1: 37–43.

Browing GG, Davis AC (1983) Clinical characterisation of the hearing adult British population. *Advances in Otorhinolaryngology* 31: 217–23.

Cacciatore F, Napoli C, Abete P, Marciano E, Triassi M, Rengo F (1999) Quality of life determinants and hearing function in an elderly population: Osservatotio Geriatrico Campano Study Group. *Gerontology* 45: 323–8.

Cooper AF (1976) Deafness and psychiatric illness. *British Journal of Psychiatry* 129: 216–26.

Dalton DS, Cruickshanks KJ, Klein BEK, Klein R, Wiley TL, Nondahl DM (2003) The impact of hearing loss on quality of life in older adults. *The Gerontologist* 43: 661–8.

Davis PB, Ives D, Traven N (1991) Hearing impairment among rural elders: characteristics and comorbidities. *Journal of the American Geriatric Society* 39: 27.

Denmark JC (1969) Management of severe deafness in adults: the psychiatrist's contribution. *Proceeding of the Royal Society of Medicine* 62: 965–7.

Eastwood MR, Corbon SL, Reed M, Nobbs H, Kedward HB (1985) Acquired hearing loss and psychiatric illness. *British Journal of Psychiatry* 147: 552–6.

Eckblad ML, Chapman LJ, Chapman JP, Mishlove M (1985) Revised Social Anhedonia Scale, 1982 (Unpublished test). Reported in M Mischlove, LJ Chapman, *Journal of Abnormal Psychology* 94: 384–96.

Folstein MF, Folstein SE, McHugh MR (1975) Mini-mental state: a practical method for grading the cognitive state of patients for the clinician. *Journal of Psychiatric Research* 12: 189–98.

Gacek RR, Schuknecht HF (1969) Pathology of presbyacusis. *International Audiology* 8: 199–209.

Gates GA, Cooper JC, Kannel WB, Miller NJ (1990) Hearing in the elderly. *Ear and Hearing* 11: 247–56.

Gilber AN, Martin R, Kemp SE (1996) Cross-modal correspondence between vision and olfaction: the color of smells. *American Journal of Psychology* 109: 335–51.

Hantouche E, Bougerol T, Chiarelli P, Lancrenon S (1996) Dépression et qualité de vie: large enquête en médecine générale. *Act. Méd. Int. Psychiatrie* 188: 3118–25.

Herbst KG, Humphrey C (1981) Hearing impairment and mental state in the elderly living at home. *British Medical Journal* 281: 903–905.

Ives DG, Bonino P, Traven ND, Kuller LH (1995). Characteristics and comorbidities of rural older adults with hearing impairment. *American Journal of Geriatric Society* 43: 803–6.

Jones DA, Victor CR, Vetter NJ (1984) Hearing difficulty and its psychological implications for elderly. *Journal of Epidemiology and Community Health* 38: 75–8.

Kalayam B, Alexopoulos GS, Merrell B, Young RC, Shindlerdecker R (1991) Patterns of hearing loss and psychiatric morbidity in elderly patients attending a hearing clinic. *International Journal of Geriatric Psychiatry* 6: 131–6.

Kalayam B, Meyers BS, Alexopoulos GS (1995) Age at onset of geriatric depression and sensorineural hearing deficits. *Biol. Psychiatry* 38: 649 58.

Karlsson K, Harris JA, Svartengren M (1997) Description and primary results from an audiometric study of male twins. *Ear and Hearing* 18: 114 20.

Kay DWK, Roth M (1961) Environmental and hereditary factors in the schizophrenias of old age. *Journal of Mental Science* 107: 649 86.

Kenneth Z, Altshuler MD (1971) Studies of the deaf: relevance to psychiatric theory. *American Journal of Psychiatry* 127: 97 102.

Khalfa S, Dubal S, Veuillet E, Perez-Diaz F, Jouvent R, Collet L, (2002) Psychometric Normalization of Hyperacusis Questionnaire. *ORL* 64: 436–42.

Kosmadakis CS, Bungener C, Pierson A, Jouvent R, Widlöcher D (1995) Traduction et validation de l'échelle révisée d'anhédonie sociale (SAS Social Anhedonia Scale, ML Eckblad, LJ Chapman et al., 1982). *L'encéphale* 21: 437–43.

McNair DM, Kahn RJ (1983) Self assessment of cognitive deficits. In T Crook et al. (eds) *Assessment in Geriatric Psychopharmacology*, New Canaan: Mark Powley Associates, 137–43.

Mahapatra SB (1974) Deafness and mental health: psychiatric and psychosomatic illness in the deaf. *Acta Psychiatrica Scandinavica* 50: 596–611.

Moore NC (1981) Is paranoid illness associated with sensory defects in the elderly? *Journal of Psychosomatic Research* 25: 69–74.

Mulrow CD, Aguilar C, Endicott JE, Velez R, Tuley MR, Charlip WS et al. (1990a) Association between hearing impairment and the quality of life of elderly individuals. *Journal of the American Geriatric Society* 38: 45–50.

Mulrow CD, Aguilar C, Endicott JE, Velez R, Tuley MR, Charlip WS et al. (1990b) Quality of life changes and hearing impairment. *Annals of Internal Medicine* 113: 188 94.

Nusbaum MD (1999) Aging and sensory senescence. *Southern Medical Journal* 92: 267–75.

Ojéda N, Dissard P, Vesson JF, Koenig O (2004) Presbyacousie, prothèse auditive et processus mnésiques. *Les cahiers de l'audition* 17: 22–30.

Pierson A, Loas G, Lesevre N (1990) Etude de potentiels évoqués cognitifs en fonction de la valence affective et de la signification des stimulus chez des sujets sain anhédoniques avec attitudes dysfonctionnelles. *Encéphale* 15: 209–16.

Prajer S, Jeste DV (1993) Sensory impairment in late-onset schizophrenia. *Schizophrenia Bulletin* 19: 755–82.

Preves D, Sammeth C, Cutting MS, Woodruff B (1995) Experimental hearing device for hyperacusis. *Hearing Instruments* 1: 37–40.

Saglier C, Perez-Diaz F, Collet L, Jouvent R (2004) Psychologie, psychopathologie des malentendants et aide auditive. *Les cahiers de l'audition* 17: 34–40.

Sheldon JH (1948) *The Social Medicine of Old Age. Report of an Inquiry in Wolverhampton.* London: Oxford University Press.

Spielberger CD (ed) (1983) *Manual for the State-trait Anxiety Inventory (Form Y) (Self-evaluation questionnaire).* Palo Alto, CA: Consulting Psychologists Press.

Stephens D, Lewis P, Davis A (2003) The influence of a perceived family history of hearing difficulties in an epidemiological study of hearing problems. *Audiological Medicine* 1: 1–4.

Stephens SDG (1970) Studies on the uncomfortable loudness level. *Sound* 4: 20–3.

Stephens SDG (1980) Evaluating the problem of the hearing-impaired. *Audiology* 19: 205–20.

Stephens SDG, Meredith R, Callaghan DE, Hogan S, Rayment A (1991) Early intervention and rehabilitation: factors influencing outcome. *Acta Otolaryngologica (suppl)* 476: 209–14.

Syka J (2002) Plastic changes in the central auditory system after hearing loss, restoration of function, and during learning. *Physiological Review* 82: 601–36.

Tesh-Romer C (1997) Psychological effects of hearing aid use in older adults. *Journal of Gerontology of the British Psychological Science Society* 52: 127–38.

Uhlmann RF, Larson EB, Koepsell TD (1986) Hearing impairment and cognitive decline in senile dementia of the Alzheimer's type. *Journal of the American Geriatric Society* 34: 207–10.

Vesterager V, Salomon G, Jagd M (1988) Age related hearing difficulties. Psychological and sociological consequences of hearing problems: a control study. *Audiology* 27: 179–92.

Weinstein BE, Ventry IM (1982) Hearing impairment and social isolation in the elderly. *ASHA* 25: 593–9.

Zeckel A (1950) Psychopathological aspects of deafness. *Journal of Nervous and Mental Disease* 138: 223–32.

III Conditions Associated with Familial Hearing Impairment

12 The Influence of a Family History of Hearing Loss, and/or of Tinnitus, on Tinnitus Annoyance and Distress

SYLVIANE CHÉRY-CROZE AND HUNG THAI-VAN

INTRODUCTION

Tinnitus is a very prevalent symptom, for which great inter-individual variability in coping is observed. Clinical observations show that, although a majority of patients (Carlsson & Erlandsson, 1991; Tyler, 1993) can habituate to tinnitus after six to twelve months, the symptom becomes less and less well-tolerated in others, leading to a state of great distress. This clearly suggests a high degree of heterogeneity in the extent of the impact of tinnitus on the individual's quality of life.

Numerous questionnaires have been designed to describe the impact of tinnitus on various aspects of the patient's life (e.g. Tyler & Baker, 1983; Halford et al., 1991; Wilson et al., 1991; Kuk et al., 1990). Problems with existing tinnitus scales include the fact that they are sometimes long, leading to incompletely answered questionnaires, and that they are generally available only in English. At the moment, only three are available for French-speaking patients, translated and validated in French by our team: the 'Tinnitus Reaction Questionnaire' (TRQ: Wilson et al., 1991; Meric et al., 1997a), the 'Subjective Tinnitus Severity Scale' (STSS: Halford et al., 1991; Meric et al., 1996) and the 'Tinnitus Handicap Questionnaire' (THQ: Kuk et al., 1990; Meric et al., 1997b). We previously described their specific targets and properties and studied the correlations of the scores obtained on each of them with those obtained on the various scales of the 'Mini-Mult', an abbreviated version (Perse and Lebeaux, 1977) of the Multiphasic Minnesota Personality Inventory (Hathaway & McKinley, 1940), a recognised questionnaire that focuses on the patient's psychological profile (Meric et al., 1998).

Recently, Kennedy et al. (2005) proposed a new scale, based on the format of the International Outcome Inventory – Hearing Aids (IOI-HA) (Cox &

Alexander, 2002). The IOI-HA is a short, user-friendly questionnaire dedicated to the assessment of the 'effectiveness of hearing aid treatment' and has proved a simple and robust tool, with unambiguous questions encouraging a high response rate and good patient compliance (Cox et al., 2002). Following Cox et al., the new questionnaire proposed by Kennedy et al., the International Tinnitus Inventory (ITI), is also short and user-friendly. Designed to assess the impact of tinnitus on quality of life, this eight-item questionnaire is based on a breakdown of the predominant complaints of tinnitus patients, and assesses the following tinnitus effects: annoyance, effect on hearing, effect on the patient's view of his/her health, effect on sleep, on peace of mind, extent of repercussions on people around, effect on daily activities, and finally on enjoyment of life (see Appendix 12.1). For each item, patients are asked to provide a score ranging from 0 to 4, and an overall score is calculated, ranging from 0 to 32. The ITI has now been validated in English and French (Kennedy et al., 2005).

Stephens et al. (2003) showed that the severity of the psychosocial impact of tinnitus as measured by the annoyance and the effect on the individuals' lives increased with the likelihood of having a family history (FH) of hearing problems, independent of any limitations on the patients' activities. The present study sought to investigate whether similar conclusions could be drawn from a sample of French tinnitus patients, despite potential cross-cultural differences. Previous studies in the literature have reported such cross-cultural differences for health status and/or disease-related concerns (Schmidtke, 1997; Levenstein et al., 2001; Morton, 2003; Voracek et al., 2003). We were particularly interested in further investigating the potential influence of family history of tinnitus and/or of hearing loss firstly on the impact of tinnitus, and secondly on the patient's psychological distress.

MATERIAL AND METHODS

QUESTIONNAIRES

Three different questionnaires were chosen and combined. The final questionnaire is shown in Appendix 12.1. First, an open-ended questionnaire comprised three demographic items. The first was a four-point scale evaluating hearing status in terms of how difficult the subject found it to follow TV programmes at a sound level comfortable to the family circle. Responses were coded 0 (not at all) to 4 (very). The remaining two items were divided into two binary (yes/no) sub-items. They were designed to identify subjects with family history of tinnitus and/or hearing-impairment and to establish whether, in the patient's opinion, this factor was relevant to his/her reaction to tinnitus. Some lines were then provided where patients could detail the various FH effects of tinnitus and/or hearing loss, according to them, on their perception

of or behaviour towards tinnitus. This enabled us to determine the actual consequences of FH on the patients' reactions to tinnitus.

Secondly, the French version of the ITI (Kennedy et al., 2005) was incorporated into the above questionnaire; it was chosen because it is simple and
patient-friendly, and provides an accurate overview of the main consequences
of tinnitus on the various aspects of an individual's life. Moreover, this inventory shows good internal consistency and can be interpreted very easily. It consists of eight five-point-scale items with responses ranging from 'never', 'not
at all' or 'better' (coded as 0) to 'all the time', 'very important' or 'very much
worse' (coded as 4), so that higher scores represent worse outcomes.

A final questionnaire – the validated French version of the TRQ (Meric
et al., 1997a) – was added on to the above. It was chosen because it focuses
predominantly on the psychosocial aspects of tinnitus and probes the various
components of tinnitus-related distress very efficiently. We predicted that any
FH effects would probably concern distress. Responses to the 26 TRQ items
were given by choosing 1 of 5 possibilities: not at all (0), a little of the time
(1), some of the time (2), a good deal of the time (3), or almost all of the time
(4). Because all items were negative descriptors, they were scored in the same
direction (>0) and summed, so that the total score lay between 0 and 104, a
higher score corresponding to a worse outcome.

PARTICIPANTS

Five hundred and eighteen subjects with tinnitus and/or hearing-loss aged
$47.1 + 14.1$ years (mean + SD; 333 males and 185 females) fully completed all
three parts of the questionnaire, distributed to patients at two meetings. The
first meeting, for individuals with tinnitus, was held in December 2003; the
other, for patients with hearing loss, was held in March 2004. Sixty completed
questionnaires (11.6%) reached us by surface mail. The remaining questionnaires of our sample (88.4%) were posted on the website of the French tinnitus association 'France Acouphènes' (www.france-acouphenes.org) between
January and September 2004. Sixteen on-line questionnaires were excluded
from the study, a majority of items not having been answered, probably either
because the on-line response procedure was not well managed or because the
subjects were not native French speakers.

STATISTICAL ANALYSIS

Discrete data, such as hearing annoyance, and overall scores on the three questionnaires as well as scores on their individual items were processed by
descriptive and analytic parametric and non-parametric statistical methods.
When they passed the normality test ($p > 0.001$), comparisons between two
groups were made by Student's t-test, while a Mann–Whitney rank sum test
was used in case of normality test failure ($p < 0.001$). The Kruskall–Wallis one-

way analysis of variance on ranks was used to test for differences between more than two (sub)groups. When the latter analysis showed significant differences (p < 0.05), paired comparisons between groups were performed to identify which group(s) explained the observed significance, using a *t*-test or Mann–Whitney test according to the result on the normality test. Spearman's rank order correlation test further enabled us to study correlations between different variables: for example, between epidemiological data from the open-ended questionnaire and item or total scores on ITI or TRQ.

RESULTS

First, data from the open-ended questionnaire enabled us to establish two groups: those having a family history of hearing troubles, and those not. Epidemiological and psychosocial data from the ITI and TRQ were then studied for each group, and compared between groups.

GROUPS DISTINGUISHED IN THE TOTAL POPULATION

The overall population appeared to be divided into two clusters. Group I comprised 283 tinnitus patients (187 male and 96 female) with no family history of hearing loss and/or of tinnitus; in contrast, Group II comprised the remaining 235 patients (146 men and 89 women) who had at least one relative affected either by hearing loss (FHHL) or tinnitus (FHT) or both (FHHLT). Table 12.1 shows the numbers of people with and without FH in the various age groups. The incidence of a family history was similar across age groups, except for the extreme groups, which comprised fewer respondents.

Group II was split into three subgroups, those respondents with a family history of hearing loss (FHHL = Group IIa; n = 114; 73 men and 41 women), of tinnitus (FHT = Group IIb; n = 41; 29 male and 12 female), or of hearing loss associated with tinnitus (FHHLT = Group IIc; n = 80; 44 men and 36 women). In each of these three subgroups, a majority of patients reported no effect of their family history (97.4% in Group IIa, 68.3% in Group IIb, and 63.75% in Group IIc).

The various demographic variables studied are summarised in Table 12.2a for the overall population and for each group or subgroup. Tables 12.2b and 12.2c shows the scores on the ITI and TRQ respectively for each group.

It is clear from Table 12.2a that the total population, Group I and Group II did not differ significantly in age, tinnitus duration or difficulty in listening to TV. Furthermore, no significant difference was found comparing these three variables between Group I and Groups IIa, IIb and IIc apart from a difference between Group I and Group IIb in tinnitus duration (p < 0.05), which was shorter in Group IIb (FHT).

Only a small percentage of FHHL subjects (Group IIa) reported any FH effect on their own tinnitus impact, in contrast to the FHT (Group IIb) and

Table 12.1 Responses to the family history question as a function of age band

Age bracket (years)	Family history		
	No	Yes	% Yes
<21	5	7	58.3
21–30	41	29	41.4
31–40	44	39	47.0
41–50	65	58	47.1
51–60	79	66	45.5
61–70	31	29	48.3
71–80	17	6	26.1
>80	1	1	50.0

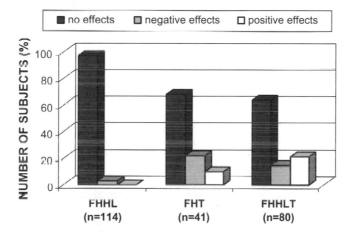

Figure 12.1 Distribution of subjects of Group I by the nature of their family history (hearing loss only, tinnitus only or hearing loss associated with tinnitus) and the nature of effects reported (no effect, positive effects, negative effects).

FHHLT subjects (Group IIc). FHHL appeared not to have a positive influence, while 4 individuals said their FHT had some positive influence on their reaction to tinnitus. Negative effects were reported in 3 and 9 individuals reporting FHHL and FHT respectively. In the FHHLT group, results were more complex: 2 people reported no effect of FHT but a negative effect of FHHL, whereas 11 reported FHT effects (8 positive and 3 negative) without any effect of FHHL, and 17 reported effects of both FHHL and FHT (9 positive and 7 negative). Overall, the observed rate of positive effects was 8.9% and that of negative effects 10.2%.

The negative and positive effects reported are respectively detailed in Tables 12.3a and 12.3b. Briefly, reported negative effects consisted of nervousness and

Table 12.2a General features observed in each group

Variable	Total population n = 518	Group I n = 283	Group II				
			Total n = 235	a n = 114	b n = 41	c n = 80
Age	47.1 ± 0.6	47.5 ± 0.9	46.7 ± 0.9	48.5 ± 1.4	45.3 ± 1.9	44.7 ± 1.4
Tinnitus duration	8.1 ± 0.4	8.1 ± 0.6	8.1 ± 0.6	9.4 ± 1.0	4.9* ± 0.8	7.8 ± 0.9
Difficulty in listening to TV	1.1 ± 1.0	1.1 ± 1.0	1.1 ± 1.0	1.1 ± 0.1	1.0 ± 0.2	1.2 ± 0.1

Values are expressed as mean ± SE
Stars indicates a comparison shown to be statistically significant by either t-test or Mann–Whitney U-test according to whether the normality test was passed (p > 0.001) or failed (p = or < 0.001) with similar values of Group I
*: p < .05; **: p < .02; ***: p < .001

Table 12.2b Mean values of ITI items in each group

Variable	Total population n = 518	Group I n = 283	Group II				
			Total n = 235	a n = 114	b n = 41	c n = 80
Item 1	2.5 ± .05	2.4 ± .07	2.5 ± .07	2.5 ± .10	2.3 ± .17	2.4 ± .12
Item 2	1.9 ± .05	3.0 ± .08	2.0 ± .08	1.9 ± .10***	2.0 ± .20***	2.0 ± .13
Item 3	1.6 ± .06	3.4 ± .08	1.5 ± .09	1.5 ± .12***	1.6 ± .21***	1.5 ± .16
Item 4	1.7 ± .06	3.1 ± .09	1.5 ± .09**	1.5 ± .13***	1.4 ± .21***	1.6 ± .15**
Item 5	2.5 ± .55	2.5 ± .07	2.5 ± .08	2.5 ± .11	2.3 ± .22	2.5 ± .14
Item 6	1.4 ± .06	3.5 ± .08	1.3 ± .08	1.3 ± .12***	1.5 ± .19***	1.2 ± .13***
Item 7	2.2 ± .05	2.8 ± .07	2.1 ± .07	2.2 ± .10***	2.1 ± .19**	2.1 ± .12***
Item 8	2.4 ± .05	2.5 ± .67	2.3 ± .07	2.4 ± .10***	2.2 ± .19	2.4 ± .14
Total score	16.3 ± 0.3	23.2 ± 0.4	15.8 ± 0.5	15.9 ± 0.7***	15.4 ± 1.2***	15.8 ± 0.8***

Values are expressed as mean ± SE
Stars indicates a comparison shown to be statistically significant by either t-test or Mann–Whitney U-test according to whether the normality test was passed (p > 0.001) or failed (p = or < 0.001) with similar values of Group I
*: p < .05; **: p < .02; ***: p < .001

Table 12.2c Mean values of TRQ items in each group

Variable	Total population n = 518	Group I n = 283	Group II			
			Total n = 235	a n = 114	b n = 41	c n = 80
Item 1	2.0 ± .05	2.1 ± .08	1.9 ± .07	2.0 ± .10	1.8 ± .18	2.0 ± .14
Item 2	2.2 ± .05	2.3 ± .07	2.1 ± .08	2.0 ± .11	1.9 ± .19	2.3 ± .14
Item 3	2.0 ± .06	2.1 ± .08	1.9 ± .079*	1.9 ± .10	1.5 ± .18*	2.0 ± .15
Item 4	1.8 ± .06	1.9 ± .08	1.6 ± .09*	1.6 ± .12	1.4 ± .20**	1.8 ± .16
Item 5	0.9 ± .05	1.0 ± .09	0.8 ± .08	0.7 ± .10	0.8 ± .17	1.0 ± .15
Item 6	1.1 ± .06	1.1 ± .08	1.0 ± .08	1.1 ± .11	1.0 ± .22	1.0 ± .14
Item 7	1.7 ± .07	1.8 ± .09	1.6 ± .10	1.6 ± .13	1.8 ± .24	1.5 ± .17
Item 8	1.6 ± .06	1.7 ± .09	1.5 ± .09	1.5 ± .13	1.5 ± .20	1.5 ± .16
Item 9	2.5 ± .05	2.6 ± .07	2.4 ± .08	2.3 ± .11	2.3 ± .20	2.6 ± .14
Item 10	1.7 ± .06	1.8 ± .08	1.6 ± .08	1.5 ± .11	1.7 ± .23	1.5 ± .14
Item 11	1.0 ± .06	1.2 ± .08	0.9 ± .07**	0.8 ± .10	0.7 ± .17	1.0 ± .15
Item 12	1.8 ± .06	1.9 ± .08	1.7 ± .08	1.8 ± .12	1.7 ± .20	1.7 ± .14
Item 13	2.2 ± .06	2.3 ± .07	2.0 ± .08	2.1 ± .12	2.0 ± .22	2.0 ± .14
Item 14	2.5 ± .05	2.6 ± .07	2.4 ± .08	2.4 ± .11	2.4 ± .21	2.4 ± .14
Item 15	1.9 ± .06	1.9 ± .08	1.8 ± .09	1.8 ± .13	1.7 ± .20	2.0 ± .16
Item 16	2.2 ± .06	2.2 ± .09	2.1 ± .10	2.0 ± .13	2.1 ± .21	2.3 ± .18
Item 17	2.0 ± .06	2.1 ± .08	2.0 ± .09	1.9 ± .12	2.0 ± .20	2.2 ± .16
Item 18	2.0 ± .06	2.1 ± .08	1.9 ± .08*	1.8 ± .12	1.9 ± .20	1.9 ± .15
Item 19	1.1 ± .06	1.2 ± .08	1.0 ± .08	0.9 ± .11	1.0 ± .18	1.2 ± .15
Item 20	2.2 ± .07	2.2 ± .09	2.2 ± .10	2.1 ± .14	2.3 ± .21	2.3 ± .18
Item 21	1.4 ± .06	1.5 ± .08	1.2 ± .09*	1.1 ± .12	1.4 ± .22	1.4 ± .16
Item 22	1.5 ± .06	1.6 ± .08	1.5 ± .09	1.3 ± .12	1.4 ± .21	1.7 ± .16
Item 23	1.9 ± .06	2.1 ± .08	1.8 ± .08*	1.7 ± .12	1.7 ± .20	2.0 ± .15
Item 24	0.8 ± .05	0.9 ± .07	0.64 ± .07	0.5 ± .09	0.6 ± .17	0.8 ± .14
Item 25	1.3 ± .06	1.4 ± .08	1.2 ± .09	1.1 ± .12	1.2 ± .20	1.3 ± .15
Item 26	1.9 ± .06	2.0 ± .09	1.8 ± .09	1.6 ± .13	1.7 ± .22	2.0 ± .15
Total score	45.4 ± 1.11	47.7 ± 1.53	42.8 ± 1.53*	41.1 ± 2.17	41.7 ± 3.68	45.7 ± 2.90

Values are expressed as mean ± SE

Stars indicates a comparison shown to be statistically significant by either t-test or Mann–Whitney U-test according to whether the normality test was passed (p > 0.001) or failed (p = or < 0.001) with similar values of Group I

*: p < .05; **: p < .02; ***: p < .001

Table 12.3a Negative effects of having a family history of hearing trouble reported by patients of Group II

Family history	Description of the effect
Group II a *(Hearing loss)*	I am afraid I will become hard of hearing in addition to having tinnitus and that will increase my tinnitus perception.
Group II b *(Tinnitus only)*	I think I am victim of a sad fate. I fear very much about my future; I often saw my father suffering a lot (or crying because of his tinnitus and thinking of committing suicide). I feel very depressed because my father (mother) suffered a lot. I am afraid because I know it is irreversible. I withdraw into myself.
Group II c *(Hearing loss* *plus tinnitus)*	I feel a lot of stress about the fact I will become as deaf as my grandmother and mother, which will increase my tinnitus. I am afraid that it will trigger some psychological disturbance. I am afraid I will become hard of hearing because my grandfather's deafness was related to his tinnitus. I am afraid my family will not understand me at all and be totally unsympathetic. My sister and my brother are hard of hearing; I know that hearing aids do not restore natural hearing and I am more worried about hearing loss than about tinnitus. The fact that my sister has also had tinnitus for a few months has increased my noises and made them troublesome.

stress; patients also referred to living in dread of an increase in their hearing loss and/or tinnitus, or to feeling pursued by fate; they described their fear of suffering from tinnitus just as their relatives did, of becoming withdrawn and cut off from communication with their family and friends and, finally, of 'cracking up'. In contrast, positive effects comprised being already informed about the symptom when it arose, being aware of what should be done or avoided to ensure favourable development, and knowing that somebody was able to understand what you are enduring. Patients also reported that knowing there was a determining family factor motivated them to understand their symptoms and accept their disability.

ITI AND TRQ RESULTS

Comparison of Group I with Group II

Scores on each item as well as total ITI and TRQ scores were compared between Groups I and II. Significant differences were found for ITI item 4 (sleep), and TRQ items 3 (irritable), 4 (angry), 11 (driven crazy), 13 (hard to concentrate), 18 (ability to work), 21 (avoid social situations), and 23 (sleep) and the total TRQ score, the higher scores being in Group I. The corresponding histograms are all shown in Figure 12.2.

Table 12.3b Positive effects of having a family history of hearing trouble reported by patients of Group II

Family history	Description of the effects
Group IIb *(Tinnitus only)*	My mind is put at ease by the fact that a relative suffered from the same health problem and got used to it. When my tinnitus appeared, I knew that I had to adopt a healthier lifestyle from now on.
Group IIc *(Hearing loss plus tinnitus)*	I have become more understanding of the suffering of sufferers but I make an effort not to react as my relatives did: i.e. isolate themselves from the others and never talk about their problems. I understand much better the hell my grandfather as well as other tinnitus sufferers had to face, but at the same time I feel relieved to know that I am not alone in enduring that and that at least one person is able to understand me. I am put at ease because I was told he suffered from tinnitus very late on and I had never noticed there was anything wrong. My uncle complained a lot about his tinnitus and as soon as my tinnitus came on I knew that I would have to deal with it by myself in order to not break down. Taking account of my family history, I knew that I should see a doctor quickly. I have the feeling of being less alone. Being aware that other people suffer from the same thing allows me to minimise my problems. My father had tinnitus and I did not understand what exactly it was. Today I want to understand. My grandmother and mother always spoke of tinnitus. They also were hard of hearing and I consider that tinnitus was inherent to their hearing loss. That's probably why I easily accepted mine when it appeared. My father had permanent tinnitus but he lived easily with it. I always considered that it is possible to live with tinnitus without being bothered. When my tinnitus came on, I knew what it was and that it was less bothersome than hearing loss. Having relatives suffering from the same problem was helpful. I heard very early on that tinnitus was caused by otosclerosis from which we have all suffered, and that there was no remedy for it and that I had to learn to live with it. My mother, who had a very positive attitude, never complained about her noises. At first, tinnitus got on my nerves but I did my best to copy her fatalism and serenity. I better accepted what happened to me and took the drama out of the situation because I knew that they stopped complaining as soon as they got hearing aids. I felt like fighting against this trouble which made my mother stronger.

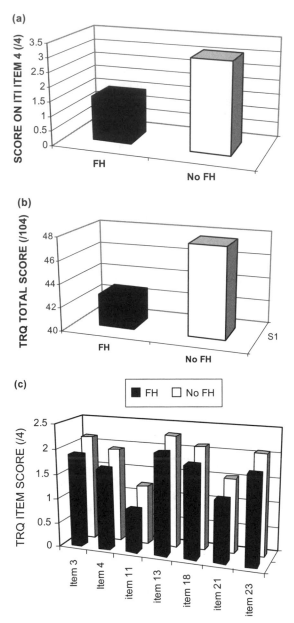

Figure 12.2 Comparison between Group I (no FH) and Group II (FH) results. (a) Mean scores on ITI item 4 observed in the two groups. They proved significantly different (Mann–Whitney test; p = 0.011). (b) Mean TRQ total scores. They proved significantly different (Mann–Whitney test; p = 0.035). (c) Comparison of the mean scores on items 3, 4, 11, 13, 18, 21 and 23 of TRQ measured in Groups I and II. Statistical significance: p < 0.045; Mann–Whitney test.

Comparison of Group I with Groups IIa, IIb and IIc

Using the Kruskal–Wallis rank-order ANOVA we analysed any possible difference between item and total scores in Group I and each subgroup of Group II. The only significant differences concerned TRQ items 3 (irritable; $p < 0.02$) and 11 (driven crazy; $p < 0.04$).

For TRQ item 3 (irritable), Mann–Whitney tests were performed between each subgroup and Group I (see Table 12.2c). These revealed that the significant difference reported above was explained by that between subgroup IIb (FHT) and Group I (no FH) (Figure 12.3; $p < 0.05$). No significant difference was found between Group I TRQ item 11 (driven crazy) and any subgroup of Group II. On the other hand, ITI item 4 scores in all Group II subgroups (a, b and c) differed significantly from those of Group I (Figure 12.4; Mann–Whitney test; $p < 0.0001$). The scores of the three subgroups of FH patients being smaller than those of Group I without FH. No significant difference was found between TRQ item 23 (sleep) in Group I and in any subgroup of Group II.

In spite of the insignificant results of ANOVA on ranks regarding data for the other items, Table 12.2c shows that, when the results of each subgroup of Group II are directly compared with those of Group I by t-test or Mann–Whitney test, significant differences emerge in all cases for ITI items 4 (sleep), 6 (other people), and 7 (effect on activities) and total ITI scores (see Figure 12.5).

In Groups IIa and b, scores on ITI items 2 (difficulty in hearing) and 3 (health problems) proved to be lower than in Group I. Scores on ITI item 8 (enjoyment of life) were only significantly lower than in Group I (no FH) in Group IIa (FHHL) (Figure 12.6; Mann–Whitney test; $p < 0.05$). TRQ items 3 (irritable) and 4 (feel angry) were lower in Group IIb (FHT) than in Group I (no FH) (see Figures 12.3 and 12.7).

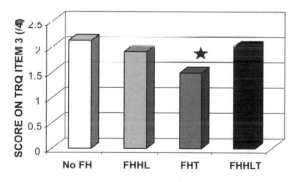

Figure 12.3 Comparison of the mean scores on TRQ item 3 (feel irritable) computed for subjects of Group I and of each subgroup of Group II. The only value which was found to be significantly different (Mann–Whitney test; $p = 0.04$) from that of Group I was that of the subgroup of subjects who had a family history of tinnitus only.

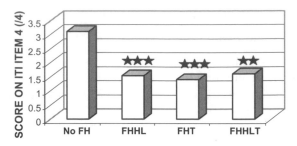

Figure 12.4 Comparison of the mean scores on ITI item 4 (sleep) computed for subjects of Group I and of each subgroup of Group II. In each subgroup of Group II, the mean score was found to be significantly different (Mann–Whitney test; p = 0.001) from that of Group I.

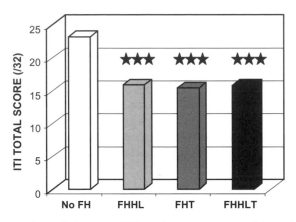

Figure 12.5 Comparison of the mean ITI total scores computed for subjects of Group I and those of each subgroup of Group II. In each subgroup, the mean score was found to differ significantly from that of Group I: *t*-test (Group IIa and IIb) or Mann–Whitney test (Group IIc; p < 0.001).

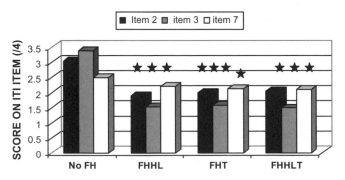

Figure 12.6 Comparison of the mean scores on ITI items 2 (difficulty hearing), 3 (health problems), 7 (affected the things you can do) computed for subjects of Group I and those of each subgroup of Group II. The mean scores on items 2, 3 and 7 were found to differ significantly (Mann–Whitney test; p < 0.001) from those of Group I in all three subgroups (Mann–Whitney test; ***p = 0.001; *p = 0.04).

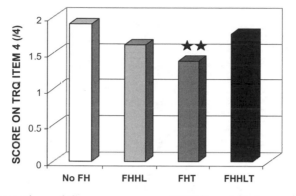

Figure 12.7 Comparison of the mean scores on TRQ item 4 (feel angry) computed for subjects of Group I and of each subgroup of Group II. The only value which was found significantly different (Mann–Whitney test; p = 0.015) from that of Group I was that of the subgroup composed of subjects who had a family history of tinnitus only.

SPECIFIC EFFECTS

Possible effects of age, tinnitus duration or difficulty in listening to TV were investigated, firstly in the overall population, Group I and Group II successively, and secondly in the three subgroups of Group II. In all these cases, Spearman rank correlation tests were run. The results obtained on all these tests are shown respectively for age, tinnitus duration and difficulty in listening to TV in Tables 12.4, 12.6 and 12.8 for the overall population, Group I and Group II, and in Tables 12.5, 12.7 and 12.9 for Groups IIa, IIb and IIc.

Effects of age

Overall population, Group I and Group II

In both the overall population and Groups I and II, age correlated positively (p < 0.05) with ITI items 1 (annoyance) and 2 (effect on hearing); negative correlations (p < 0.05) were observed between age and total TRQ score, which can be explained by the negative correlations (p < 0.05) found between age and numerous TRQ items: 4 (angry), 5 (cry), 15 (distressed), 16 (helpless), 17 (frustrated), 19 (despair), 23 (sleep), 24 (thoughts of suicide) and 25 (feel panicky).

In the overall population only, age correlated negatively (p < 0.05) with TRQ items 2 (tense), 10 (confused) and 12 (enjoyment of life).

In the overall population and Group II, but not in Group I, there were significant negative correlations (p < 0.05) between age and TRQ items 6 (avoid quiet situations), 7 (going out), 9 (annoyance), 14 (hard to relax), 18 (work), 22 (hopeless about future) and 26 (feel tormented).

Table 12.4 Results of Spearman rank correlation tests between age, score on each item and total scores of ITI and TRQ for the overall population, Group I and Group II

Questionnaire ITI item	Total n = 518		Group I n = 283		Group II n = 235	
	T	p	T	p	T	p
1: how often it is found annoying	.09	.004	.14	.002	.15	.021
2: difficulty caused in the situation where you most wanted to hear	0.13	0.004	.12	.04	.15	.019
3: caused or aggravated health problems	.023	NS	-.03	NS	-.02	NS
4: affected sleep	-.15	.0001	-.20	.0001	-.11	NS

Questionnaire TRQ item	Total n = 518		Group I n = 283		Group II n = 235	
	T	p	T	p	T	p
1: made unhappy	-.08	NS	-.07	NS	-.15	.018
2: feel tense	-.12	.007	-.07	NS	-.14	.026
3: feel irritable	-.08	NS	-.01	NS	-.06	NS
4: feel angry	-.15	.0001	-.18	.003	-.18	.005
5: made to cry	-.17	.0001	-.23	.0001	-.24	.0001
6: made to avoid quiet situations	-.10	.025	-.10	NS	-.15	.021
7: less interested in going out	-.12	.006	-.08	NS	-.15	.019
8: feel depressed	-.07	NS	-.05	NS	-.05	NS
9: feel annoyed	-.15	.0001	-.02	NS	-.17	.011
10: feel confused	-.10	.027	-.07	NS	-.10	NS
11: driven crazy	-.16	.0001	-.20	.0001	-.12	NS
12: interfered with enjoyment of life	-.09	.0001	-.03	NS	-.11	NS

	5: affected peace of mind	6: affected other people	7: affected the things you can do	8: changed enjoyment of life	Total score
13: hard to concentrate			-.10 *.012*	-.05 *NS*	-.06 *NS*
14: hard to relax			-.06 *NS*	-.10 *.029*	-.17 *.008*
15: feel distressed			-.20 *.0001*	-.15 *.0001*	-.19 *.004*
16: feel helpless			-.18 *.0001*	-.18 *.0001*	-.24 *.0001*
17: feel frustrated with things			-.16 *.002*	-.13 *.002*	-.17 *.001*
18: interfered with ability to work			-.03 *.005*	-.10 *.002*	-.16 *.016*
19: led to despair			-.12 *NS*	-.17 *.0001*	-.24 *.0001*
20: avoid noisy situations			-.06 *.049*	-.08 *NS*	-.12 *NS*
21: avoid social situations			.06 *NS*	-.04 *NS*	-.04 *NS*
22: feel hopeless about the future			-.07 *NS*	-.13 *.004*	-.21 *.001*
23: interfered with my sleep			-.16 *.006*	-.14 *.002*	-.14 *.029*
24: led to think about suicide			-.13 *.023*	-.15 *.0001*	-.19 *.003*
25: feel panicky			-.17 *.004*	-.20 *.0001*	-.27 *.0001*
26: feel tormented			-.09 *NS*	-.13 *.002*	-.20 *.002*
Total score			-.14 *.019*	-.17 *.0001*	-.22 *.0001*

	5: affected peace of mind	6: affected other people	7: affected the things you can do	8: changed enjoyment of life	Total score
5: affected peace of mind	-.11 *.010*	-.14 *NS*	.02 *NS*	-.09 *NS*	-.05 *NS*
6: affected other people	-.01 *NS*	-.04 *NS*	.02 *NS*	.02 *NS*	-.04 *NS*
7: affected the things you can do	-.02 *NS*	-.02 *NS*	.02 *NS*	-.05 *NS*	-.05 *NS*
8: changed enjoyment of life	-.00 *NS*	-.05 *NS*	-.09 *NS*	-.05 *NS*	-.04 *NS*
Total score	-.05 *NS*	-.04 *NS*	.01 *NS*	-.04 *NS*	-.05 *NS*

Table 12.5 Results of Spearman rank correlation tests between age of patients, scores on each item and total scores of ITI and TRQ for Group IIa, Group IIb and Group IIc

Questionnaire ITI item	Group IIa n = 114		Group IIb n = 41		Group IIc n = 80	
	T	p	T	p	T	p
1: how often it is found annoying	.17	NS	.24	NS	.06	NS
2: difficulty caused in the situation where you most wanted to hear	.28	.002	.02	NS	.03	NS
3: caused or aggravated health problems	-.000	NS	.07	NS	-.09	NS
4: affected sleep	-.02	NS	-.23	NS	-.22	.045

Questionnaire TRQ item	Group IIa n = 114		Group IIb N = 41		Group IIc n = 80	
	T	p	T	p	T	p
1: made unhappy	-.07	NS	-.12	NS	-.27	.001
2: feel tense	-.10	NS	-.04	NS	-.27	.014
3: feel irritable	-.01	NS	-.20	NS	-.09	NS
4: feel angry	-.09	NS	-.19	NS	-.30	.007
5: made to cry	-.18	NS	-.12	NS	-.36	.001
6: made to avoid quiet situations	-.10	NS	-.08	NS	-.31	.006
7: less interested in going out	-.19	.042	-.23	NS	-.08	NS
8: feel depressed	.01	NS	-.16	NS	-.08	NS
9: feel annoyed	-.21	.028	-.02	NS	-.14	NS
10: feel confused	-.08	NS	.17	NS	-.28	.001
11: driven crazy	-.10	NS	.07	NS	-.20	NS
12: interfered with enjoyment of life	-.07	NS	-.04	NS	-.23	.037

Item	(r)	(p)	(r)	(p)	(r)	(p)
5: affected peace of mind	-.05	NS	-.09	NS	-.16	NS
6: affected other people	.11	NS	.08	NS	-.12	NS
7: affected the things you can do	.00	NS	.17	NS	-.12	NS
8: changed enjoyment of life	-.03	NS	.09	NS	-.22	.023
Total score	.09	NS	.05	NS	.05	NS
13: hard to concentrate	-.03	NS	.08	NS	-.23	.044
14: hard to relax	-.18	NS	-.16	NS	-.15	NS
15: feel distressed	-.10	NS	-.19	NS	-.27	.015
16: feel helpless	-.22	.021	-.01	NS	-.33	.003
17: feel frustrated with things	-.15	NS	-.09	NS	-.16	NS
18: interfered with ability to work	-.20	.003	.16	NS	-.23	.042
19: led to despair	-.17	NS	-.24	NS	-.30	.008
20: avoid noisy situations	-.09	NS	-.18	NS	-.10	NS
21: avoid social situations	.00	NS	-.06	NS	-.06	NS
22: feel hopeless about the future	-.18	.005	-.25	NS	-.17	NS
23: interfered with my sleep	-.10	NS	-.23	NS	-.15	NS
24: led to think about suicide	-.16	NS	-.21	NS	-.19	NS
25: feel panicky	-.26	.004	-.13	NS	-.31	.006
26: feel tormented	-.19	.046	-.02	NS	-.30	.007
Total score	-.20	.004	-.15	NS	-.28	.012

Table 12.6 Results of Spearman rank correlation tests between tinnitus duration, scores on each item scores and total scores of ITI and TRQ for the overall population, Group I and Group II

Questionnaire ITI item	Total n = 518		Group I n = 283		Group II n = 235	
	T	p	T	p	T	p
1: how often it is found annoying	.89	.043	.10	NS	.10	NS
2: difficulty caused in the situation where you most wanted to hear	.13	.004	.07	NS	.18	.004
3: caused or aggravated health problems	.02	NS	.02	NS	.01	NS
4: affected sleep	-.11	.001	-.13	.029	-.09	NS

Questionnaire TRQ item	Total n = 518		Group I n = 283		Group II n = 235	
	T	p	T	p	T	p
1: made unhappy	-.01	NS	-.03	NS	.07	NS
2: feel tense	-.02	NS	-.03	NS	-.02	NS
3: feel irritable	-.00	NS	-.01	NS	.03	NS
4: feel angry	-.04	NS	-.05	NS	.02	NS
5: made to cry	-.91	.038	-.11	NS	.10	NS
6: made to avoid quiet situations	-.07	NS	-.06	NS	.08	NS
7: less interested in going out	.01	NS	.01	NS	.03	NS
8: feel depressed	.03	NS	.03	NS	.05	NS
9: feel annoyed	-.06	NS	-.05	NS	-.08	NS
10: feel confused	-.01	NS	-.02	NS	.01	NS
11: driven crazy	-.07	NS	-.10	NS	-.04	NS
12: interfered with enjoyment of life	.00	NS	.02	NS	-.00	NS

Item						
5: affected peace of mind	−.10	.0229	−.13	032	−.08	NS
6: affected other people	−.01	NS	−.02	VS	.02	NS
7: affected the things you can do	−.02	NS	−.03	NS	−.01	NS
8: changed enjoyment of life	−.00	NS	.02	NS	−.03	NS
Total score	−.00	NS	−.01	NS	.02	NS

Item						
13: hard to concentrate	.01	NS	.01	NS	.05	NS
14: hard to re ax	−.03	NS	.00	NS	−.07	NS
15: feel distressed	.02	NS	.03	NS	.00	NS
16: feel helpless	−.06	NS	−.02	NS	−.10	NS
17: feel frustrated with things	−.01	NS	.04	NS	−.07	NS
18: interfered with ability to work	.05	NS	.05	NS	.08	NS
19: led to despair	−.02	NS	.00	NS	−.08	NS
20: avoid noisy situations	.04	NS	.02	NS	.03	NS
21: avoid social situations	.07	NS	.14	NS	−.04	NS
22: feel hopeless about the future	−.04	NS	−.04	NS	−.06	NS
23: interfered with sleep	−.15	.0001	−.16	.007	−.11	NS
24: led to think about suicide	−.03	NS	−.04	NS	−.01	NS
25: feel panicky	−.09	.036	−.11	NS	−.09	NS
26: feel tormented	−.02	NS	.000	NS	−.06	NS
Total score	−.03	NS	−.02	NS	−.05	NS

Table 12.7 Results of Spearman rank correlation tests between tinnitus duration, scores on each item and total scores of ITI and TRQ for Group IIa, Group IIb and Group IIc

Questionnaire ITI item	Group IIa n = 114		Group IIb n = 41		Group IIc n = 80	
	T	p	T	p	T	p
1: how often it is found annoying	.17	NS	.02	NS	.01	NS
2: difficulty caused in the situation where you most wanted to hear	.19	.048	.03	NS	.29	NS
3: caused or aggravated health problems	.11	NS	-.06	NS	-.08	NS
4: affected sleep	.09	NS	-.46	.002	-.19	NS

Questionnaire TRQ item	Group IIa n = 114		Group IIb n = 41		Group IIc n = 80	
	T	p	T	p	T	p
1: made unhappy	.11	NS	-.11	NS	-.08	NS
2: feel tense	.05	NS	-.06	NS	-.08	NS
3: feel irritable	.03	NS	-.11	NS	.03	NS
4: feel angry	-.01	NS	-.21	NS	.03	NS
5: made to cry	-.07	NS	-.21	NS	-.04	NS
6: made to avoid quiet situations	-.05	NS	-.20	NS	-.09	NS
7: less interested in going out	.07	NS	-.04	NS	.02	NS
8: feel depressed	.19	.046	-.20	NS	-.03	NS
9: feel annoyed	-.04	NS	-.35	NS	.01	NS
10: feel confused	.07	NS	.06	NS	-.01	NS
11: driven crazy	-.05	NS	.06	NS	-.04	NS
12: interfered with enjoyment of life	.10	NS	-.16	NS	-.08	NS

Item						
5: affected peace of mind	.01	NS	−.26	NS	−.13	NS
6: affected other people	.04	NS	.02	NS	.02	NS
7: affected the things you can do	.02	NS	.06	NS	−.05	NS
8: changed enjoyment of life	.15	NS	.09	NS	−.22	.05
Total score	.14	NS	−.01	NS	−.13	NS
13: hard to concentrate	.12	NS	.06	NS	.02	NS
14: hard to relax	−.00	NS	−.28	NS	−.04	NS
15: feel distressed	.03	NS	−.14	NS	.03	NS
16: feel helpless	−.13	NS	−.15	NS	−.04	NS
17: feel frustrated with things	.01	NS	−.27	NS	−.05	NS
18: interfered with ability to work	.13	NS	.15	NS	.00	NS
19: led to despair	.05	NS	−.24	NS	−.16	NS
20: avoid noisy situations	.00	NS	−.03	NS	.15	NS
21: avoid social situations	.00	NS	−.02	NS	.27	NS
22: feel hopeless about the future	−.01	NS	−.23	NS	.03	NS
23: interfered with my sleep	.04	NS	−.46	.002	−.15	NS
24: led to think about suicide	.04	NS	−.32	.044	.00	NS
25: feel panicky	−.02	NS	−.19	NS	−.19	NS
26: feel tormented	.05	NS	−.17	NS	.06	NS
Total score	.03	NS	−.24	NS	.08	NS

Table 12.8 Results of Spearman rank correlation tests between 'difficulty in listening to TV', scores on each item and total scores of ITI and TRQ for the overall population, Group I and Group II

Questionnaire ITI item	Total n = 518		Group I n = 283		Group II n = 235	
	T	p	T	p	T	p
1: how often it is found annoying	.16	.0001	.223	.0001	.093	NS
2: difficulty caused in the situation where you most wanted to hear	.46	.0001	.51	.0001	.38	.0001
3: caused or aggravated health problems	.10	.017	.08	NS	.14	.003
4: affected sleep	-.04	NS	-.05	NS	-.02	NS

Questionnaire TRQ item	Total n = 518		Group I n = 283		Group II n = 235	
	T	p	T	p	T	p
1: made unhappy	.03	NS	.04	NS	.01	NS
2: feel tense	.05	NS	.05	NS	.07	NS
3: feel irritable	.12	.004	.13	.03	.12	NS
4: feel angry	.04	NS	.06	NS	.02	NS
5: made to cry	.00	NS	.02	NS	-.02	NS
6: made to avoid quiet situations	-.05	NS	-.00	NS	-.11	NS
7: less interested in going out	.14	.002	.16	.006	.11	NS
8: feel depressed	.08	NS	.06	NS	.10	NS
9: feel annoyed	.06	NS	.09	NS	.03	NS
10: feel confused	.15	.0001	.16	.007	.14	.003
11: driven crazy	.07	NS	.06	NS	.11	NS
12: interfered with enjoyment of life	.16	.0001	.21	.0001	.11	NS

Item	r	p	r	p	r	p
5: affected peace of mind	.03	NS	.04	NS	.01	NS
6: affected other people	.19	.0001	.16	.007	.23	.0001
7: affected the things you can do	.16	.0001	.19	.001	.12	NS
8: changed enjoyment of life	.05	NS	.08	NS	.01	NS
Total score	.19	.0001	.22	.0001	.17	.009

Item	r	p	r	p	r	p
13: hard to concentrate	.19	.0001	.23	.0001	.15	.022
14: hard to relax	.12	.0061	.16	.007	.07	NS
15: feel distressed	.08	NS	.07	NS	.08	NS
16: feel helpless	.08	NS	.10	NS	.00	NS
17: feel frustrated with things	.11	.009	.13	.028	.10	NS
18: interfered with ability to work	.25	.0001	.28	.0001	.21	.001
19: led to despair	.03	NS	.06	NS	.01	NS
20: avoid noisy situations	.19	.0001	.19	.001	.20	.002
21: avoid social situations	.28	.0001	.28	.0001	.30	.0001
22: feel hopeless about the future	.06	NS	.10	NS	.01	NS
23: interfered with my sleep	.06	NS	-.04	NS	-.06	NS
24: led to think about suicide	-.05	NS	-.02	NS	.02	NS
25: feel panicky	-.00	NS	-.00	NS	-.10	NS
26: feel tormented	-.08	NS	.09	NS	.08	NS
Total score	.12	.005	.15	.013	.10	NS

Table 12.9 Results of Spearman rank correlation tests between 'difficulty in listening to TV', scores on each item and total scores of ITI and TRQ for Group IIa, Group IIb and Group IIc

Questionnaire TRQ item	Group IIa n = 114		Group IIb n = 41		Group IIc n = 80	
	T	p	T	p	T	p
1: made unhappy	-.00	NS	.03	NS	.02	NS
2: feel tense	.06	NS	.17	NS	-.02	NS
3: feel irritable	.07	NS	.17	NS	.16	NS
4: feel angry	-.01	NS	-.10	NS	.12	NS
5: made to cry	-.07	NS	.00	NS	.02	NS
6: made to avoid quiet situations	-.07	NS	.02	NS	-.22	NS
7: less interested in going out	.11	NS	.21	NS	.08	NS
8: feel depressed	.14	NS	.12	NS	.02	NS
9: feel annoyed	.00	NS	.01	NS	.06	NS
10: feel confused	.12	NS	.44	.004	.01	NS
11: driven crazy	.14	NS	.28	NS	-.03	NS
12: interfered with enjoyment of life	.15	NS	.27	NS	-.02	NS

Questionnaire ITI item	Group IIa n = 114		Group IIb n = 41		Group IIc n = 80	
	T	p	T	p	T	p
1: how often it is found annoying	.19	.042	-.04	NS	.01	NS
2: difficulty caused in the situation where you most wanted to hear	.40	.0001	.09	NS	.51	.0001
3: caused or aggravated health problems	.07	NS	.30	NS	.15	NS
4: affected sleep	.06	NS	-.24	NS	-.03	NS

	r	p	r	p	r	p
5: affected peace of mind	.11	NS	-.16	NS	-.03	NS
6: affected other people	.33	.0001	.10	NS	.13	NS
7: affected the things you can do	.26	.005	-.07	NS	.02	NS
8: changed enjoyment of life	.14	NS	-.15	NS	-.04	NS
Total score	.27	.004	-02	NS	-.02	NS
13: hard to concentrate	.17	NS	.24	NS	.08	NS
14: hard to relax	.06	NS	.19	NS	.01	NS
15: feel distressed	.04	NS	.13	NS	.11	NS
16: feel helpless	-.02	NS	-.01	NS	.15	NS
17: feel frustrated with things	.05	NS	.08	NS	.13	NS
18: interfered with ability to work	.13	NS	.22	NS	.30	.007
19: led to despair	.00	NS	.19	NS	-.07	NS
20: avoid noisy situations	.18	NS	.10	NS	.26	.020
21: avoid social situations	.30	.001	.33	.034	.27	.014
22: feel hopeless about the future	-.01	NS	.03	NS	.03	NS
23: interfered with my sleep	.00	NS	-.07	NS	-.15	NS
24: led to think about suicide	.03	NS	.03	NS	.00	NS
25: feel panicky	-.07	NS	.00	NS	-.19	NS
26: feel tormented	.06	NS	.10	NS	.06	NS
Total score	.07	NS	.18	NS	.08	NS

Group II differed from the overall population and Group I with a significant negative correlation ($p < 0.05$) found between age and TRQ item 1 (unhappy) and by the fact that no negative correlation was found between age and either ITI item 4 (effect on sleep) or 5 (peace of mind).

Groups IIa, IIb and IIc

In Group IIb there were no significant correlations with age. On the other hand, many significant correlations were found in Group IIc: negative correlations with age were found for ITI items 4 (sleep) and 8 (enjoyment of life) and for total TRQ score and TRQ items 1 (unhappy), 2 (tense), 4 (angry), 10 (confused), 12 (enjoyment of life), 13 (hard to concentrate), 15 (distressed), 16 (helpless), 18 (work), 19 (despair), 25 (feel panicky) and 26 (feel tormented).

In Group IIa, ITI Item 2 (hearing difficulties) and TRQ items 7 (going out), 9 (annoyed), 16 (helpless), 18 (work), 22 (hopeless about future), 25 (feel panicky), 26 (feel tormented) and total TRQ score correlated significantly with age.

Effects of tinnitus duration

Overall population, Group I and Group II

There were no significant correlations that were common to all three groups (overall population, Group I and Group II).

In the overall population only, tinnitus duration correlated positively ($p < 0.05$) with ITI item 1 (annoyance; $p < 0.04$) and negatively ($p < 0.05$) with TRQ items 5 (tears) and 25 (feel panicky).

Except in Group I, ITI item 2 (hearing difficulties) correlated positively with tinnitus duration ($p < 0.005$).

In Group I, unlike Group II, tinnitus duration was negatively ($p < 0.05$) related to ITI items 4 (sleep), and 5 (peace of mind) and TRQ item 23 (sleep).

Groups IIa, IIb and IIc

In Group IIa, the only significant correlations with tinnitus duration ($p < 0.05$) found were a positive correlation with ITI item 2 (hearing difficulties) and a negative one with TRQ item 8 (depressed).

In Group IIb, ITI item 4 (sleep) and TRQ items 23 (sleep) and 24 (thoughts about suicide) correlated negatively with tinnitus duration.

Only one negative correlation – with ITI item 8 (enjoyment of life) – was found in Group IIc.

Effects of difficulty in listening to TV

Overall population, Group I and Group II

In all the three groups (overall population, Group I and Group II), difficulty in listening to TV correlated positively ($p < 0.05$) with the total ITI score, scores on ITI items 2 (hearing difficulties) and 6 (other people) and scores on TRQ items 10 (confused), 13 (hard to concentrate), 18 (work), 20 (avoid noisy situations) and 21 (avoid social situations). In the overall population and in Group I, difficulty hearing TV correlated positively with ITI items 1 (annoyance) and 7 (activities) on the one hand, and with total TRQ score and scores on TRQ items 3 (irritable), 7 (going out) and 17 (frustrated with things) on the other.

In the overall population and Group II, unlike Group I, difficulty in listening to TV correlated significantly ($p > 0.05$) with ITI item 3 (health problems).

Subgroups IIa, IIb and IIc

One positive correlation was found between difficulty in listening to TV and TRQ item 21 (avoid social situations) in all three subgroups of Group II. In addition, in subgroup IIa this variable showed significant correlations ($p < 0.05$) with total ITI score and ITI items 1 (annoyance), 2 (hearing difficulties), 6 (other people) and 7 (going out). In subgroup IIc, it is positively correlated with ITI item 2 (hearing difficulties) and TRQ items 18 (work) and 20 (avoid noisy situations).

DISCUSSION

Tinnitus is known to affect 10–17% of the population in western countries (Coles, 1984; Jastreboff, 2000). However, the impact of this symptom can vary greatly. Recent epidemiological studies conducted in Germany (Pilgramm et al., 1999) and in Poland (Fabijanska et al., 1999) reported different rates of severe-to-unbearable tinnitus (2% and 9.7%, respectively). It is of epidemiological interest that having a family history of a disabling symptom can greatly affect the patient's perception of and reaction to the symptom. This was highlighted by previous studies focusing on various somatic disorders (Thyrum et al., 1995; Esplen et al., 2001). Focusing on ENT symptoms, a British survey came to the conclusion that, independently of the degree of hearing loss, the emotional impact of hearing loss and tinnitus is linked to the likelihood of having a family history of hearing loss (Stephens et al., 2003). Given that cross-cultural differences are frequently involved in health problems (Levenstein et al., 2001; Morton, 2003), the validity of this finding may depend on the patient's culture and background.

RESULTS FROM THE OPEN-ENDED QUESTIONNAIRE

The present findings showed that about 45% of respondents had relatives with hearing problems: 48.5% with hearing loss, 34.1% with hearing loss plus tinnitus and 17.4% with tinnitus alone. A very small percentage of people (2.6%) having a family history of hearing loss reported it as having an effect on tinnitus impact, while a majority (respectively 68.3% and 63.7%) of those having a family history of tinnitus or tinnitus associated with hearing loss reported it as having an effect on tinnitus annoyance and on the impact on the individual's life.

Overall, the negative effects of FH (10.2%) outnumbered the positive effects (8.9%), although the difference was small. The reported negative effects were essentially emotional and linked to the stressful aspects of this disability. The fact that a majority of FH effects were negative is in agreement with the results reported by Stephens et al. (2003) showing that the probability of a patient having an FHHL increases with the annoyance caused by the tinnitus, independently of the limitation in the patient's activity.

DATA FROM THE ITI AND TRQ

Data from the ITI and TRQ shed more light on the above effects and how FH influences the impact of and reaction to tinnitus; they also reveal consequences specific to the type of FH (i.e. hearing loss, tinnitus, or hearing loss associated with tinnitus) on this impact and reaction.

Differences between Group I and Group II

Tinnitus effects on sleep (ITI item 4 and TRQ item 23), irritability (TRQ item 3), feelings of anger (TRQ item 4), or of being driven crazy (TRQ item 11), on difficulty in concentrating (TRQ item 13), the ability to work (TRQ item 18), and avoidance of social situations (TRQ item 21) proved to differ significantly between the two groups. Likewise, the overall reaction to tinnitus (total TRQ score) was found to be lower in those with a family history of hearing troubles.

Thus, a family history of hearing troubles generally alleviates the individual's reactions to tinnitus. It may be that sharing the life or a good part of the life of a person with hearing problems familiarises the subject with such disability, making him/her aware, by simple observation as well as from shared experience, of what to do or not to do in order to cope.

The effects of age, tinnitus duration and difficulty in listening to TV which characterised Group I (without a FH) are listed below:

The older a subject without a FH, the less sleep (ITI item 4) and peace of mind (ITI item 5) were affected by tinnitus and the less he/she was 'driven crazy' (TRQ item 11), whereas these effects of age were absent in Group II (with FH). Tables 12.2b and 12.2c show higher mean scores for ITI item 4 and TRQ item 11 in Group I (without FH) than in Group II. These results probably indicate that, in Group I, age compensates in part, for the lack of beneficial effects resulting from a FH.

Similar conclusions can be drawn concerning tinnitus duration, since, in subjects with no FH, the longer the duration, the less tinnitus affected sleep (ITI item 4, and TRQ item 23) or peace of mind (ITI item 5), while these correlations were not found in subjects with a FH.

Again, the correlations with the increased difficulty in listening to TV found in subjects without a FH, i.e. aggravation of the effect on how often per day tinnitus was found annoying (ITI item 1), the things the subject could do (ITI item 7), irritability (TRQ item 3), interest in going out (TRQ item 7), enjoyment of life (TRQ item 12), difficulty relaxing (TRQ item 14), a feeling of frustration with things (TRQ item 17), and finally, the overall reaction to tinnitus (total TRQ score) were not found in those with a FH. What might explain these results? It may be that, in absence of a FH, some consequences of increasing hearing loss are falsely attributed to tinnitus. FH subjects, being better informed as to the actual consequences of hearing loss, would be less liable to make such a misattribution. However, from Table 12.9 it can be seen that only the FHHL subgroup showed any significant correlation between difficulty in listening to TV and the positive benefit of having a family history.

Some correlations were specific to Group II (with a FH). A majority of these corresponded to positive consequences and concerned age effects. Thus, the older a subject with a FH, the less he/she felt unhappy (TRQ item 1), the less the tinnitus led him/her to avoid quiet situations (TRQ item 6), the less he/she felt uninterested in going out (TRQ item 7), and the less tinnitus made him/her feel annoyed (TRQ 9), made it hard to concentrate (TRQ item 14), interfered with the ability to work (TRQ item 18), or made him/her feel hopeless about the future (TRQ item 22) or tormented (TRQ item 26). On the other hand, a FH had negative consequences, related to tinnitus duration and difficulty in listening to TV: the longer the tinnitus duration of an FH subject, the more tinnitus made it difficult to hear in situations where he/she most wanted to hear (ITI item 2), and the greater an FH subject's difficulty in listening to TV, the more his/her tinnitus 'caused' or 'aggravated' health problems (ITI item 3).

Observations common to the subgroups of Group II

The only effect found in all three FH subgroups concerned difficulty in listening to TV. The more severe this was (whatever the FH: FHHL, FHT or FHHLT), the more tinnitus led the subject to avoid social situations (TRQ item 21). One may wonder in this regard whether it is actually the tinnitus that is causing the subject to avoid social situations, inasmuch as worsening hearing loss itself would tend to have the same effect. At the same time, as hearing loss increases, the tinnitus comes to stand out more strongly against the background noise, and would thus indeed tend to hamper social interaction more.

Some other effects were observed in subgroups IIa and IIc only. Thus, the older a subject with a FHHL or a FHHLT, the less tinnitus made him/her feel helpless (TRQ item 16), interfered with the ability to work (TRQ item 18), or made him/her feel panicky (TRQ item 25) or tormented (TRQ item 26), and, finally, the less the overall reaction to tinnitus (total TRQ score). Living or having lived with a relative affected by hearing loss and/or tinnitus would thus seem to enable tinnitus subjects to obtain a perspective on the impact of ageing on these emotional reactions to tinnitus, and on tinnitus's disabling impact on the capacity to work; in tinnitus subjects whose relatives were, on the other hand, afflicted with tinnitus but not hearing loss, no such sense of perspective is on offer. A family history of hearing loss – associated with tinnitus or not – would thus seem to act as a safeguard against age-linked worsening of these particular aspects of the reaction to tinnitus.

Specific findings in Group IIa

The older a subject with FHHL, the more tinnitus caused difficulty in hearing in situations where he/she most wanted to hear (ITI item 2), the less it made him/her uninterested in going out (TRQ item 7), or feel annoyed (TRQ item 9) or hopeless about the future (TRQ item 22).

The longer the tinnitus duration in a subject with a FHHL, the more tinnitus caused difficulty in hearing in situations where they most wanted to hear (ITI item 2) and made them feel depressed (TRQ item 8).

The greater a FHHL subject's difficulty in listening to TV, the greater the impact of tinnitus as measured by the ITI (total score), the more often tinnitus was found annoying (ITI item 1), and the more it affected other people (ITI item 6) and the things the person could do (ITI item 7).

Except for the lessening of their interest in going out, these findings are the logical consequence of hearing loss increasing with age and hindering communication. It is noticeable that only in this group having no FH of tinnitus, age displayed the unexpected effect of making the subjects more interested in going out in spite of absence of difference in age and TRQ item 7 scores between Groups IIa, IIb and IIc. However, the longer tinnitus has lasted and the more it is seen as hindering good hearing, the more it causes subjects with a family history of hearing loss to feel depressed. Both of these findings may reflect how tinnitus is seen as a further problem coming on top of the familiar (because familial) ones brought on by hearing deteriorating with age: the longer it has lasted, the more depressing tinnitus becomes, as the subject gets even more tired of this symptom as the hearing loss, which it only aggravates, gets worse.

Specific findings in Group IIb

In Group IIb, unlike Groups IIa and IIc, no effect of age emerged from ITI and TRQ items or total scores. The longer the tinnitus duration in FHT subjects, the less tinnitus affected sleep (ITI item 4 and TRQ item 23) or led him/her to think about suicide (TRQ item 24). The greater an FHT subject's difficulty in listening to TV, the more tinnitus made him/her feel confused (TRQ item 10).

It would thus seem that having or having had relatives afflicted by tinnitus but without hearing loss prevents age having the positive and negative effects described above, with regard to tinnitus impact and reactions to tinnitus. The observed reduction in tinnitus impact on sleep with increasing tinnitus duration, specific to Group IIb, shows how awareness of tinnitus-specific effects drawn from observation of affected relatives, likewise specific to this subgroup, is probably a necessary condition for such a positive effect to occur. The same goes for the alleviation of suicidal thoughts. The increasing feeling of confusion caused by tinnitus with increasing hearing difficulty, on the other hand, seems logical inasmuch as, on top of the acoustical interference due specifically to the presence of tinnitus, there come difficulties of understanding and misunderstanding relating to the severity of the hearing deficit.

Specific findings in Group IIc

The following effects proved specific to Group IIc. The older a FHHLT subject, the less tinnitus affected sleep (ITI item 4) and enjoyment of life (ITI item 8 and TRQ item 12), made him/her feel unhappy (TRQ item 1), tense (TRQ item 2), angry (TRQ item 4), confused (TRQ item 10), or distressed (TRQ item 15), made it hard to concentrate (TRQ item 13), or led him/her to despair (TRQ item 19).

The longer the tinnitus duration in a FHHLT subject, the less tinnitus changed his/her enjoyment of life (ITI item 8). The greater a FHHLT subject's difficulty in listening to TV, the more tinnitus interfered with their ability to work (TRQ item 18) and led him/her to avoid noisy situations (TRQ item 20).

The group of subjects with a family history of tinnitus associated with hearing loss experienced the beneficial effects of ageing on reactions to tinnitus. Having witnessed the cumulative aggravating effect of hearing loss and tinnitus in relatives probably accounts for how increasing severity of hearing problems entails a greater impact of tinnitus on the capacity to work in this group, as in Group IIa.

CONCLUSION

Although some subjects were of the opinion that having or having had relatives with hearing troubles had negative effects for them, overall our findings showed that not having a family history of hearing troubles led to a greater deterioration in the quality of life and caused a stronger reaction to their tinnitus. To some extent, these results contradict those of the MRC Survey of Ear Nose and Throat problems (Stephens et al., 2003), which found that the likelihood of having a FH of hearing problems increased with the annoyance caused by tinnitus. However, our observations and Stephens' were not obtained from similarly defined samples. Our population was self-selected and comprised predominantly members of a support group or, at least, people searching for specific information via the Internet; as a consequence, they probably came from the more severe end of tinnitus spectrum. On the other hand, the MRC–ENT survey was a population study which included mainly people with normal hearing and the FH criteria chosen were quite severe. In addition, in the present study, the nature of the family history of each participant was determined precisely (hearing loss only, tinnitus only, or hearing loss associated with tinnitus) whereas Stephens et al. considered only the possibility of having a FHHL, but this probability was calculated globally from data obtained from people who might also have had tinnitus in addition to their hearing loss. Moreover these discrepancies may also be a matter of cross-cultural differences, although the precise nature of these has yet to be determined.

REFERENCES

Bauch CD, Lynn SG, Williams DE, Mellon MW, Weaver AL (2003) Tinnitus impact: three different measurement tools. *Journal of the American Academy of Audiology* 14: 181–7.

Carlsson SG, Erlandsson SI (1991) Habituation and tinnitus: an experimental study. *Journal of Psychosomatic Research* 35: 509–14.

Coles RR (1984) Epidemiology of tinnitus: (1) prevalence. *Journal of Laryngology and Otology Suppl.* 9: 7–15.

Cox RM, Alexander GC (2002) The International Outcome Inventory for Hearing Aids (IOI-HA): psychometric properties of the English version. *International Journal of Audiology* 41: 30–5.

Cox RM, Stephens D, Kramer SE (2002) Translations of the International Outcome Inventory for Hearing Aids (IOI-HA). *International Journal of Audiology* 41: 3–26.

Esplen MJ, Madlensky L, Butler K, McKinnon W, Bapat B et al. (2001) Motivations and psychosocial impact of genetic testing for HNPCC. *American Journal of Medical Genetics* 103: 9–15.

Fabijanska A, Rogowski M, Bartnik G, Skarzynski H (1999) Epidemiology of tinnitus and hyperacusis in Poland. In J Hazell (ed) Proceedings of the Sixth International Tinnitus Seminar, Cambridge UK, pp. 569–71.

Halford JBS, Stewart M, Anderson D (1991) Tinnitus severity measured by a subjective scale, audiometry and clinical judgment. *Journal of Laryngology and Otology* 105: 89–93.

Hallam R, Rachman S, Hinchcliffe R (1984) Psychological aspects of tinnitus. In S. Rachman (ed) *Contributions to Medical Psychology*. Oxford: Pergamon Press, pp. 31–4.

Harvey-Berino J, Casey Gold E, Smith West D, Shuldiner AR, Walston J et al. (2001) Does genetic testing for obesity influence confidence in the ability to lose weight? A pilot investigation. *JADA* 101: 1351–3.

Hathaway SR, Jakes SC, Hinchcliffe R (1988) Cognitive variables in tinnitus annoyance. *British Journal of Psychology* 27: 213–22.

Henry JL, Kangas M, Wilson PH (2001) Development of the psychological impact of the tinnitus interview: a clinician-administered measure of tinnitus-related distress. *International Tinnitus Journal* 7: 20–6.

Hiller W, Goebel G (1992) A psychometric study of complaints in chronic tinnitus. *Journal of Psychosomatic Research* 36: 337–48.

Jakes SC, Hallam RS, Chambers C, Hinchcliffe R (1985) A factor analytical study of tinnitus complaint behaviour. *Audiology* 24: 195–206.

Jastreboff PJ, Jastreboff MM (2000) Tinnitus Retraining Therapy (TRT) as a method for treatment of tinnitus and hyperacusis patients. *Journal of the American Academy of Audiology* 11(3): 162–77.

Kennedy V, Chéry-Croze S, Stephens D, Kramer S, Thai Van H, Collet L (2005) Development of the International Tinnitus Inventory (ITI). a patient-directed problem questionnaire. *Audiological Medicine* 3: 228–37.

Kuk FK, Tyler RS, Russel D et al. (1990) The psychometric properties of a tinnitus handicap questionnaire. *Ear and Hearing* 11.

Levenstein S, Li Z, Almer S, Barbosa A, Marquis P et al. (2001) Cross-cultural variation in disease-related concerns among patients with inflammatory bowel disease. *American Journal of Gastroenterology* 96: 1822–30.

Meric C, Gartner M, Collet L, Chéry-Croze S (1998) Psychopathological profile of French tinnitus sufferers: evidence concerning the relationship between tinnitus features and impact on life. *Audiology and Otoneurology* 3: 240–52.

Meric C, Pham E, Chéry-Croze S (1996) Traduction et validation de l'échelle subjective de mesure de la sévérité de l'acouphène (Subjective Tinnitus Severity Scale, JBS Halford et al., 1991) *Journal Français d'ORL* 45: 409–12.

Meric C, Pham E, Chéry-Croze S (1997a) Traduction et validation de l'échelle subjective de mesure de la détresse de l'acouphène (Tinnitus Reaction Questionnaire, Wilson et al., 1991). *L'encéphale* 23: 442–6.

Meric C, Pham E, Chéry-Croze S (1997b) Traduction et validation du questionnaire 'Mesure du handicap lié à l'acouphène' (Tinnitus Handicap Questionnaire, 1990) *Journal of Otolaryngology* 26: 167–70.

Meric C, Pham E, Chéry-Croze S (2000) Validation assessment of a French version of the Tinnitus Reaction Questionnaire: a comparison between data from English and French versions. *Journal of Speech, Language, and Hearing Research* 43: 184–90.

Morton RP (2003) Studies in the quality of life of head and neck cancer patients: results of a two-year longitudinal study and a comparative cross-sectional cross-cultural survey. *Laryngoscope* 113: 1091–103.

Perse J, Lebeaux MO (1977) Manuel du Mini-Mult. Paris: Centre de Psychologie Appliquée.

Pilgramm M, Rychlick R, Lebisch H, Siedentop H, Goebel G, Kirchoff D (1999) Tinnitus in the Federal Republic of Germany: a representative epidemiological study.

In J Hazell (ed) Proceedings of the Sixth International Tinnitus Seminar Cambridge, UK, pp. 64–7.

Schmidtke A (1997) Perspective suicide in Europe. *Suicide Life Threatening Behaviour* 27: 127–36.

Stephens D, Lewis P, Davis A (2003) The influence of a perceived family history of hearing difficulties in an epidemiological study of hearing problems. *Audiological Medicine* 1: 1–4.

Thyrum ET, Blumenthal JA, Madden DJ, Siegel W (1995) Family history of hypertension influences neurobehavioral function in hypertensive patients. *Psychosomatic Medicine* 57: 496–500.

Tyler RS (1993) Tinnitus disability and handicap questionnaires. *Seminars in Hearing* 14: 377–84.

Tyler RS, Baker L (1983) Difficulties experienced by tinnitus sufferers. *Journal of Speech and Hearing Disorders* 48: 150–4.

Voracek M, Fisher ML, Marusic A (2003) The Finno-Ugrian suicide hypothesis: variation in European suicide rates by latitude and longitude. *Perceptual and Motor Skills* 97: 401–6.

Wilson PH, Henry J, Bowen M, Haralambous G (1991) Tinnitus reaction questionnaire: psychometric properties of a measure of distress associated with tinnitus. *Journal of Speech, Language and Hearing Research* 34: 197–201.

APPENDIX 12.1

ENGLISH VERSION OF THE ON-LINE QUESTIONNAIRE

A preliminary study has shown that effects of tinnitus may differ depending on the presence or not of a family history of hearing problems.

Our objective is, first, to confirm this result in the framework of a European multicentre study (Amsterdam – Cardiff – Lyon) and, second, to assess the severity of your tinnitus.

To this aim, we would like to submit to you the following three questionnaires. Thank you in advance for your cooperation.

Please, first answer the following questions in capitals. The corresponding information will be kept secret.

Last name: First name:

Age:

Gender:

Address:

Email:

For how many years and months has your tinnitus lasted?

A. *Open-ended questionnaire*

1. *Do you have difficulty following TV programmes at a volume others find acceptable without any aid to your hearing?*

none   slight   moderate   severe

☐   ☐   ☐   ☐

2. *Do or did other members of your family (brothers, sisters, parents, grand parents, etc) have problems with <u>tinnitus</u>?*

yes   no

☐   ☐

⇒ *If yes, has this influenced your reaction to your own tinnitus?*

yes   no

☐   ☐

⇒ *If yes, please list any ways this knowledge has affected you. Write down as many effects as you can think of.*

3. *Do or did other members of your family (brothers, sisters, parents, grandparents, etc) have problems with their <u>hearing</u>?*

yes   no

☐   ☐

⇒ *If yes, has this influenced your reaction to your own tinnitus?*

yes   no

☐   ☐

⇒ *If yes, please list any ways this knowledge has affected you. Write down as many effects as you can think of.*

B. *International Tinnitus Inventory*

1. *Think about your tinnitus over the past two weeks. On an average day, how often have you found it annoying?*

all the   most of   some of   occasionally   never
the time   the time   the time

☐   ☐   ☐   ☐   ☐

2. *Think about the situation where you most wanted to hear. Over the past two weeks, how much difficulty has the tinnitus caused in that situation?*

very much   quite a lot   moderate   slight   no difficulty
difficulty   of difficulty   difficulty   difficulty

☐   ☐   ☐   ☐   ☐

3. *How much has your tinnitus caused or aggravated other health problems?*

very much	quite a lot	moderately	slightly	not at all
☐	☐	☐	☐	☐

4. *Over the past two weeks, how much has your tinnitus affected your sleep?*

very much	quite a lot	moderately	slightly	not at all
☐	☐	☐	☐	☐

5. *Over the past two weeks, how much has your tinnitus affected your peace of mind?*

very much	quite a lot	moderately	slightly	not at all
☐	☐	☐	☐	☐

6. *Over the past two weeks, how much do you think your tinnitus has affected other people?*

very much	quite a lot	moderately	slightly	not at all
☐	☐	☐	☐	☐

7. *Overall, how much has your tinnitus affected the things you can do?*

very much	quite a lot	moderately	slightly	not at all
☐	☐	☐	☐	☐

8. *Considering everything, how much has your tinnitus changed your enjoyment of life?*

very much worse	quite a lot worse	slightly worse	not at all	better
☐	☐	☐	☐	☐

C. Tinnitus Reaction Questionnaire

Among the list shown below, some sentences can apply to you and some others do not. In order to answer each question, please tick the number which applies the best to you during the past week.

1. *My tinnitus has made me unhappy*

Not at all	A little of the time	Some of the time	A good deal of the time	Almost all of the time
☐	☐	☐	☐	☐

2. *My tinnitus has made me feel tense*

Not at all	A little of the time	Some of the time	A good deal of the time	Almost all of the time
☐	☐	☐	☐	☐

3. *My tinnitus has made me feel irritable*

Not at all	A little of the time	Some of the time	A good deal of the time	Almost all of the time
☐	☐	☐	☐	☐

4. *My tinnitus has made me feel angry*

Not at all	A little of the time	Some of the time	A good deal of the time	Almost all of the time
☐	☐	☐	☐	☐

5. *My tinnitus has led me to cry*

Not at all	A little of the time	Some of the time	A good deal of the time	Almost all of the time
☐	☐	☐	☐	☐

6. *My tinnitus has led me to avoid quiet situations*

Not at all	A little of the time	Some of the time	A good deal of the time	Almost all of the time
☐	☐	☐	☐	☐

7. *My tinnitus has made me feel less interested in going out*

Not at all	A little of the time	Some of the time	A good deal of the time	Almost all of the time
☐	☐	☐	☐	☐

7. *My tinnitus has led me to feel depressed*

Not at all	A little of the time	Some of the time	A good deal of the time	Almost all of the time
☐	☐	☐	☐	☐

8. *My tinnitus has made me feel annoyed*

Not at all	A little of the time	Some of the time	A good deal of the time	Almost all of the time
☐	☐	☐	☐	☐

9. *My tinnitus has made me feel confused*

Not at all	A little of the time	Some of the time	A good deal of the time	Almost all of the time
☐	☐	☐	☐	☐

11. *My tinnitus has 'driven me crazy'*

Not at all	A little of the time	Some of the time	A good deal of the time	Almost all of the time
☐	☐	☐	☐	☐

12. *My tinnitus has interfered with my enjoyment of life*

Not at all	A little of the time	Some of the time	A good deal of the time	Almost all of the time
☐	☐	☐	☐	☐

13. *My tinnitus has made it hard for me to concentrate*

Not at all	A little of the time	Some of the time	A good deal of the time	Almost all of the time
☐	☐	☐	☐	☐

14. *My tinnitus has made it hard for me to relax*

Not at all	A little of the time	Some of the time	A good deal of the time	Almost all of the time
☐	☐	☐	☐	☐

15. *My tinnitus has made me feel distressed*

Not at all	A little of the time	Some of the time	A good deal of the time	Almost all of the time
☐	☐	☐	☐	☐

16. *My tinnitus has made me feel helpless*

Not at all	A little of the time	Some of the time	A good deal of the time	Almost all of the time
☐	☐	☐	☐	☐

17. *My tinnitus has made me feel frustrated with things*

Not at all	A little of the time	Some of the time	A good deal of the time	Almost all of the time
☐	☐	☐	☐	☐

18. *My tinnitus has interfered with my ability to work*

Not at all	A little of the time	Some of the time	A good deal of the time	Almost all of the time
☐	☐	☐	☐	☐

19. *My tinnitus has led me to despair*

Not at all	A little of the time	Some of the time	A good deal of the time	Almost all of the time
☐	☐	☐	☐	☐

20. *My tinnitus has led me to avoid noisy situations*

Not at all	A little of the time	Some of the time	A good deal of the time	Almost all of the time
☐	☐	☐	☐	☐

21. *My tinnitus has led me to avoid social situations*

Not at all	A little of the time	Some of the time	A good deal of the time	Almost all of the time
☐	☐	☐	☐	☐

22. My tinnitus has led me to feel hopeless about the future

Not at all	A little of the time	Some of the time	A good deal of the time	Almost all of the time
☐	☐	☐	☐	☐

23. My tinnitus has interfered with my sleep

Not at all	A little of the time	Some of the time	A good deal of the time	Almost all of the time
☐	☐	☐	☐	☐

24. My tinnitus has led me to think about suicide

Not at all	A little of the time	Some of the time	A good deal of the time	Almost all of the time
☐	☐	☐	☐	☐

25. My tinnitus has made me feel panicky

Not at all	A little of the time	Some of the time	A good deal of the time	Almost all of the time
☐	☐	☐	☐	☐

26. My tinnitus has made me feel tormented

Not at all	A little of the time	Some of the time	A good deal of the time	Almost all of the time
☐	☐	☐	☐	☐

13 Tinnitus: The Impact of Family History

VERONICA KENNEDY AND DAFYDD STEPHENS

INTRODUCTION

Tinnitus is a commonly experienced sensation. In the United Kingdom, approximately one-third of adults report that they have experienced tinnitus (Davis, 1995). About 10% of all adults report tinnitus lasting at least 5 minutes with approximately 5% experiencing tinnitus most if not all the time. The perception of annoyance or adverse effect on quality of life attributed to tinnitus occurs to a much lesser extent. About 2.6% reported that their tinnitus was severely annoying and 6.9% felt that their tinnitus interfered with their sleep. 0.4% of the adults in that study reported that tinnitus severely affected their quality of life. Axelsson and Ringdahl (1989) reported that 14.2% of adults in a Swedish population study reported having tinnitus 'often' or 'always'. 2.4% of this population had severe intrusive tinnitus. Simple awareness of tinnitus, therefore, is not automatically associated with adverse quality of life effects.

A recent epidemiological study in the United Kingdom (Stephens et al., 2003) noted an increased prevalence in tinnitus in those individuals reporting a family history of hearing problems than in those not doing so (18.6% and 10.0% respectively). This prevalence was noted to increase with the reported severity of the psychosocial impact of tinnitus with greater annoyance reported in those individuals with a positive family history. There was a larger effect on life for those with a family history with each reported level of tinnitus, even after allowing for the degree of annoyance.

The effect of tinnitus on the quality of an individual's family life was assessed by El Refaie et al. (1999). They noted that the coping strategies of the families and the extent to which they felt restricted in their day-to-day activities involving the individual with tinnitus were affected by the perceived severity of the tinnitus. Little work appears to have been done to investigate the impact of a family history of tinnitus on an individual with tinnitus other than the epidemiological study by Stephens et al. (2003).

The genetic aspects of many illnesses including heart disease, cancers, diabetes and depression have been well documented. To a lesser, but increasing, extent, studies have looked at the psychological impact of the awareness of a family history of a number of both life-threatening and non-life-threatening illnesses. The diverse range of non-life-threatening illnesses studied include Parkinson's disease (Schrag et al., 2004), familial risk of major depression or panic disorder (Maier et al., 1993) and depression (Sullivan et al., 1996; Sobieraj et al., 1998). Those with depression and panic disorders were noted to have a higher rate of that condition within family members than did the control groups (Maier et al., 1993; Sullivan et al., 1996) with an elevated risk to relatives of developing depression (Kupfer et al., 1989). Depression was also noted to be associated with increased physical morbidity in the families of those with depression (Sobieraj et al., 1998).

Other studies have looked at the perceived impact of a family history of illness on an individual with a similar illness. Edwards et al. (1985) reported a relationship between the type of pain model to which the individual has been exposed and the individual's experience of pain as well as a gender effect with a greater impact on females. Kanazawa et al. (2004) noted that a parental history of bowel problems is a significant risk factor for development of irritable bowel syndrome and that those with such a family history showed more psychological distress than other patients. There are also papers which describe a sense of burden experienced by the family of an individual with problems. Schrag et al. (2004) explored the fears and anxiety experienced by the children of patients with Parkinson's disease. Apart from a higher perceived risk of developing a disease where there is a family history of that disease, having a friend with an illness also appears to have an impact, increasing an individual's perceived risk of developing that illness (Montgomery et al., 2003).

The aim of this present study was to explore further the suggestion proposed by Stephens et al. (2003) that there is an association between having a family history of hearing loss and an individual's emotional response to tinnitus. We also looked at the association between a family history of tinnitus and the individual's response to his/her own tinnitus. In order to exclude any national bias, as well as exploring the characteristics of different populations, this study was designed as a European multi-centre study (Cardiff-Amsterdam-Lyon). The results from the Cardiff centre are discussed here and compared with the results from the Lyon centre which are reported in the previous chapter; the data from Amsterdam are still being collected.

METHOD

PARTICIPANTS

One hundred and two consecutive adult patients attending a designated tinnitus clinic at the Welsh Hearing Institute in Cardiff were involved. The age of the participants ranged from 42 to 73 years. The mean age was 57.7 (SD = 15.7). There was a slight male predominance with 56 men (54.9%) and 46 (45.1%) women. Both new and follow-up patients took part in the study. Sixty-eight of the participants (66.7%) were new attenders at the clinic, while 34 (33.3%) were follow-up patients. The duration of tinnitus was reported by 94 of the 102 participants. The median duration reported was 5 years (interquartile range: 3–12 years).

MEASURES

We used a set of questions which sought demographic information, duration of the individual's tinnitus, the presence or absence of a family history of both hearing difficulties and tinnitus, with open-ended questions seeking the perceived impact of any reported family history. (These questions are shown in Appendix 12.1, previous chapter.)

Also included in this set were two closed questionnaires – the International Tinnitus Inventory (ITI) (Kennedy et al., 2005) and the Tinnitus Reaction Questionnaire (TRQ) (Wilson et al., 1991). The International Tinnitus Inventory was designed as a short, unifactorial and user-friendly scale of tinnitus impact based on the commonest perceived difficulties reported in open-ended questionnaires (Tyler & Baker, 1983; Sanchez & Stephens, 1997). It provides a quick assessment of the impact of tinnitus across a range of the most commonly reported tinnitus effects. Each question is phrased simply, based on the format of the International Outcome Inventory – Hearing Aids (IOI-HA) (Cox et al., 2002) and has five response choices ranging from the least favourable to most favourable impact. All items are scored in the same direction. Each item of the inventory is scored from 1 to 5, with 1 indicating great difficulty with tinnitus and 5 indicating no difficulty. Scores to the left, i.e. low scores, reflects a more intrusive perception of tinnitus. It has been shown to have a good response rate and high internal consistency, and is easy to interpret. Preliminary results indicate that it also translates well into other languages. Both the English and French versions showed similarly high Cronbach's alpha coefficients and item-total correlations. The International Tinnitus Inventory has also been translated into Dutch. (The English version of the International Tinnitus Inventory is shown in Appendix 12.1 (previous chapter) and the French translation is shown in Appendix 13.1 (this chapter).

The Tinnitus Reaction Questionnaire was used to evaluate the psychological distress attributed to an individual's tinnitus. It is a 26-item questionnaire with again five responses, all scored in the same direction but here a high score reflects a more negative psychosocial impact of tinnitus, 0 indicating no distress or difficulty and 4 difficulty or distress almost all the time. The French version of this questionnaire has been previously validated (Meric et al., 1998). These two measures show a positive correlation when the overall total scores of these two questionnaires were assessed using Kendall's tau correlations (r = 0.68, p < 0.05 (two-tailed)). This questionnaire is shown in Appendix 12.1 (previous chapter).

RESPONSE RATE

In the Cardiff arm of the study all 102 questionnaires were returned with a variable response rates for the different sections of between 76.5% and 100%.

HEARING DIFFICULTY/IMPAIRMENT

Perceived hearing difficulty was assessed by the question 'Do you have difficulty following TV programmes at a volume others find acceptable without any aid to your hearing?' with the choice of answers provided being 'none', 'slight', 'moderate' or 'severe'. This question was posed in both the Cardiff and Lyon arms of the study.

In the Cardiff arm of the study both the better ear hearing level (BEHL) and worse ear hearing level (WEHL) were assessed by taking the mean pure tone audiometric results for each ear at the frequencies 500, 1000, 2000 and 4000 Hz.

STATISTICAL ANALYSES

The distribution and inter-relationships of the different items were analysed. Since the Kolmogorov–Smirnov normality test revealed a non-normal distribution of the inventory scores for some of the individual items, Kendall's tau correlation coefficients were calculated to assess inter-item correlations. A Mann–Whitney rank sum test was used to compare the results between the groups with and without a positive family history.

The influence of demographic variables (age, gender), duration of tinnitus, hearing status, presence and impact of family history of tinnitus and/or hearing loss on the patient as reflected by the response to the open question, International Tinnitus Inventory and Tinnitus Reaction Questionnaire were assessed.

RESULTS OF CARDIFF STUDY

DESCRIPTIVE DATA

Presence of family history and reported effects

Twenty-five (24.5%) of the participants were aware of a family history of tinnitus, of whom 3 had a family history of tinnitus alone, while 71 had no known family history of tinnitus. Of those with a family history of tinnitus, 7 participants (28%) felt that this had an impact on their perception of their own tinnitus while 18 (72%) felt that there was no effect. The numbers of individuals reporting the presence or absence of a family history of tinnitus and/or hearing difficulty are outlined in Table 13.1.

Fifty-one of the participants had a known family history of hearing difficulties; 29 of these had a family history of hearing difficulties alone. Eleven (23%) of the participants with a family history of hearing difficulties felt that this family history had affected their perception of their own difficulty and 37 (77%) felt that their family history had no effect.

Twenty-two of the 102 participants reported a family history of both tinnitus and hearing difficulties. It was noted that 6 of these participants reported that the awareness of this family history had an effect on their perception of tinnitus.

Of the 75 participants with a family history of tinnitus and/or hearing difficulty, 14 outlined the effects they perceived this to have on their tinnitus. There was an even split of individuals reporting the presence of a family history of tinnitus with or without hearing impairment and those reporting the presence of a family history of hearing impairment without tinnitus. Each individual reported between one and six effects, some were positive, some negative while other reported effects were neutral or were not related to the question of the effect of a family history on the individual's tinnitus. The range of these effects is shown in Table 13.2.

Thirty-seven effects on the individual's tinnitus attributed to the presence of a family history were described, of which 20 were positive and 12 were negative. Six reported effects were not considered to be related to the effect on the individual's tinnitus. The effects as reported by each individual are listed in Table 13.3.

Table 13.1 Number of individuals with a family history

	Number of participants
Family history of tinnitus	25
Family history of tinnitus only	3
Family history of hearing difficulty	51
Family history of hearing difficulty only	29
Family history of both	22
Family history of neither	48

Table 13.2 Number of individuals reporting perceived effects of family history of tinnitus and/or hearing difficulty on the individual's tinnitus

Effects reported	Number of individuals reporting effects	Mean number of effects reported
Positive effect	8	2.4
Negative effect	6	2.2
Non-tinnitus related effect	5	1.4
TOTAL	14	2.6

Table 13.3 Reported effects on perception of tinnitus attributed to the presence of a family history of tinnitus or hearing difficulty

Individuals reporting effect	Where family history of **tinnitus**, responses to: 'Please list any ways this knowledge influenced your reaction to your own tinnitus'	Where family history of **hearing difficulty**, responses to: 'Please list any ways this knowledge influenced your reaction to your own tinnitus'
1	N 'mother has suffered for years' N/T 'learned within past few months that my brother has also suffered with tinnitus for a number of years'	P 'brother with tinnitus who had not sought help obviously took my advice'
2		P 'more relaxed about problem as can see it is not as debilitating as may have once thought'
3		N 'worry that tinnitus will lead to severe or complete deafness'
4	P 'knowledge that pitch and volume of tinnitus will vary' P 'that tinnitus will lessen/disappear of it's own accord' P 'having been advised of success of approach of focusing on something else' P 'observing that tinnitus is a condition that can be lived with' P 'not as distressed by tinnitus as other sufferers who lack family support' P 'have observed other family member living and coping with condition, thus more likely have adopted a positive attitude'	
5	P 'I could understand the symptoms as my father used to tell me about them, i.e. feeling disorientated, feeling cut off from everything (as if I am in world of my own) and not being able to join in conversations in noisy places' P 'have observed other family member living and coping with condition, thus more likely have adopted a positive attitude' P 'I now understand what he was going through'	
6	N 'it has made me more concerned and worried that it could be inherited'	N 'worried' N 'scared' N 'very concerned' N 'paranoid'

Table 13.3 *Continued*

Individuals reporting effect	Where family history of **tinnitus**, responses to: 'Please list any ways this knowledge influenced your reaction to your own tinnitus'	Where family history of **hearing difficulty**, responses to: 'Please list any ways this knowledge influenced your reaction to your own tinnitus'
7	N/T 'when flying it (tinnitus) goes!' N/T 'I am used to it, when I have my hearing aid on all day it is bad in my other ear, much better when I take my hearing aid off'	
8	N/T 'causing me to fall sideways'	
9	N 'I have seen and experienced how annoyed people can get when you have hearing problems'	N/T 'I see my aunt virtually switch off to any conversation other than one to one'
10		N/T 'learned to project my voice' P 'sensitive to loss of hearing in others' P 'aware of slight changes in my own hearing'
11		P 'made me think about my grandmother's deafness and how she coped'
12		N 'thinking it's hereditary'
13		P 'to be more understanding of mother's defective hearing'
14	N 'heard how unpleasant tinnitus could be' N 'heard of progressive course' P 'heard of other symptoms yet to come but heard of some "tricks" you can use to live with it' P 'provided a possible answer to a symptom which bothers me a great deal'	N 'it worries me because I can see myself moving in that direction'

P: Positive perceived effect   N: Negative effect   N/T: Non-tinnitus effect

Impact of family history on International Tinnitus Inventory and Tinnitus Reaction Questionnaire items

Due to the small numbers of participants reporting a family history of tinnitus alone, in order to assess the impact on the individual TRQ and ITI items, the participants were grouped into those with a family history of tinnitus and hearing difficulty and those with a family history of neither for Mann–Whitney analysis.

When the results of the questionnaires were analysed there was no significant difference noted with the overall Tinnitus Reaction Questionnaire or

Table 13.4 Comparison of the impact of a family history of tinnitus and hearing problems on the affected individual International Tinnitus Inventory items

Individual ITI items	Annoyance (item 1)	Peace of mind (item 5)	Effect on enjoyment (item 8)
Significance	0.026	0.03	0.004
Z	2.22	2.17	2.85
Mean (i) no FH	2.43	3	2.55
(ii) FH both tinnitus and hearing problem	3.1	3.77	3.27

Table 13.5 Impact of family history of tinnitus and hearing problems on affected individual Tinnitus Reaction Questionnaire items

Affected TRQ items	Drive crazy (item 11)	Enjoyment interference (item 12)	Avoidance of noise (item 20)
FH both tinnitus and hearing problems: – significance	0.02	0.046	0.024
– z	2.33	2.00	2.26
Mean (i) absent FH	1.36	1.79	1.91
(ii) FH both tinnitus and hearing problem	0.68	1.09	1.05

International Tinnitus Inventory scores and the presence or absence of a family history of tinnitus and hearing impairment.

Individual features of both the ITI and TRQ, however, related to the presence of a family history using a Mann–Whitney analysis. The impact of a family history on particular ITI items is outlined in Table 13.4. this shows that 'Annoyance', 'Peace of mind' and 'Enjoyment' were less affected by the tinnitus in those with a family history of tinnitus. There were no significant effects in those with a family history of hearing problems.

The TRQ items affected by reported family history are outlined in Table 13.5. There was a decreased tinnitus-related effect noted with those ITI items referring to 'being driven crazy', 'affecting enjoyment of life' and 'desire to avoid noise' where there was a family history of both tinnitus and hearing difficulty. The TRQ also showed a decreased impact of tinnitus in those with a family history. There were no overall effects in those with a family history of hearing difficulty alone.

Age and gender

There was no relationship between the new or follow-up status of the patients and the impact of their tinnitus in either of the groups with or without a family history of tinnitus or hearing difficulty when the overall International Tinnitus Inventory (ITI) and Tinnitus Reaction Questionnaire (TRQ) scores are examined. There was a significant negative correlation (tau = −0.24; p < 0.05) with increasing age indicating a worsening impact of tinnitus in those without a family history with ITI item 2 (hearing difficulty attributed to tinnitus). There was also a positive correlation noted with age and TRQ question 18 (interference with ability to work) (tau = 0.28; p < 0.05) in those both with and without a family history, again indicating a worsening impact of tinnitus. There was no significant gender effect.

Duration of tinnitus

The duration of tinnitus did not significantly relate to the perceived impact of tinnitus as assessed by the International Tinnitus Inventory (ITI) or the Tinnitus Reaction Questionnaire (TRQ) total scores.

When the individual items were examined, duration was noted to correlate only with item 2 (hearing difficulty attributed to tinnitus) of the ITI (tau = −0.23; p < 0.05) in those with no family history of hearing loss or tinnitus indicating that, for this group, the effect of tinnitus on the perception of hearing ability is greater the longer the tinnitus has been present. There was no significant correlation noted with any of the individual TRQ items, nor was there a significant difference in the reported duration of tinnitus between those individuals with or without a family history of tinnitus or hearing difficulty.

There was no significant difference in the reported impact of tinnitus as noted by the results of these questionnaires between those individuals presenting for the first time with tinnitus or attending for follow-up visits post-treatment.

Severity of hearing difficulty

In the Cardiff arm of this European study, hearing problems were assessed subjectively, as in the Lyon study, according to a perceived difficulty in listening to TV and also objectively, according to audiometric thresholds. These results were then compared both with each other and with the tinnitus measures. There was good spread of self-reported hearing difficulties across the different levels of severity; this distribution is shown in Table 13.6.

The perceived difficulty in listening to television correlated significantly with the audiometric thresholds of both better ear hearing level (BEHL) and worse

Table 13.6 The distribution of self-reported hearing difficulties

Degree of difficulty watching television	None	Slight	Moderate	Severe
Number of participants	25	29	27	20

ear hearing level (WEHL) (tau = 0.58 and 0.59; p < 0.01). The subjective and objective hearing levels are outlined in Table 13.7.

There was no relationship between the presence or absence of a family history and better ear hearing levels but there were increased worse ear hearing levels where there was no family history. When the impact of hearing level, both self-reported and audiometric thresholds, on the results of the questionnaire was analysed, perceived TV difficulty negatively correlated with the total ITI score (tau = −0.2; p < 0.05), indicating a worse impact attributed to tinnitus in the presence of increasing hearing difficulty. The effect of hearing difficulty on the individual items of the ITI is shown in Table 13.8.

There was no significant correlation of hearing difficulty with the total TRQ score. The affected individual TRQ items are shown in Table 13.9 showing an

Table 13.7 Relationship between the subjective perception of hearing difficulties and the audiometric thresholds

Degree of difficulty watching television	None	Slight	Moderate	Severe
Better ear hearing level – mean	12.8 dB	20 dB	28.5 dB	48.9 dB
(standard deviation):	(10.7 dB)	(9.9 dB)	(10.3 dB)	(19.7 dB)
Worse ear hearing level – mean	20.4 dB	26.6 dB	35.5 dB	66.1 dB
(standard deviation):	(20.9 dB)	(12.8 dB)	(11.8 dB)	(25.3 dB)

Table 13.8 Relationship between ITI items and perceived TV difficulty (Kendall's tau at p < 0.01 level (**) and p < 0.05 level (*) (two-tailed)

ITI items:	Annoyance (item 1)	Effect on hearing (item 2)	Effect on health (item 3)	Effect on sleep (item 4)	Peace of mind (item 5)	Effect on others (item 6)	Effect on activities (item 7)	Effect on enjoyment (item 8)
Perceived TV difficulty	NS	−0.44**	NS	NS	NS	−0.28**	−0.19*	NS

Table 13.9 Relationship between perceived TV difficulty and TRQ items affected (Kendall's tau at p < 0.05 level (*) (two-tailed))

TRQ items	Unhappy (item 1)	Irritable (item 3)	Enjoyment of life interference (item 12)	Avoid social situations (item 21)
Perceived TV difficulty	0.17*	0.17*	0.18*	0.22*

increased difficulty with social interaction and effect on mood where there was a perceived hearing difficulty.

DISCUSSION

The effect of tinnitus may vary with each individual as may coping styles. The aim of this study was to determine whether any trends could be seen within different specific groups – those with a family history of tinnitus, of hearing difficulty or of both. As with many studies on tinnitus there is a selection bias as it involves individuals who have problems with their tinnitus rather than those many individuals who do not seek help for their tinnitus. Similarly an unreported family history does not exclude its presence but, rather, may reflect a lack of awareness of such a family history. The ability of an individual to adjust to tinnitus may be related to his/her own coping style but may also be influenced by how others around him/her are seen to cope with tinnitus. The effectiveness (or ineffectiveness) of the adopted coping style may be related to the perceived severity of tinnitus and the associated emotional distress (Dudd & Pugh, 1996). Tinnitus may also impact on the quality of family life of an individual (El Refaie et al., 1999) depending on the coping strategies of the family. As an awareness of a family history may impact on an individual's perception of his/her own tinnitus, we wanted to investigate whether such awareness would have a similar impact across different population groups. Sociocultural factors have been shown to impact on the perception of illness and the perceived quality of life (Levenstein et al., 2001; Morton, 2003).

The Cardiff study involved consecutive patients attending a specific tinnitus clinic having been referred by their primary care practitioners, ENT or other specialties because of tinnitus. The Lyon study targeted a self-selected patient group, recruiting participants via the website of 'France Acouphènes' (French tinnitus association) and meetings of tinnitus or hard of hearing patients' groups. There was a difference in the demographics of the study population in both studies. The Cardiff population was older (mean 57.7 years + 15.7) with a slight male preponderance (54.9%); the mean age of the Lyon population was 47.1 years (standard deviation: 14.1), 64.3% were male. The number of participants reporting a family history in both arms of the study is

Table 13.10 Number of participants reporting a family history

	Cardiff participants	Lyon participants
Family history of either tinnitus or hearing difficulty	54 (52.9%)	235 (45.4%)
Family history of tinnitus only	3 (2.9%)	41 (8%)
Family history of hearing difficulty	29 (28.4%)	114 (22%)
Family history of both together	22 (21.6%)	80 (15.4%)
Family history of neither	48 (47%)	283 (54.6%)

outlined in Table 13.10. In the Cardiff arm of the study 54 of the 102 participants (52.9%) were aware of a family history of tinnitus and/or hearing difficulty. Of these, 3 participants (2.9%) were aware of a family history of tinnitus alone, 51 (50%) of hearing impairment and 22 (21.6%) of both. In the Lyon arm of the study 235 of the 518 participants (45.4%) reported a family history of hearing impairment and/or tinnitus. 114 (22%) reported a family history of hearing impairment, 41(8%) reported a family history of tinnitus and 80 (15.4%) reported a family history of both. The overall difference between the groupings for the two studies was significant ($\chi^2 = 8.79$; 3 df; p = 0.032). This difference related specifically to the small number of patients in the Cardiff group reporting a family history of tinnitus but not of hearing problems. Such a difference in the reported family history may be related to awareness rather than true presence of a family history.

The overall mean duration of tinnitus was similar in both groups (8.7 ± 0.9 years in the Cardiff population and 8.0 ± 0.4 years in the total Lyon population). However, when the presence of a family history was considered, an effect on reported duration was noted in the Lyon study: the duration was reported as 4.95 ± 0.8 years in those aware of a family history of tinnitus, 9.4 ± 1.0 in those with a family history of hearing difficulty and 7.8 ± 0.9 years in those aware of a family history of both tinnitus and hearing difficulty. There was no significant difference in the Cardiff population when the presence of a family history was considered. It is not certain whether this difference is due to the difference in sample size or to the selection process, or whether it reflects cultural differences.

When the participants were asked to volunteer the effect which the presence of a family history of tinnitus, with or without hearing impairment, had on their perception of tinnitus, a difference was noted between both centres with more negative results reported in the Lyon group. Of the 121 participants who reported a family history, 10.2% felt it had a negative impact on their perception of tinnitus while 8.9% felt it had a positive effect. In the Cardiff population, of the 54 participants reporting a family history of tinnitus with or without hearing impairment, 10.7% report a positive impact of this on their perception of their tinnitus while 6.7% report negative effects.

The attitudes of role models can impact on an individual's attitude to problems. Lockwood et al. (2005) explored the cultural effect of role models and the preferential motivation of positive or negative role models depending on the culture. In our study the way in which the affected family member portrayed their experience of tinnitus seemed to be associated with either a positive or a negative attitude to the individual's own tinnitus. The positive effects of a family history were mainly related to positive coping strategies of the affected family member and therefore a greater acceptance by the individual of his/her own tinnitus. These also included an increased empathy with and tolerance of others with problems. The negative effects tended to be related to the emotional and stressful perception of tinnitus and the perceived association with hearing-related difficulties. The increased negative effects in the Lyon population may reflect the self-selection process among members of a self-help group and the nature of the target population rather than the general French population.

We also looked at whether the presence of a family history had on an effect on the perception of tinnitus of which the individual was unaware. Specific effects of tinnitus were assessed using the closed questionnaires, the International Tinnitus Inventory to look at the degree of impact of the commonest reported range of problems and the Tinnitus Reaction Questionnaire to look at the emotional and psychological impact of tinnitus. A difference was noted between the two centres. In the Cardiff population no difference was noted between the total scores for ITI or TRQ in the groups with or without a family history. There was, however, a reduced impact of tinnitus noted in those items related to annoyance and enjoyment in both measures where there was a family history. In the Lyon study a lower total TRQ score was seen in the group with a family history of hearing difficulties indicating a lower reaction to tinnitus in this group. (There was no significant correlation of a family history of tinnitus with any of the individual components of the TRQ.) The total ITI score, however, was lower in the groups with any family history. (With ITI a lower score indicates a greater severity of those problems associated with tinnitus.) This may reflect a wider range of problems attributed to tinnitus present in those with a family history in the Lyon population but with less of a negative emotional impact of the tinnitus.

When the individual TRQ items were considered, again there was a difference in the items found to be significant. In the Lyon population TRQ 3 (feeling irritable) and TRQ 4 (feeling angry) were significantly less affected in the tinnitus and overall family history groups. TRQ items 11 (driven crazy), 18 (interference with ability to work), 21 (avoidance of social situations) and 23 (interference with sleep) were also significantly less affected in the overall family history group.

When the individual ITI items were considered between the groups with and without a family history, the only significant item within the family history group overall in the Lyon study compared with the group without a family history of tinnitus or hearing difficulty was ITI item 4 (effect on sleep). There was no significant difference in the tinnitus effect on sleep between the groups with or without a family history in the Cardiff population. When the responses from each of the different family history groups in Lyon were analysed, other individual items were noted to be significant. ITI items 6 (effect on others) and 7 (affect activities) were significantly less affected in the groups with either or both a family history of tinnitus or hearing difficulty, while ITI item 8 (effect on enjoyment of life) was significantly only in those with a family history of hearing difficulty. The duration of tinnitus was related to a larger effect of tinnitus on hearing (ITI item 2) in those with a reported family history of hearing impairment and/or tinnitus. However, the duration of tinnitus positively correlated with the sleep item (ITI item 4) and peace of mind item (ITI item 5) of the International Tinnitus Inventory, with those with a longer duration reporting less effect.

Interestingly the items differing between groups in the Cardiff population were not the same. In this population ITI items 1 (annoyance), 5 (peace of mind) and 8 (effect on enjoyment of life) showed a significantly smaller effect in those with a family history of tinnitus. The only item which correlated with duration in the Cardiff group was ITI item 2 (hearing difficulty).

It is difficult to say why the response to tinnitus is so different in the two tinnitus groups. There may be a cultural effect involved. However, it is more likely due to the nature of the groups recruited, whether the individual goes through a referral process to be assessed or seeks help through more informal means. It may be that the nature and severity of the perceived effect of tinnitus determines where an individual seeks help.

In the Lyon group it was noted that, in those individuals without a family history, the older an individual and the longer the reported duration of tinnitus the less it affected sleep and peace of mind, whereas age was not an influential factor in those with a family history. While there was no difference in the age of the participants across the different groups, there was a difference noted in the effect of tinnitus with age between the groups with and without a family history in the Lyon arm of the study. Age was noted to positively correlate with annoyance (ITI 1) and effect on hearing (ITI 2) in both those with and without a family history, i.e. it was associated with a reduced impact. A negative correlation, i.e. reduced impact, was also noted between age and the TRQ total score ($r = 0.22; p = 0.0001$) in those with a family history. A positive correlation was noted with age and tinnitus-related effect on sleep (ITI 4) and peace of mind (ITI 5) in those without a family history. In the Cardiff group there was a negative correlation with age and TRQ 18 (interference with ability to work) in all the groups.

When the hearing-related effect of tinnitus was assessed across family groups, the perceived severity of hearing difficulty negatively correlated with the International Tinnitus Inventory total score in both those with and those without a family history in both the Cardiff and Lyon arms of the study. The effect on the individual items varied. The perceived severity of hearing difficulty negatively correlated with the items concerned with annoyance (ITI 1), hearing effect (ITI 2), effect on other people (ITI 6) and effect on activities (ITI 7) in those individuals who had no reported family history. In those with a family history, the severity of hearing difficulty negatively correlated with the items concerned with effect on hearing (ITI 2), effect on health (ITI 3) and effect on other people (ITI 6). A positive correlation was noted with the severity of hearing difficulty and items of the Tinnitus Reaction Questionnaire (confused (TRQ 10), hard to concentrate (TRQ 13), work (TRQ 18), avoids noisy situations (item 20), and avoids social situations (TRQ 21)) in those with a family history. The impact of a family history on the various effects attributed to tinnitus is summarised in Tables 13.11 and 13.12 for the Cardiff and

Table 13.11 Effect of a family history on complaints attributed to tinnitus (Lyon findings)

No family history	Family history of tinnitus and/or hearing problems	Family history of tinnitus	Family history of hearing problems
Decreased interest in going out	**With increased age:** Decreased unhappiness due to tinnitus	**With increased duration:** Decreased effect on sleep Decreased thoughts about suicide	**With increased age:** Increased hearing difficulty attributed to tinnitus Decreased in disinterest in going out
Increased irritability attributed to tinnitus			
Increased frequency of annoyance Decreased enjoyment of life	Decreased avoidance of quiet situations	**With increased hearing difficulty:** Increased feeling of confusion	Decreased annoyance Decreased hopelessness about the future
Increased difficulty relaxing Increased feeling of frustration	Decreased annoyance Decreased in disinterest in going out Decreased difficulty concentrating Decreased hopelessness about the future Decreased feelings of torment, helplessness, panic Decreased overall reaction to tinnitus		**With increased duration:** Increased hearing difficulty attributed to tinnitus Increased feeling of depression
With either increased age or duration of tinnitus: Decreased effect of tinnitus on sleep Decreased effect on peace of mind Less 'driven crazy'	**With increased duration:** Increased difficulty hearing Increased difficulty listening to TV Increased effect on hearing and health **With increased hearing difficulty:** Increased avoidance of social situations		**With increased hearing difficulty:** Increased frequency of annoyance Increased effect on others Increased effect on what subject can do

Table 13.12 Effect of a family history on complaints attributed to tinnitus
(Cardiff findings)

No family history	Family history of tinnitus and hearing problems	Family history of hearing problems
Gender effect:	Less annoyance	Less feeling of being
Females: Increased desire	Less interference with	tormented
to cry	enjoyment of life	Less interference with
	Less 'driven crazy'	enjoyment of life
With increased age:	Less desire to avoid noise	Less 'driven crazy'
Increased interference	Less interference with	
with ability to work	peace of mind	
With either increased age	**With increased duration:**	
or duration of tinnitus:	Increased hearing difficulty	
Increased hearing difficulty	attributed to tinnitus	
attributed to tinnitus		

Lyon groups respectively. As the numbers in the group concerning a family history of tinnitus only are small, this group within the Cardiff population have been added to the group with a family history of both hearing difficulty and tinnitus.

CONCLUSIONS

As the prevalence of tinnitus is high, one would expect that there is also a high prevalence of family members with tinnitus. The awareness of such a family history, however, may not reflect this prevalence. Considering how common tinnitus is, it may be that, where a family member was untroubled by or coping well with tinnitus, the individual did not consider the tinnitus worthy of discussion. When we asked about the presence of a family history, we did not explore the effect of tinnitus on the affected family member. The findings of this study indicate that the positive or negative approach of that family member to tinnitus may be an influential factor in the awareness of a family history rather than the presence of tinnitus within the family and that the perception of impact of a family history on an individual's tinnitus appears to be related to how well or poorly the family member dealt with his/her own difficulty. The age of the individual and duration of tinnitus were also noted to be influential factors on the psychosocial impact of tinnitus and were associated with a decrease in tinnitus-related problems, regardless of whether there was a family history of hearing loss or tinnitus. Similarly there was an effect of hearing difficulty on the perceived impact of tinnitus with increased difficulty with tinnitus noted with worsening hearing. This impact has certainly been recognised in the literature (McKinney et al., 1999).

There was a wider range of effects reported in the Lyon population with more differences noted between those with and those without a family history. As different population groups are used in both centres, the differences in the results are more likely to reflect this rather than any cultural difference. Within both populations, however, those with a family history of tinnitus and/or hearing difficulties were seen to show a lesser adverse reaction to tinnitus but a greater impact of hearing difficulty.

REFERENCES

Axelsson A, Ringdahl A (1989) Tinnitus: a study of its prevalence and characteristics. *British Journal of Audiology* 23: 53–62.

Budd RJ, Pugh R (1996) Tinnitus coping style and its relationship to tinnitus severity and emotional distress. *Journal of Psychosomatic Research* 4: 327–35.

Coles R, Davis A, Smith P (1990) Tinnitus: its epidemiology and management: presbycusis and other age related aspects. In Jensen JH (ed) *Presbycusis and Other Age Related Aspects.* København: Jensen, pp. 377–402.

Cox RM, Alexander GC (2002) The International Outcome Inventory for Hearing Aids (IOI-HA): psychometric properties of the English version. *International Journal of Audiology* 41: 30–5.

Davis AC (1995) *Hearing in Adults.* London: Whurr.

Edwards PW, Zeichner A, Kuczmierczyk AR, Boczkowski J (1985) Familial pain models: the relationship between family history of pain and current pain experience. *Pain* 21: 379–84.

El Refaie A, Davis A, Kayan A, Baskill JL, Lovell E, Taylor A et al. (1999) Quality of family life of people who report tinnitus. Sixth International Tinnitus Seminar, Cambridge, UK, pp. 45–50.

Kanazawa M, Endo Y, Whitehead WE, Kano M, Hongo M, Fukudo S (2004) Patients and nonconsulters with irritable bowel syndrome reporting a parental history of bowel problems have more impaired psychological distress. *Digestive Diseases and Sciences* 49: 1046–53.

Kennedy V, Chéry-Croze S, Stephens D, Kramer S, Thai-Van H, Collet L (2005) Development of the International Tinnitus Inventory (ITI): a patient-directed problem questionaire. *Audiological Medicine* 3: 228–37.

Kupfer DJ, Frank E, Carpenter LL, Neiswanger K (1989) Family history in recurrent depression. *Journal of Affective Disorders* 17: 113–19.

Levenstein S, Zhiming L, Almer S, Barbosa A, Marquis P, Moser G et al. (2001) Cross-cultural variation in disease-related concerns among patients with inflammatory bowel disease. *American Journal of Gastroenterology* 96: 1822–30.

Lockwood P, Marshall TC, Sadler P (2005) Promoting success or preventing failure: cultural differences in motivation by positive and negative role models. *Personality & Social Psychology Bulletin* 31: 379–92.

McKinney CJ, Hazell JWP, Graham RL (1999) The effects of hearing loss on tinnitus. In Proceedings of the Sixth International Tinnitus Seminar, Cambridge, UK, pp. 407–14.

Maier W, Lichtermann D, Minges J, Oehrlein A, Franke P (1993) A controlled family study in panic disorder. *Journal of Psychiatric Research* 27(Supplement 1): 79–87.

Meric C, Gartner M, Collet L, Chery-Croze S (1998) Psychopathological profile of tinnitus sufferers: evidence concerning the relationship between tinnitus features and impact on life.' *Audiology and Neurootology* 3: 240–52.

Montgomery G, Erblich J, DiLorenzo T, Bovbjerg D (2003) Family and friends with disease: their impact on perceived risk. *Preventive Medicine* 37: 242–9.

Morton RP (2003) Studies in the quality of life of head and neck cancer patients: results of a two-year longitudinal study and a comparative cross-sectional cross-cultural survey, *Laryngoscope* 113: 1091–1103.

Sanchez L, Stephens D (1997) A tinnitus problem questionnaire in a clinic population. *Ear and Hearing* 18: 210–17.

Schrag A, Morley D, Quinn N, Jahanshahi M (2004) Impact of Parkinson's disease on patients' adolescent and adult children. *Parkinsonism and Related Disorders* 10: 391–7.

Sindhusake D, Golding M, Newall P, Rubin G, Jakobsen K, Mitchell P (2003) Risk factors for tinnitus in a population of older adults: the Blue Mountains Hearing Study. *Ear and Hearing* 24: 501–7.

Sobieraj M, Williams J, Marley J, Ryan P (1998) The impact of depression on the physical health of family members. *British Journal of General Practice* 48(435): 1653–5.

Stephens D, Lewis P, Davis A (2003) The influence of a perceived family history of hearing difficulties in an epidemiological study of hearing problems. *Audiological Medicine* 1: 228–31.

Sullivan PF, Wells JE, Joyce PR, Bushnell JA, Mulder RT, Oakley-Browne MA (1996) Family history of depression in clinic and community samples. *Journal of Affective Disorders* 40: 159–68.

Tyler R, Baker L (1983) Difficulties experienced by tinnitus sufferers. *Journal of Speech and Hearing Disorders* 48: 150–4.

Wilson PH, Henry JL, Bowen M, Haralambous G (1991) Tinnitus Reaction Questionnaire: psychometric properties of a measure of distress associated with tinnitus. *Journal of Speech and Hearing Research* 34: 197–201.

APPENDIX 13.1

INTERNATIONAL TINNITUS INVENTORY – FRENCH VERSION

1. Si vous pensez à vos acouphènes durant ces 2 dernières semaines, combien de temps êtes vous gêné(e) par vos acouphènes par jour?

tout le temps   **la plupart du temps**   **assez souvent**   **parfois**   **jamais**

☐ ☐ ☐ ☐ ☐

2. *Pensez à la situation dans laquelle il est pour vous le plus important d'entendre. Durant les 2 dernières semaines, quelle difficulté avez-vous ressenti dans cette situation à cause de vos acouphènes?*

beaucoup difficulté	**de pas mal de difficulté**	**difficulté moyenne**	**légère**	**aucune**
☐	☐	☐	☐	☐

3. *Pensez-vous que vos acouphènes ont causé ou aggravé d'autres problèmes de santé?*

beaucoup	**assez**	**moyennement**	**un peu**	**pas du tout**
☐	☐	☐	☐	☐

4. *Durant les 2 dernières semaines, est-ce que vos acouphènes ont perturbé votre sommeil?*

beaucoup	**assez**	**moyennement**	**un peu**	**pas du tout**
☐	☐	☐	☐	☐

5. *Durant les 2 dernières semaines, dans quelle mesure vos acouphènes ont-ils altéré votre tranquillité d'esprit?*

beaucoup	**assez**	**moyennement**	**un peu**	**pas du tout**
☐	☐	☐	☐	☐

6. *Durant les 2 dernières semaines, pensez-vous que vos acouphènes ont perturbé votre entourage?*

beaucoup	**assez**	**moyennement**	**un peu**	**pas du tout**
☐	☐	☐	☐	☐

7. *De façon générale, quel est l'impact de vos acouphènes sur vos activités quotidiennes?*

très important	**assez important**	**moyennement important**	**peu important**	**pas important du tout**
☐	☐	☐	☐	☐

8. *Tout bien considéré, dans quelle mesure vos acouphènes ont-ils affecté votre plaisir de vivre?*

de façon très importante	**de façon assez importante**	**moyennement**	**peu**	**pas du tout**
☐	☐	☐	☐	☐

14 Psychosocial Aspects of Neurofibromatosis Type 2 Reported by Affected Individuals

**WANDA NEARY, DAFYDD STEPHENS,
RICHARD RAMSDEN AND GARETH EVANS**

INTRODUCTION

Neurofibromatosis type 2 (NF2) is a dominantly inherited genetic condition caused by a defect on chromosome 22 (Roulcau et al., 1987). It is genotypically and phenotypically distinct from neurofibromatosis type 1 (previously known as von Recklinghausen's disease), where the defect is located on chro mosome 17 (Barker et al., 1987). Approximately 50% of cases have a family history of NF2 and show clearly dominant transmission. In the remaining cases the condition arises as a result of a spontaneous mutation.

The hallmark of NF2 is the presence of bilateral vestibular Schwannomas, but meningiomas, gliomas and ependymomas are associated with the disorder. Schwannomas may occur in the spinal canal and on peripheral nerves. Total deafness is likely in most cases as a result of the bilateral vestibular Schwannomas or the surgery to remove them. In the most severely affected individuals premature death is common, but in some patients the progression of the condition is slow and the patients retain hearing into their seventies (Evans et al., 1992a).

There is a high probability of lens abnormalities in individuals with NF2, and slit-lamp examination of the lenses through dilated pupils may reveal presenile lenticular opacities and cortical opacities. Cutaneous examination may reveal the presence of café-au-lait macules, but nearly always less than six in number, together with skin tumours.

The incidence of tumours of the central and peripheral nervous systems, together with the cutaneous and ophthalmological findings from three large studies of patients affected with NF2 (Evans et al., 1992b; Parry et al., 1994; Mautner et al., 1996), is documented in Table 14.1.

There is no published literature regarding the specific psychosocial impact of NF2 on the affected individual and family (Neary et al., 2005). Individuals

The Effects of Genetic Hearing Impairment in the Family. Edited by D. Stephens and L. Jones.
Copyright © 2006 by John Wiley & Sons, Ltd.

Table 14.1 The age at onset, frequency of tumour types and cutaneous and ocular features in NF2

	Evans et al., 1992b	Parry et al., 1994	Mautner et al., 1996
Number of cases	120	63	48
Number of families	75	32	Not stated
Isolated cases	45	17	44
Age at onset (years)	22.2	20.3	17
Meningiomas	45%	49%	58%
Spinal tumours	25.8%	67%	90%
Skin tumours	68% (of 100 cases)	67%	64%
More than 10 skin tumours	10% (of 100 cases)	Not known	Not known
Café-au-lait macules	43% (of 100 cases)	47%	42%
Cataracts	38% (of 90 cases)	81%	62%
Astrocytoma	4.1%	1.6%	15%
Ependymoma	2.5%	3.2%	6%
Optic sheath meningioma	4.1%	4.8%	8%

affected with NF2 may be expected to experience an impact on their lives as a result of difficulties in four major areas, hearing impairment, facial disfigurement, loss of mobility and loss of vision. Deafness may or may not be aidable, and an increasing number of NF2 patients are being offered auditory brainstem implants (ABIs) at the time of tumour removal. A small number are suitable for cochlear implantation. Cosmetic effects may result from facial paralysis after vestibular Schwannoma surgery, from cutaneous tumours or from orbital tumours. Mobility may be impaired as a result of bilateral loss of vestibular function, the effects of spinal tumours, or the consequences of peripheral neuropathy. Peripheral neuropathy is a well recognised feature of NF2, although it is often misdiagnosed as poliomyelitis in childhood (Evans et al., 1999). Vision may be affected by orbital tumours, cataracts and amblyopia from oculomotor neuropathy and as a result of damage to the facial and trigeminal nerves, usually from surgery.

The diagnosis of NF2 may be expected to impact not only on the patient, but also on their partner and family. The effects of clear, informed and comprehensive genetic counselling need to be considered, together with the additional support which may be received from specific voluntary organisations.

In order to address the deficit in information regarding the psychosocial aspects of NF2, we carried out a pilot study using an open-ended questionnaire for the patient and a separate open-ended questionnaire for the significant other. The advantage of the open-ended questionnaire is that it allows individuals to volunteer problems themselves, and is therefore likely to be more representative of what the individuals are actually experiencing (Barcham & Stephens, 1980; Bateman et al., 2000; Bem et al., 2004).

Within this chapter we discuss the findings when such a questionnaire was administered to affected individuals, and the next chapter reports the results obtained from significant others.

METHODS

Ethical approval for the study to proceed was obtained from the North Manchester Local Research Ethics Committee in July 2003, and the study commenced in August 2003. Home visiting of the patients was completed by the end of April 2004.

SUBJECTS

Twenty-two adult individuals affected with NF2, including seven patients who had participated in a previous audiological and genetic study (Neary et al., 1993), were invited to take part. Fifteen subjects consecutively attending the NF2 Clinic at Manchester Royal Infirmary were asked to participate. Two patients declined to take part. The Multidisciplinary NF2 Clinic at the Manchester Royal Infirmary, was set up along the lines recommended by Evans et al. (1993, 2005). The team members include a neuro-otologist, a neurosurgeon, a geneticist, a neuroradiologist, an ophthalmologist, an audiologist and an NF2 support worker. The clinic receives referrals from all over the United Kingdom (UK). Patients have often undergone multiple previous operations at other institutions, and may present with many difficulties. The Manchester Royal Infirmary is the UK centre for the insertion of ABIs.

Nineteen patients were visited at home, where they completed a three-page open-ended questionnaire. One patient returned the questionnaire in the post. The open-ended questionnaire sought to define the effects of NF2 on the patient's life. The patients were not selected on the basis of the severity of their condition and included individuals with a full range of manifestations of the disorder. The patients included those diagnosed by genetic methods because of a family history of NF2 and who were currently asymptomatic as well as those with total hearing loss, facial palsy, visual impairment and severe mobility and balance problems. These patients were broadly representative of the patients seen in the Manchester Multidisciplinary NF2 Clinic.

QUESTIONNAIRES

The questionnaire used is shown in Appendix 14.1. When the patient and significant other had completed the questionnaires, one of the authors (WN) conducted a semi-structured interview, probing into detailed aspects of NF2. The results of these interviews will be presented elsewhere.

ANALYSIS OF OPEN-ENDED QUESTIONNAIRES

The responses were categorised by the researcher (WN), and then independently by two senior researchers, who are experienced in the analysis of open-ended questionnaires. The conclusions of all three researchers were compared, and the final categorisation was decided upon by the most senior member of the team.

RESULTS

Twenty patients affected with NF2 consented to complete an open-ended questionnaire. There were 9 males in the study, and 11 females. The average age at diagnosis of NF2 was 36 years (range 12–52 years). The average age at the time of the study was 46 years (range 23–57 years). There was a family history of NF2 in a previous generation or in a sibling in 5 patients. Six patients presented as the first family member to be diagnosed. Subsequent evaluation of their families identified further affected members. Five patients had undergone insertion of an ABI. This included one patient who had undergone insertion, but not activation of the device. This general information regarding the study population is shown in Table 14.2.

QUESTION 1

The first question on the patient questionnaire asked '*What effects has having NF2 had on your life?*' Not every patient responded to the question. Forty-eight responses were received from 18 patients. The responses were designated positive, negative or neutral. Five *positive* responses were recorded from five separate patients. One response reported that 'It had not stopped her and her husband from doing things'. Another response related to how the patient felt that after surgery, when she had lost all her hearing, she felt emotionally relieved and felt she could 'get on with her life'. Two responses indicated that the patients

Table 14.2 An overview of the patients included in the study

Number of NF2 patients	20
Males	9 (45%)
Females	11 (55%)
Mean age at diagnosis of NF2 (years)	36 (range 12–52)
Mean age at time of study (years)	46 (range 23–57)
Family history of NF2 in previous generation or sibling	5 (25%)
Family history of NF2 now, but patient was first family member to be diagnosed	6 (30%)
Number of patients with ABIs (including one inserted but not activated)	5 (25%)

thought that having NF2 had made them more caring and understanding people. The fifth response indicated that the patient felt that she was very positive in her outlook and so made sure that NF2 did not affect her life too much.

Forty-three *negative* responses were recorded. Six patients recorded negative responses related to their deafness and five patients to balance and mobility problems. Five patients also indicated negative responses related to the genetic nature of NF2, with the 50% risk of transmission of the condition to their children. Others reported a range of effects on their education, employment and a variety of activities. Several of the patients gave more than one response to the question. Table 14.3 shows the responses reported by two or more patients.

Seven individual negative responses were given. One patient described the need for home adaptations. A further patient reported reduced ambition in life. One patient noted problems with vision. A further patient described how she missed music, both listening to music and playing music. She also missed not chatting on the phone. A further patient documented the need to learn to live a new life because of NF2. This patient also described the need for ongoing hospital visits to monitor her condition.

QUESTION 2

The next question asked '*Which of the following is the biggest problem: hearing difficulties, facial weakness, mobility problems, visual difficulties or others?*' All

Table 14.3 Negative responses made by two or more NF2 patients to question 1, '*What effects has having NF2 had on your life?*' (18 out of 20 patients answered this question)

Response	Number of responses	Number of patients responding (percentage of those who responded to this question)
Problems because of deafness	6	6 (33%)
Problems because of balance and mobility	5	5 (28%)
Problems because of genetic nature of NF2	5	5 (28%)
Had to give up further education or work because of NF2	4	4 (22%)
Limitations to hobbies and social life	4	4 (22%)
Psychological problems	3	3 (17%)
Fear of the unknown	3	3 (17%)
Difficulties with driving, or having to give up driving	2	2 (11%)
Communication problems	2	2 (11%)
Loss of independence	2	2 (11%)

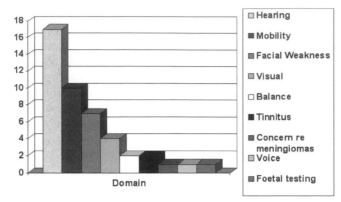

Figure 14.1 Biggest problems listed (n).

20 patients answered this question. Some patients noted that more than one area was causing them equal difficulties.

Overall, the largest number of patients (17) described hearing difficulties as being the biggest problem in NF2. Ten patients indicated that mobility problems were the most significant. Seven patients described facial weakness. Four patients described visual difficulties as being the most problematic. One patient poignantly described the emotional difficulties for himself and his wife during the testing of their foetuses for NF2 mutations. These and the other responses to question 2 are shown in Figure 14.1.

QUESTION 2(a)

The next question asked '*How has having hearing difficulties, if any, affected your life?*' Fifty-one responses were received from the 20 patients with NF2. Thirty-three of the responses were given by at least two patients. The remaining 18 responses were individual responses.

Hearing difficulties were reported to be making communication, both socially and at work, more difficult by eight patients, and five patients specified that communication in their marriage and within their family was becoming progressively more difficult. Others reported a range of activity limitations and psychological effects, including isolation and loss of confidence. Two patients stated that they might not respond to people, as they had not heard them speaking. The responses to this question documented by two or more patients are presented in Table 14.4.

There were 18 individual responses to question 2(a) from 12 individual subjects These are shown in Table 14.5. One asymptomatic patient said that he had concerns for the future.

Table 14.4 Responses received from NF2 patients to question 2(a), *'How has having hearing difficulties, if any, affected your life?'* and reported by two or more patients

Effect	Number of responses	Number of patients responding	Percentage of series
Communication socially and at work progressively difficult	8	8	40%
Communication in marriage and family progressively difficult	5	5	25%
Difficulties with listening in crowded places	4	4	20%
Loss of confidence	3	3	15%
Loss of music/film sound track/ nature sounds – upsetting	3	3	15%
Feeling left out of conversation and social life	2	2	10%
Mishearing – leading to misunderstandings	2	2	10%
Difficulties with everyday dealings	2	2	10%
May not respond as do not hear	2	2	10%
Cannot localise sounds	2	2	10%

Table 14.5 Individual responses received from NF2 patients to question 2(a), *'How has having hearing difficulties, if any, affected your life?'* Responses bracketed together came from the same individual

Individual response

1. As hearing loss has progressed, tend to withdraw myself from conversations involving more than one person
2. Forced to give up work because of deafness
{ 3. Felt isolated, lonely and angry
4. Lost confidence
5. Stopped visiting friends
6. Improvement after learning BSL
{ 7. Impossible to understand lectures
8. Cannot ask questions
9. Difficulty with using telephone
10. Feeling depressed at knowledge of complete deafness in future
11. Have to be more proactive if involved in conversations
{ 12. No 'new' music
13. Listening hard is exhausting
14. Feeling vulnerable – can't hear smoke alarm
15. Can't hear traffic
16. Concern for future
{ 17. Not able to use telephone
18. Have to have someone with you, even when it is personal

QUESTION 2(b)

This question asked '*How has your facial weakness, if any, affected your life?*' Six of the 20 patients had no facial weakness. Twenty-five responses were obtained from 14 patients with facial weakness. Three patients, with varying degrees of facial weakness, reported that it was not a big problem to them. The remainder of the responses fell into five categories; appearance, difficulties with eating and dental hygiene, eye problems, impact on speech and psychological impact. The breakdown of these responses is shown in Table 14.6.

QUESTION 2(c)

This asked '*How have your mobility problems, if any, affected your life?*' Thirty-seven responses were received from 19 patients. Seven patients reported non-specific problems with their balance. Six patients said that they needed someone to lean on, or a stick when outside of the house. These and the other responses reported by more than one respondent are shown in Table 14.7.

Eleven specific responses to question 2(c) by eight patients are shown in Table 14.8.

Table 14.6 Responses received from NF2 patients to question 2 (b), '*How has your facial weakness, if any, affected your life?*' Number affected with facial weakness = 14. Twenty-five responses were obtained

Not a big problem	Problem with appearance	Problem with eating and dental hygiene	Problem with eye	Impact on speech	Psychological impact
N = 3	N = 10	N = 6	N = 4	N = 1	N = 1
	'Embarrassment'	Food tends to get trapped.	Eye dries out quickly	Slurred speech with face cold	Less confident when meeting people for the first time
	'Conscious of facial weakness'				
	'Children often stare – not nice'	Oral problems	Painful eye in windy conditions		
	'People think I'm stupid'	Difficulty eating with mouth shut			
	'I dislike cameras'		Sore eye		
	'Has not enhanced my appearance as I approach 60!'	'I cannot chew on the affected side'	Unable to close eye		
	'Don't like looking in mirrors'				
	'Miss being able to smile at people'	'Can't eat properly on one side'			
	'I'm very upset at not having a proper smile'	Dental problems because of difficulties with cleaning teeth			
	'Made me more self-conscious of my appearance'				

Table 14.7 Responses received from NF2 patients to question 2(c), *'How have your mobility problems, if any, affected your life?'* Responses received from more than two patients. Nineteen patients answered this question

Response	Number of responses	Number of patients responding
Problems with balance	7	7 (37%)
Need someone to lean on or a stick when outside of the house	6	6 (31%)
Mobility problems	4	4 (21%)
People might think I'm drunk	3	3 (16%)
Can't go out in the dark or if it's been snowing	3	3 (16%)
Falls with injury	2	2 (11%)

Table 14.8 Specific individual responses received from NF2 patients to question 2(c), *'How have your mobility problems, if any, affected your life?'* Nineteen patients answered the question. Responses bracketed together came from the same individual

Response
Not being able to go out on my own
My husband worried when I was out alone
Loss of confidence
⌠Can't jog
⌡Can swim and go to the gym
⌠Feel vertiginous on occasions
⌡Feel dizzy on occasions
⌠Movement around the house is the most difficult in every conceivable way
⌡Have to plan journeys
Care needed in wind and rain
No problems now – concern for the future

QUESTION 2(d)

Question 2(d) on the patient questionnaire asked *'How have your visual difficulties, if any affected your life?'* Sixteen out of the 20 patients answered this question. Six patients reported that they did not have any visual difficulties. A further 6 patients said that they were affected with a painful, dry eye and experienced problems outside in the wind. The various responses to question 2(d) on the patient questionnaire are shown in Table 14.9.

QUESTION 3

The next question asked *'Are there any positive effects that the diagnosis has had on your life?'* Seventeen patients with NF2 answered this question. Two of them stated that there were no positive effects. The positive responses

Table 14.9 Responses received from NF2 patients to question 2(d), '*How have your visual difficulties, if any, affected your life?*' Responses received from 16 patients

Response	Number of responses	Number of patients responding
Painful dry eye, problems outside in wind	6	6 (38%)
Problems with judging distances	2	2 (13%)
Blurred vision with lacrilube	2	2 (13%)
'I can't drive at night'	1	1 (6%)
'It's painful to watch TV with subtitles for long'	1	1 (6%)
'I can't read for long'	1	1 (6%)
Concern for the future	1	1 (6%)

Table 14.10 Responses received from 17 patients with NF2 to question 3, '*Are there any positive effects that the diagnosis of NF2 has had on your life?*'

Effect	Number of responses	Number of patients responding
'It has made me more considerate, caring and sensitive towards other people'	5	5 (29%)
'Has made me more deaf and disability aware'	3	3 (18%)
'It has drawn us closer together'	2	2 (12%)
'Gained confidence from having a diagnosis'	2	2 (12%)
'It has helped me widen my circle of friends'	2	2 (12%)

Table 14.11 Individual positive responses received from patients with NF2 to question 3, '*Are there any positive effects that the diagnosis has had on your life?*' Responses bracketed together came from the same individual

Effect
'Having to deal with the effects has helped me to cope with the difficulties'
'I enjoy a sleep in the afternoon'
['I learned BSL with my husband and family' / 'I made new friends in the Deaf congregation' / 'I am lucky to have NF2 mildly']
['I find that other people show so much kindness and patience towards me' / 'I want to achieve so much in my personal life to show everyone that having a disability doesn't mean your life stops']
'I have been able to ensure that for my family this ends with me. My children do not have NF2, and I find that comforting, knowing that they have a chance at a normal life'

where two or more patients reported the same positive effects are shown in Table 14.10.

Eight individual responses were received from five patients with NF2 to question 3. These responses to question 3 in the patient questionnaire are shown in Table 14.11. Where more than one response came from the same individual, they are bracketed together.

QUESTION 4

The fourth question on the patient questionnaire asked '*Are there any other effects that NF2 has had on your life?*' Thirty-eight responses were received from 19 patients. The responses were designated positive, negative and neutral. Six positive responses were received from 5 patients. Twenty-seven negative responses were given by 14 patients, as well as five neutral responses by 5 patients. The positive responses to question 4 are shown in Table 14.12. Where responses came from the same individual, they are bracketed together.

Twenty-seven negative responses to question 4 were received from 14 patients. Responses were subdivided into psychological effects, effects on personal relationships and marriage, general effects, effects related to hearing loss, effects related to work and employment and effects related to appearance. These are shown in Figure 14.2.

The seven responses related to psychological effects and the six responses related to personal relationships and marriage are shown in Table 14.13.

Five negative responses were related to general effects. One patient described slight imbalance when he was tired or stressed. A further patient stated that he had gone through all the effects of NF2 apart from depression. Another was affected with weakness in the right arm and hand, and noted that her writing was awful on some occasions. One patient noticed pain at the site of her Schwannomas, and had to take analgesics. The fifth patient noticed tiredness.

Four negative responses were specifically related to loss of hearing. One patient described the difficulties in trying to listen to music and current affairs on the radio. A further patient underlined the danger of hearing loss – he had stepped out in front of a bus as he had not heard it. Another patient commented that hearing loss, specifically, can be limiting. A further patient reported his sadness in being unable to hear his children's voices.

Table 14.12 Positive responses recorded by five NF2 patients to question 4, '*Are there any other effects that NF2 has had on your life?*' Responses bracketed together came from the same individual

Response
(6 responses from total number of 38 responses)

['Being deafened made me think more of others and appreciate more my quality of
  life'
'I learned I could do things I never thought possible'
'The way in which I've managed to deal with the problems it has caused me has
  meant I have gained a great deal of respect from my friends/colleagues'
'I have retired from work which I feel has been a great benefit for me – not having
  to get up rushing around on a morning to go to a stressful job'
'I feel fortunate that I could have a very more severe version or progression I
  work, I continue to study, and I am well-supported'
'Learned that there is so much else in life that we take for granted'

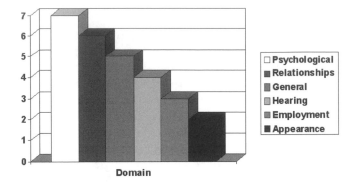

Domain

Figure 14.2 Grouping of negative responses to question 4 (n).

Table 14.13 Negative responses relating to psychological effects and effects on personal relationships and marriage recorded by NF2 patients to question 4, '*Are there any other effects that NF2 has had on your life?*' Responses bracketed together came from the same individual

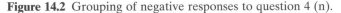

Response	Number of responses
Psychological effects	
Depression and anxiety	1
Panic attacks	2
⌠'The illness takes up so much of our time'	1
⌡'The illness never goes away'	1
Loss of independence	1
Loneliness and isolation	1
Personal relationships and marriage	
Strain on marital partner and family because of diagnosis	2
Concerns because of inherited nature of NF2	1
Did not marry, nor have children because of NF2	1
Guilt because of transmitting condition to children	1
Worry about how children will cope with a deaf father	1

Three negative effects were related to work and employment. One patient said that he had been less ambitious in his career because of being affected with NF2. Another patient stated that he was unable to obtain employment because of his NF2. A further patient, who was asymptomatic, voiced his insecurity about the future and the need for financial planning.

Two further negative effects were related to appearance. One patient stated that in earlier life he found difficulties in making relationships with the opposite sex. A further patient said that people thought that she had suffered from a stroke.

Five neutral responses were made to question 4. One patient reported surgery for other Schwannomas. Another patient said that she was looking after her mother who was quite severely affected with NF2. A further patient said that she had been fitted with a hearing aid on her better ear, and she needed a loop system to be fitted in her home. Another patient said that people were unaware of NF2 as it is such a rare condition, and could be suspicious when she started to describe her problems. The fifth patient said that 'Early diagnosis is good for family planning, but it leaves you knowing for years that you have a ticking time bomb – it's a double-edged sword'.

QUESTION 5

This asked '*If you have had a brainstem implant (ABI), how do you think that it has helped?*' Five patients had undergone the insertion of an ABI, including one patient in whom the device had been inserted but not activated. Fifteen patients had not undergone insertion of an ABI.

All four patients answered question 5. Three patients reported benefit from their devices. The fourth patient reported that she had undergone insertion of an ABI in 1994, but unfortunately it had never worked. The four patients' comments regarding their ABIs are documented in Table 14.14.

QUESTION 6

The final question asked '*If you have a family history of NF2, do you think that this has had an effect on your reaction to it?*' Five patients had a family history of NF2. Three of these confirmed that the family history had certainly had an effect on their reaction to it. One patient said that she was more prepared. A further patient said that seeing his father dealing positively with NF2 had made him more determined not to let it alter his lifestyle. The third patient said that he is fully aware of what the condition is capable of, which is good because he is prepared, but he feels the weight of carrying this knowledge with him.

Table 14.14 Patients' responses to question 5, '*If you have had a brainstem implant (ABI), how do you think that it has helped?*' Four patients answered this question

Response
'It helps with lip-reading my partner. There are far less misunderstandings with the ABI'
'I did have one fitted in 1994 but it never worked, which is such a shame. I am therefore totally deaf'
'A lot, especially in a one to one situation. If there is a lot of background noise, it is not very useful at all'
'I had my implant in July 2003. It has completely changed my life. I wouldn't be without it. Being able to "hear" has made me feel less vulnerable and more normal again'

Table 14.15 Patients' responses to question 6, 'If you have a family history of NF2, do you think that this has had an effect on your reaction to having it?' Five patients answered this question

Response
'We learned our daughter had the defective gene of NF2. I was upset for her. Also I felt I had let her down. Now I don't worry'
'Yes, I think I was more prepared'
'Yes, seeing my father dealing positively with it has made me more determined not to let it alter my lifestyle'
'It has depressed me to learn that I have passed this disorder to at least one of my children'
'Yes – I am fully aware of what the condition is capable of which is good because you are prepared – but you feel the weight of carrying this knowledge with you'

Two patients did not comment on how knowledge of the family history had affected their own reactions to the diagnosis, but they said they were upset when their children were diagnosed with NF2. One of these patients said that when her daughter was confirmed to be affected with NF2, she was upset for her. The other patient said that it had depressed him to learn that he had passed NF2 on to at least one of his children. Patients' responses to question 6 are documented in Table 14.15.

DISCUSSION

There is no published literature regarding the psychosocial impacts of NF2 on the affected individual and their family at the present time. Bateman et al. (2000), reported on the measurements of patients' health-related quality of life, using an open-ended questionnaire, following surgery for a sporadic unilateral vestibular Schwannoma. They sent out open-ended questionnaires to 70 consecutive patients who had undergone surgery for a sporadic unilateral vestibular Schwannoma. They found that patients most commonly reported problems relating to auditory dysfunction. The next most common grouping of symptoms was vestibular dysfunction, and eye problems. Neary et al. (2005), suggested that patients affected with NF2 would have difficulties in four major areas, hearing impairment, facial disfigurement, impaired mobility and eye problems.

It was not initially appreciated that patients might report positive responses as an effect of NF2 on their lives. Five very positive responses were obtained from the twenty patients – two relating to NF2 making the patients more caring individuals, another two underlining that the condition had not prevented them from engaging in everyday activities. One response related to how the patient felt that after surgery when she lost all her hearing she felt emotionally relieved and was then able to 'get on with her life'.

In a similar open-ended study on positive experiences associated with hearing impairment, Kerr and Stephens (2000) identified the specific finding of less disturbance by unwanted noise. Kerr and Stephens also identified a number of areas similar to those found in the present study, including improved communication strategies, affinity with other deaf and disabled groups, perceived self-development, and aids to communication such as hearing aids, assistive listening devices and typing machines. They also identified the use of hearing loss to self advantage. Other areas to emerge from a structured study (Stephens & Kerr, 2003) were changes in self-perception and resignation. These authors also emphasised the fact that positive experiences had also been reported in HIV/AIDS (Folkman et al., 1997) as well as various forms of neoplastic conditions such as Hodgkin's disease (Cella & Tross, 1986).

As in the case of patients with sporadic unilateral vestibular Schwannomas described by Bateman et al. (2000), patients with NF2 reported problems because of deafness and because of difficulties with balance and mobility. Six patients (33%) reported negative responses relating to their deafness, four (22%) having to give up work or further education. Four patients (22%) pointed out the limitations to their hobbies and social life and two patients (11%) underlined their communication problems. Five patients (28%) noted problems because of balance and mobility. Unlike the situation with sporadic unilateral vestibular Schwannomas, where there are no genetic sequelae for the offspring and family, in the case of NF2 particular difficulties in this respect, because of the genetic nature of the condition, were highlighted.

Bateman et al. also reported that psychosocial morbidity was very significant in their series of patients who had undergone surgery for a sporadic unilateral vestibular Schwannoma. Thirty-four per cent of their patients reported a variety of related symptoms such as depression, anxiety and loss of confidence. The authors suggested that, for some patients, early involvement of a clinical psychologist could be useful. In the present series of NF2 patients, six patients (34%) reported psychological problems, and fear of the unknown as negative effects of NF2 on their lives. Although the point was not specifically addressed in the questionnaire, our experience in the Multidisciplinary NF2 Clinic suggests that the psychological impact of the diagnosis differs depending on whether the patient represents a new mutation, or is a member of an already diagnosed family. In the latter group there is often, as revealed by this study, a reluctant preparedness for the diagnosis. In the case of the new mutation, however, who may have presented with relatively trivial symptoms in teenage years or in early twenties, all the implications of the diagnosis both for the individual and for future generations may have a devastating effect. These individuals need considerable support.

Patients affected with NF2 were specifically asked what was their biggest problem – hearing difficulties, facial weakness, mobility problems, visual difficulties or others. Some patients felt several areas to be equally problematic. Eighty-five per cent in this series identified hearing difficulties as their biggest problem. Fifty per cent felt that mobility problems were their biggest problem. Thirty-five per cent identified facial weakness as their biggest problem. In the 'other' category, two patients (10%) felt that tinnitus was their biggest problem. Bateman et al., reported that tinnitus seemed to have a very small impact on the lives of patients with unilateral vestibular Schwannomas, being reported in 4% of their series. Two patients identified balance problems as their biggest problem and one patient poignantly described how the testing of foetuses for NF2 mutations had been his biggest problem.

Progressive hearing loss resulting in total deafness causes severe difficulties with communication. An affected person should be encouraged to attend speechreading classes as soon as it is feasible, while he/she still has hearing and may be wearing a hearing aid. Speechreading will enhance the use of an ABI, once the latter is necessary. For patients with no hearing and no ABI, a typing communicator (Lightwriter) may be recommended. Some patients and their families may decide to learn British Sign Language.

Support in the way of environmental aids (Assistive Devices) is essential, starting with an assessment of patients' particular needs in the home. Flashing light doorbells, vibrating mattress alarm clocks, television subtitles, walking sticks, Zimmer frames and wheelchairs may be required. Patients should be made aware that they can communicate by telephone if they can use text phones. A vibrating function to alert the patient to a text message can be made available.

Patients troubled with a dry eye should be reminded to use lubricating drops such as hypromellose or lacrilube on a regular basis each day. Patients wearing spectacles and having difficulty outside in the wind may be fitted with a protective side-arm to their spectacles.

The similarities in the figures relating to the areas of deafness, balance and mobility, psychosocial morbidity and tinnitus, when the present study is compared with that of Bateman et al., are noteworthy. The patients in the present study of a dominantly transmitted genetic condition report very similar problems in these areas to those described by patients with a sporadic unilateral vestibular Schwannoma. The latter condition has no genetic implications, and therefore genetic aspects are not mentioned in the study of Bateman et al. The particular difficulties because of the genetic nature of NF2 are highlighted by the patients in the present study. Despite all the negative effects described by the patients in this study, it is of note that they also described positive consequences of their condition.

The question of disfigurement following treatment for head and neck cancer and the resulting psychosocial impact was reviewed by Owen et al. (2001). They pointed out that patients might be particularly vulnerable to psychosocial problems following treatment because social interaction and emotional expression greatly depend on the structure and functional integrity of the head and neck region. In the present study of patients affected with NF2 it was of particular note that when patients were asked about the effects of NF2 on their life none of the patients mentioned facial weakness. It was only when the patients were specifically asked about facial weakness that 35% said that this was their biggest problem. When patients were asked about the ways in which their facial weakness had affected their lives they then specified full details. They reported ten negative responses related to their facial appearance, ranging from a feeling of embarrassment and self-consciousness, to being upset at being unable to smile at people and six negative responses related to problems with eating and dental hygiene. One patient reported slurred speech with a cold face and another described loss of confidence when meeting people for the first time.

The question of informing patients of the results of predictive testing in serious, and indeed lethal conditions was addressed by Wiggins et al. (1992) and by Hayes (1992). They discussed the psychological impact of such information on patients at risk of Huntington's disease, which like NF2 is a dominantly transmitted genetic condition, but which unlike NF2 invariably has a lethal outcome. Wiggins et al. concluded that predictive testing had potential benefits for the psychological health of those who receive the results that indicate either an increase or decrease in the risk of inheriting the gene for the disease.

Hayes gave a personal insight as an 'at risk' individual. She recommended that the test should be approached by all parties with the utmost caution, and should not be undertaken without safeguards. She stated that, for most individuals, an answer helps by eliminating the daily worrying and allows time for planning. She urged more open communication among medical professionals, families and voluntary organisations, which can serve as a bridge between the other two groups. In the present study, several patients had undergone presymptomatic DNA testing while asymptomatic. In fact the first positive MRI scan had more impact than the positive DNA test. Uptake of DNA presymptomatic testing in NF2 is high in both adults and 10–12-year-olds (Evans et al., 1997). Prenatal diagnosis was carried out by one patient, who wished to avoid passing on the NF2 gene mutation to his offspring. Patients with NF2 described the strain on the marital partner and family, the concerns because of the inherited nature of the condition, and the guilt because of transmitting the genetic condition.

CONCLUSIONS

NF2 is is a dominantly inherited genetic condition which has a particularly marked impact on four areas of the affected patient's life, those of hearing loss, mobility, facial disfigurement and vision. A further area identified by patients in this study is that of psychological problems and fear of the unknown. The importance of careful management and support of the patient and family by a Specialist Multdisciplinary NF2 Team cannot be overstated. An experienced otolaryngologist and neurosurgeon require to assess the optimal time for surgery. The consultant in clinical genetics is an important member of the team, explaining the transmission of the condition and the molecular genetic tests for mutations in the NF2 gene. The patient and family should be assigned an NF2 Keyworker, who sits in on the Multidisciplinary NF2 Clinic and can act as a bridge of information and ongoing support between the specialist staff and the patients and families. The patient should be given contact details of other patients with NF2, consent for release of contact details having been given by the other patients. Details of voluntary organisations, and appropriate website addresses should be made available. Follow-up of the affected patient by the Multidisciplinary Team is required on a lifelong basis.

REFERENCES

Barcham LJ, Stephens SDG (1980) The use of an open-ended problems questionnaire in auditory rehabilitation. *British Journal of Audiology* 14: 49–54.

Barker V, Wright E, Nguyen K, Cannon L, Fain P, Goldgar D et al. (1987) Gene for von Recklinghausen neurofibromatosis is in the pericentromeric region of chromosome 17. *Science* 236: 1100–2.

Bateman N, Nikolopoulos TP, Robinson K, O'Donoghue GM (2000) Impairments, disabilities, and handicaps after acoustic neuroma surgery. *Clinical Otolaryngology* 25: 62–5.

Bem C, Lee C, Dawson R, Watkinson J (2004) Is Clinical Otolaryngology publishing patient-centred research? *Clinical Otolaryngology* 29: 84–93.

Cella DF, Tross S (1986) Psychological adjustment to survival from Hodgkin's disease. *Journal of Consulting and Clinical Psychology* 54: 616–22.

Evans DGR, Baser ME, O'Reilly B, Rowe J, Gleeson M, Saeed S et al. (2005) Management of the patient and family with neurofibromatosis 2: A Consensus Conference Statement. *British Journal of Neurosurgery* 19:1 5–12.

Evans DGR, Birch JM, Ramsden RT (1999) Paediatric presentation of type 2 neurofibromatosis. *Archives of Disease in Childhood* 81: 496–9.

Evans DGR, Huson SM, Donnai D, Neary W, Blair V, Teare D et al. (1992a) A genetic study of type 2 neurofibromatosis in the United Kingdom. 1. Prevalence, mutation rate, fitness and confirmation of maternal transmission effect on severity. *Journal of Medical Genetics* 29: 841–6.

Evans DGR, Huson SM, Donnai D, Neary W, Blair V, Newton V et al. (1992b) A clinical study of type 2 neurofibromatosis. *Quarterly Journal of Medicine* 84(304): 603–18.

Evans DG, Maher ER, Macleod R, Davies DR, Crauford D (1997) Uptake of genetic testing for cancer predisposition. *Journal of Medical Genetics* 34: 746–8.

Evans DGR, Ramsden R, Huson SM, Harris R, Lye R, King TT (1993) Type 2 neurofibromatosis: the need for supraregional care? *Journal of Laryngology and Otology* 107: 401–6.

Folkman S, Moskowitz JT, Ozer EM, Park CL (1997) Positive meaningful events and coping in the context of HIV/AIDS. In B Gottlieb (ed) *Coping with Chronic Stress.* New York: Plenum Press, pp. 293–314.

Hayes CV (1992) Genetic testing for Huntington's disease – a family issue (Editorial). *New England Journal of Medicine* 327: 1449–51.

Kerr P, Stephens D (2000) Understanding is the nature and function of positive experiences in living with auditory disablement. *Scandinavian Journal of Disability Research* 2: 21–38.

Mautner VF, Lindenau M, Baser ME, Hazim W, Tatagiba M, Haase W et al. (1996) The neuroimaging and clinical spectrum of neurofibromatosis 2. *Neurosurgery* 38: 881–5.

Neary WJ, Newton VE, Vidler M, Ramsden RT, Lye RH, Dutton JEM et al. (1993) A clinical, genetic and audiological study of patients and families with bilateral acoustic neurofibromatosis. *Journal of Laryngology and Otology* 107: 6–11.

Neary WJ, Ramsden RT, Evans DGR, Baser ME (2005) Psychosocial aspects of NF2. In D Stephens, L Jones (eds) *The Impact of Genetic Hearing Impairment.* London: Whurr, pp. 201–18.

Owen C, Watkinson JC, Pracy P, Glaholm J (2001) The psychological impact of head and neck cancer (Editorial). *Clinical Otolaryngology* 26: 351–6.

Parry DM, Eldridge R, Kaiser-Kupfer MI, Bouzas EA, Pikus A, Patronas N (1994) Neurofibromatosis 2 (NF2): clinical characteristics of 63 affected individuals and clinical evidence for heterogeneity. *American Journal of Medical Genetics* 52: 450–61.

Rouleau GA, Wertelecki W, Haines JL, Hobbs WJ, Trofatter JA, Seizinger BR et al. (1987) Genetic linkage of bilateral acoustic neurofibromatosis to a DNA marker on chromosome 22. *Nature* 329: 246–8.

Stephens D, Kerr P (2003) The role of positive experiences in living with acquired hearing loss. *International Journal of Audiology* 42: S118–127.

Wiggins S, Whyte P, Huggins M, Adam S, Theilmann J, Bloch M et al. (1992) The psychological consequences of predictive testing for Huntington's disease. *New England Journal of Medicine* 327: 1401–5.

APPENDIX 14.1

QUESTIONNAIRE 1

TITLE: PSYCHOSOCIAL ASPECTS OF NEUROFIBROMATOSIS TYPE 2
PATIENT QUESTIONNAIRE

This is a confidential questionnaire to try and find out about the effects of NF2 on your daily life. We are trying to find out what is most important to you. There is no right or wrong answer to questions – we would like you to let us know as many things as you think are important. We would like you to put a star (*) by the most important things.

1. What effects has having NF2 had on your life?

2. Which of these is your biggest problem?
   - Hearing difficulties
   - Facial weakness
   - Mobility problems
   - Visual difficulties
   - Others (please list)

2a How has having hearing difficulties, if any, affected your life?

2b How has your facial weakness, if any, affected your life?

2c How have your mobility problems, if any, affected your life?

2d How have your visual difficulties, if any, affected your life?

3. Are there any POSITIVE effects that the diagnosis has had on your life?

4. Are there any other effects that NF2 have had on your life?

5. If you have had a brainstem implant (ABI), how do you think that it has helped?

6. If you have a family history of NF2, do you think this has had an effect on your reaction to having it?

Thank you for your help with this. We hope it will be useful in improving the service to patients with NF2.

15 Psychosocial Aspects of Neurofibromatosis Type 2 Reported by Relatives and Significant Others

**WANDA NEARY, DAFYDD STEPHENS,
RICHARD RAMSDEN AND GARETH EVANS**

INTRODUCTION

Neurofibromatosis type 2 (NF2) is a dominantly inherited genetic condition caused by a defect on chromosome 22 (Rouleau et al., 1987). It is phenotypically and genotypically distinct from NF1, previously known as von Recklinghausen's disease, which is caused by a defect on chromosome 17 (Barker et al., 1987). The hallmark of NF2 is the presence of bilateral vestibular Schwannomas, but other tumours of the central and peripheral nervous systems are associated with the disorder. Total deafness is likely in most cases as a result of the bilateral vestibular Schwannomas or the surgery to remove them. The incidence of tumours of the central and peripheral nervous systems, together with the cutaneous and ophthalmological findings from three large studies of patients affected with NF2 (Evans et al., 1992; Parry et al., 1994; Mautner et al., 1996) is shown in Table 14.1 (Chapter 14).

There is no published literature regarding the psychosocial impact of NF2 on the relatives of affected patients (Neary et al., 2005). In order to address this deficit in information, we carried out a study using an open-ended questionnaire to be completed by the NF2 patient's significant other. The advantage of the open-ended questionnaire is that it allows individuals to volunteer problems themselves, and is therefore more likely to be representative of what the individuals are actually experiencing (Barcham & Stephens, 1980).

This approach to the impact of their partner's hearing loss has previously been used in significant others of patients with hearing problems by Stephens et al. (1995). Meehan et al. (2002) reported on the use of an open-ended questionnaire with parents of hearing-impaired teenagers. In addition, Stephens

The Effects of Genetic Hearing Impairment in the Family. Edited by D. Stephens and L. Jones.
Copyright © 2006 by John Wiley & Sons, Ltd.

et al. (2004) used it to explore the positive experiences reported by significant others of patients with hearing impairments.

METHODS

Twenty adult individuals affected with NF2 consented to take part in the study. The patients were not selected on the basis of the severity of their condition and included individuals with a full range of manifestations of the disorder. Thus they included a range from those diagnosed by genetic methods because of a family history of NF2 and presently asymptomatic, to those with total hearing loss, facial palsy, visual impairment and severe mobility and balance problems. These patients were broadly representative of the patients seen in the Manchester Multidisciplinary NF2 Clinic. Nineteen patients were visited at home, where they completed a three-page open-ended questionnaire. One patient returned the questionnaire in the post.

The patient's partner/significant other was invited to complete a separate two-page open-ended questionnaire regarding the effects of the diagnosis of NF2 on themselves.

QUESTIONNAIRE

The open-ended questionnaire completed by the partner/significant other is shown in Appendix 15.1. It comprised two questions, enquiring about life effects and positive effects.

Analysis of open-ended questionnaire

The responses were categorised by the researcher (WN) and independently by a senior researcher (DS), who is experienced in the analysis of open-ended questionnaires. The conclusions of the two researchers concurred.

RESULTS

Fifteen relatives/significant others of patients affected with NF2 consented to complete an open-ended questionnaire. Eight female partners, and one mother, whose affected daughter lived at home, completed the questionnaire. The six other respondents were male partners. Two female patients were visited at home while their partners were away. Questionnaires were left for the relatives to complete, but they did not return the questionnaires. Three patients did not have a partner. Two of these patients, one female and the other male, were in their early twenties and unmarried. The third patient was aged 50 years, and was divorced from her husband.

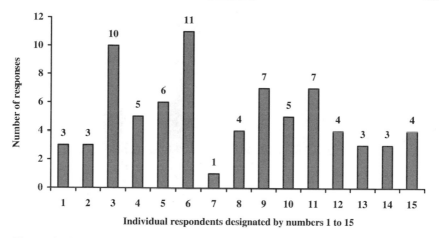

Figure 15.1 The number of responses to question 1 by individual respondents.

Seventy-six responses were received from 15 relatives to question 1, '*Please could you tell me about the ways in which your partner being diagnosed with NF2 has affected your life?*' The number of responses given by individual respondents to question 1 are shown in Figure 15.1.

Sixteen responses from 14 respondents related to difficulties directly concerning the patients' hearing loss and frustrations relating to difficulties with communication. Fourteen responses from 9 relatives identified the need to support the patient physically or emotionally, and worries about their partner's and children's future health. Five responses from 4 relatives underlined the loss or limitation to social life. Five responses from 4 relatives noted the difficulties relating to the genetic nature of NF2. These responses to question 1 are shown in Figure 15.2.

A number of responses were made by two individuals. These are shown in Table 15.1, together with two responses made by one further individual.

The remaining 15 responses were individual responses. One relative reported that the fact that her partner had been diagnosed with NF2 had made no difference to her life as she was a carer by occupation. She said that she had nursed her terminally ill mother in the past, and did not find illness too difficult to manage. A response from a further relative described the fact that her husband's tinnitus made him irritable. The same relative reported that she was constantly aware if her children did not hear what she was saying. A third relative said that he felt loss of self-esteem. He also said that he used to drink quite a lot at one stage, but he found that this only made things twice as bad. Another relative reported that communication was better with sign language. However, he stated that communication could still be frustrating in situations such as when travelling in the car. Another relative gave eight individual responses to question 1. She said that her husband being diagnosed with NF2 had made her more

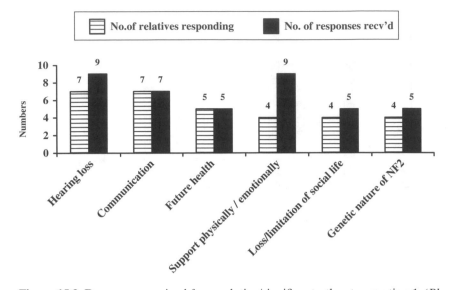

Figure 15.2 Responses received from relative/significant other to question 1, *'Please could you tell me about the ways in which your partner being diagnosed with NF2 has affected your life?'* The figure shows response groups given by four or more respondents.

Table 15.1 Responses received from relative/significant other to question 1, *'Please could you tell me about the ways in which your partner being diagnosed with NF2 has affected your life?'* The table shows categories of responses reported by two individuals in italics, together with two responses reported by one individual

Response	Number of respondents	Number of responses recorded
Misunderstanding because of mishearing	2	2
'I would rather have this illness than my partner/children'	2	2
'I feel isolated'	2	2
Problems because of stress and/or depression	2	2
Always having to answer phone	2	2
Needing to take time off work for hospital appointments	2	2
My children's lack of understanding of NF2	1	1
Other people's lack of understanding of NF2		1

independent. She had developed a separate group of friends whom she could chat to and go to the cinema with. She said that it had made her quieter. She noted that she rarely gets angry, as her husband is unable to lip-read her when she is cross. She said that she has to consider what she is saying and be succinct.

She reported that she has to be at home when he is 'on call' for his work to answer the telephone and relay information. She noted that until text phones were available, she was unable to contact her husband if she was away. This relative considered the fact that her husband had been diagnosed when they were 25 years old and just married. She said that they had both matured and changed in the 27 years since diagnosis, and it was impossible to be sure how much was due to NF2, and how much to increasing maturity and the passage of time.

Seven individual responses were obtained from five further relatives. One mother said that her daughter's epilepsy was terrible until it was controlled. She also underlined the enormous effect that NF2 had had on her daughter's life. Another relative said that vertigo could be a real problem, and he and his partner could no longer enjoy fairground rides together. A further relative described her concern because of her partner's lack of mobility, and a sudden onset in the deterioration of his condition. A husband said that he felt guilty if he had an argument with his wife. He stated that he admired the way in which she coped with her illness, but he said that it did affect everything. The last response from a husband related to giving up work to care for his wife.

Question 2 on the questionnaire asked *'Are there any positive effects that the diagnosis of NF2 in your partner has had on your life?'* Respondents reported increased respect towards people with disabilities and said that they had become closer to their partner. Responses were given regarding the genetic aspects of NF2. One relative was appreciative of the genetic counselling and genetic testing that the family had received. A further relative highlighted the effect of being aware of and being able to avoid passing on the NF2 mutation to their children. Other respondents underlined that the positive attitude of the patient had a positive effect on the situation. Two relatives stated that their families had developed non-aural communication modes. Two respondents emphasised how they had discovered the need to enjoy life. One mother of a patient gave two separate responses regarding the benefit that her family had received from voluntary organisations. Three respondents stated that they had not experienced any positive effects on their life from their partner being diagnosed with NF2. These responses are shown in Figure 15.3.

Ten individual responses from seven relatives were received to question 2, *'Are there any positive effects that the diagnosis of NF2 in your partner has had on your life?'* These individual responses from the relatives/significant others to question 2 are shown in Table 15.2.

DISCUSSION

The use of the open-ended questionnaire in highlighting the main problems volunteered by patients has been recommended for the past 25 years (Barcham & Stephens, 1980). This approach to the impact of their partner's hearing loss has been used in significant others of patients with hearing

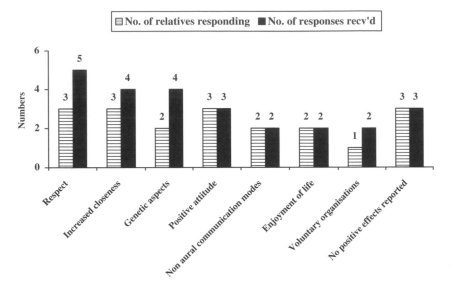

Figure 15.3 Responses received from relative/significant other to question '*Are there any positive effects that the diagnosis of NF2 in your partner has had on your life?*'

Table 15.2 Individual responses received from relative/ significant other to question 2 in questionnaire 2, '*Are there any positive effects that the diagnosis of NF2 in your partner has had on your life?*' Individual responses from the same relative/ significant other are bracketed together

Response
'I feel sympathy towards my husband'
'My life has been enriched by my partner'
⎡'When attending NF meetings and seeing others who suffer from NF2 more ⎢ seriously than my wife helps us appreciate the quality of life we do have' ⎨'We have learned sign language and attend a Church congregation for the Deaf. We ⎣ have made many dear friends, both Deaf and hearing'.
⎡'Made me feel stronger and more independent' ⎨'Made me consider ways to make us happy rather than just be upset at what we ⎣ had lost'
'He has been issued with a hearing aid'
'My daughter is such an able girl, very talented in so many ways. Everything she   does, she does well'
⎡'We all go out to see other people with NF2' ⎨'We go to other parts of the country to see people which is good because it helps ⎣ us to understand what goes on in NF2'

problems by Stephens et al. (1995) and by Meehan et al. (2002), with parents of hearing-impaired teenagers. In addition, Stephens et al. (2004) used it to explore the positive experiences reported by the significant others of patients with hearing impairments.

The most commonly listed problems in the present study of significant others of patients with NF2 related to difficulties directly resulting from the patient's hearing loss, with misunderstandings due to mishearing and frustrations regarding communication. Stephens et al. (1995), found that the significant others of patients with hearing loss most often listed problems with live conversation, and particularly that the relatives had to repeat conversation for the patient. Meehan et al. (2002), carried out a study of parents of hearing-impaired teenagers with the use of an open-ended questionnaire. They found that two major categories of difficulties were elicited, those associated with psychosocial difficulties and live speech difficulties. Many relatives in the present study underlined the fact that they felt responsible for supporting the patients physically and emotionally, and they remarked that they often felt isolated themselves, as they felt unable to discuss their fears with their partners lest they caused them to feel guilty or become upset. Some relatives said that they would prefer to be affected with NF2 themselves, rather than their partner and children being affected. Many relatives noted the loss and limitation to their social lives because of their partner's NF2.

Several relatives voiced concerns about their partner's and children's future health, with particular difficulties relating to the genetic nature of NF2. One relative said that her partner being affected with NF2 had made her question her priorities in life.

A number of relatives said that they noted that they had increased respect towards people with disabilities as a result of their experiences with their partner being affected with NF2. Two noted problems because of stress and depression, as a result of their partners being affected with NF2. Two relatives underlined how they always had to answer the phone, as their partners were unable to use it. Two relatives said that they needed to take time off work, because of their affected partners' hospital appointments. One relative said that she was concerned because of her children's and other people's lack of understanding of NF2.

Many relatives gave individual responses. These responses were wide-ranging, from the statement that it made no difference to the relative's life as she was a carer by occupation, to detailed accounts of the emotional and practical effects of NF2 on the relatives' lives. It is of note that relatives considered their affected partners' and children's needs above their own, making every attempt to improve methods of communication by being succinct and clear when speaking, to learning British Sign Language as a family. Moreover the relatives underlined as to how they attended to their partners' and children's physical and emotional needs as the first priority, but developed strategies to help them to manage the ongoing situation.

Stephens et al. (2004), probed into positive experiences reported by significant others of patients with hearing loss. They found that 45% of respondents were able to report at least one positive experience. They found that children, nieces and grandchildren comprised 50% of those reporting positive responses, whereas they amounted to only 33% of the total respondents. Spouses and partners on the other hand comprised 51% of the total respondents, but only 37% of those giving positive responses. In this study when the significant other was asked whether there had been any positive effects that the diagnosis of NF2 had had on their lives, it is of particular note that 80% indicated one or more positive effects. The perspective of children, nieces and grandchildren had not been sought in this study. Relatives highlighted that they had learned to be more respectful towards other people with disabilities, including deafness. They also noted an increased closeness to their partner.

The importance of careful management of the patient and family by a Specialist Multidisciplinary NF2 Team has been emphasised by Evans et al. (1993; in press). The significant other should be offered genetic counselling together with the affected patient. There should be a named NF2 support worker, who can be contacted by telephone, to speak to the relative and family members, and offer information and support as required. The names of voluntary support agencies, other NF2 patients who have given consent to being contacted, and NF2 websites should be made available to the relatives and families. Relatives in this study reported that they had appreciated the information from genetic counselling and testing, to diagnose or exclude NF2 in an offspring, or to be able to avoid passing the NF2 mutation on to their children. Help received from voluntary organisations was described as a positive effect.

Other relatives commented that their affected partners had a positive attitude to the diagnosis, and this made the situation easier to manage. The development of non-aural communication modes was reported as a positive effect. Enjoyment of life was highlighted as a positive effect, and relatives also gave individual responses to question 2. These ranged from emotional to practical issues. One relative commented on the sympathy she felt towards her partner; another commented on how her life had been enriched by her partner; another relative said that she had become more independent, and the diagnosis of NF2 had made her consider ways to make the family happy, rather than just be upset at what they had lost; two further relatives commented on how they attended NF2 meetings, and realised that some other patients were more seriously affected than their partners. One relative commented on the practical benefit of her affected husband being issued with a hearing aid.

It is of note that the significant others of patients affected with NF2 considered their partners' and children's needs above their own, making every effort to improve methods of communication, and attempting to attend to their partner's physical and emotional needs. Moreover 80% of relatives were able to report one or more positive effects resulting from the diagnosis of NF2 in their partner.

Finally, it is of interest to compare the most commonly listed problems of relatives/significant others of patients with NF2 with the most commonly listed problems identified by the patients themselves. Both relatives and patients identified problems because of deafness and communication difficulties as the most significant in their lives. Both relatives and patients identified the loss or limitation to their hobbies and social lives as difficulties. They also both highlighted the particular difficulties that they had to consider due to the genetic nature of NF2.

In considering the positive aspects identified by the relatives and patients in this study, both felt that they had become more considerate, caring and sensitive people as a result of the diagnosis of NF2, and they considered that they were more deaf and disability aware. They both felt that the condition had brought them closer to their partners. In addition, both relatives and patients commented that the condition had resulted in them widening their circle of friends.

CONCLUSIONS

There are particular difficulties for the relatives of patients affected with NF2, relating to difficulties with communication, the need to support the patient both physically and emotionally, and the dominantly inherited genetic nature of the condition. The patient and significant other should be referred to a multidisciplinary team with expertise in the management of NF2, where it is recognised that the patient's relative requires a considerable amount of practical and emotional support, to avoid their feeling a sense of isolation in the ongoing everyday care of the patient affected with NF2.

REFERENCES

Barcham LJ, Stephens SDG (1980) The use of an open-ended problems questionnaire in auditory rehabilitation. *British Journal of Audiology* 14: 49–54.

Barker V, Wright E, Nguyen K, Cannon L, Fain P, Goldgar D et al. (1987) Gene for von Recklinghausen neurofibromatosis is in the pericentromeric region of chromosome 17. *Science* 236: 1100–2.

Evans DGR, Baser ME, O'Reilly B, Rowe J, Gleeson M, Saeed S et al. (in press) Management of the patient and family with neurofibromatosis type 2: A Consensus Conference Statement. *British Journal of Neurosurgery*.

Evans DGR, Huson SM, Donnai D, Neary W, Blair V, Newton V et al. (1992) A clinical study of type 2 neurofibromatosis. *Quarterly Journal of Medicine* 84(304): 603–18.

Evans DGR, Ramsden R, Huson SM, Harris R, Lye R, King TT (1993) Type 2 neurofibromatosis: the need for supraregional care? *Journal of Laryngology and Otology* 107: 401–6.

Mautner VF, Lindenau M, Baser ME, Hazim W, Tatagiba M, Haase W et al. (1996) The neuroimaging and clinical spectrum of neurofibromatosis 2. *Neurosurgery* 38: 881–5.

Meehan T, France EA, Stephens SDG (2002) The use of an open-ended questionnaire with parents of hearing-impaired teenagers; an exploratory study. *Journal of Audiological Medicine* 11: 46–59.

Neary WJ, Ramsden RT, Evans DGR, Baser ME (2005) Psychosocial aspects of NF2. In D Stephens, L Jones (eds) *The Impact of Genetic Hearing Impairment*. London: Whurr, pp 201–18.

Parry DM, Eldridge R, Kaiser-Kupfer MI, Bouzas EA, Pikus A, Patronas N (1994) Neurofibromatosis 2 (NF2): clinical characteristics of 63 affected individuals and clinical evidence for heterogeneity. *American Journal of Medical Genetics* 52: 450–61.

Rouleau GA, Wertelecki W, Haines JL, Hobbs WJ, Trofatter JA, Seizinger BR et al. (1987) Genetic linkage of bilateral acoustic neurofibromatosis to a DNA marker on chromosome 22. *Nature* 329: 246–8.

Stephens D, France L, Lormore K (1995) Effects of hearing impairment on the patient's family and friends. *Acta Otolaryngologica* 115: 165–7.

Stephens D, Kerr P, Jones G (2004) Positive experiences reported by significant others of patients with hearing impairments. *Audiological Medicine* 2: 134–8.

APPENDIX 15.1

QUESTIONNAIRE 2

TITLE: PSYCHOSOCIAL ASPECTS OF NEUROFIBROMATOSIS TYPE 2

Relative/Significant Other

This is a confidential questionnaire to try and find out about the effects of the diagnosis of NF2 in a family. We are trying to find out what is the most important to family members. There is no right or wrong answer, but what you feel is important to you.

1. *Please could you tell me about the ways in which your partner being diagnosed with NF2 has affected your life. Please could you put a star(*) by the ones you feel are most important.*

2. *Are there any **POSITIVE** effects that the diagnosis of NF2 in your partner has had on your life? Could you write them down.*

Thank you for completing this questionnaire. We hope it will be useful in improving the service to families with NF2.

16 Attitudes of Adults with Otosclerosis towards Issues Surrounding Genetics and the Impact of Hearing Loss

ANNA MIDDLETON, IOANNIS MOUMOULIDIS,
GRAEME CROSSLAND, MALLAPPA RAGHU,
PRANAY KUMAR SINGH, EVAN REID AND PATRICK AXON

INTRODUCTION

Otosclerosis is a condition that causes hearing loss. It is different from many other causes of hearing impairment in that the loss can often be corrected by surgery, resulting in a restoration of hearing. The psychological impact of this condition has largely been ignored due to the perception that the disability from the condition can be easily 'fixed' (Lemkens, 2005). However, the impact of having a hearing loss cannot be underestimated, particularly if the patient chooses not to have any intervention or if the intervention is inappropriate or unsuccessful. This chapter focuses on the attitudes of people with otosclerosis towards their hearing loss and the impact of this on their lives.

Otosclerosis is a condition that results when the stapes within the middle ear becomes fixed. Typically, the resultant hearing loss is progressive over several years leading to a mild, moderate and sometimes severe or profound loss. Approximately 70% of cases are bilateral and the hearing loss may typically start to become apparent in the late teens or early twenties, with a clinical hearing loss usually picked up in the 20s or 30s. Otosclerosis initially causes a conductive hearing loss, but the latter stages of the disease can affect the inner ear so causing a mixed loss. Surgery and hearing aids are used as effective methods to restore hearing. If the otosclerosis is very far advanced and associated with a profound hearing loss, treatment with a cochlear implant may also be appropriate (House & Cunningham, 2005).

Otosclerosis is thought to have a prevalence of 3 per 1000 in the Caucasian population (Declau et al., 2001). It is also thought, in some families, to have

The Effects of Genetic Hearing Impairment in the Family. Edited by D. Stephens and L. Jones.
Copyright © 2006 by John Wiley & Sons, Ltd.

an autosomal dominant pattern of inheritance with reduced penetrance and expression, although the majority of cases of otosclerosis appear to be sporadic (Lemkens, 2005).

The study documented in this chapter considers the attitudes of a group of patients with suspected otosclerosis, who have not yet had surgery. They presented to an ENT clinic with diagnostic signs of the condition and more than half of the group had a family history of the condition in other relatives. They therefore had knowledge and experience of coping with otosclerosis and, as this had not been corrected yet by surgery, they were in a position to report the impact of this condition on their lives.

METHODS

A structured questionnaire was designed including 12 closed questions, based around work previously piloted (Middleton, 1999). The questions assessed attitudes towards genetics, having a genetic test for deafness, burden of hearing loss, success of communication and need for support. The questionnaire was offered to patients with otosclerosis attending an ENT clinic in Cambridge, UK, in 2003. Completed questionnaires were received from 205 participants in total, 62% of whom had already had successful surgery for their otosclerosis. The data presented here relates to the 71 participants who had not yet had surgery or for whom surgery was not appropriate, i.e patients currently living and coping with the condition. Socio-demographic data relating to the sample is given in Table 16.1.

Table 16.1 Socio-demographic data

Total participants with otosclerosis (n = 71)	%
Married	75%
Female	66%
Age ranges:	
20–39	28%
40–59	52%
60–79	20%
Degree of hearing loss:	
Mild (21–40 dB)	52%
Moderate (41–60 dB)	47%
Severe (61–80 dB)	1%
Has a family history of otosclerosis	53%
Social class 1–2 (manager, senior official, professional)	35%
Social class 3–7 (Assoc. professional, technical, administration, secretarial, skilled trade, sales, customer services)	41%
Social class 8–9 (Plant and machinery operatives, elementary occupations)	24%

Table 16.2 Responses to each question documenting attitudes towards issues surrounding genetics and impact of deafness

Question	% response
If there was a cure or treatment for deafness, would you want to have it?	
Yes	75%
No	1%
Not sure	24%
If you could have had a genetic test (blood test) when you were younger that would have predicted whether you were likely to develop a hearing loss when you were older, would you have wanted such a test?	
Yes	76%
No	10%
Not sure	14%
If you answered yes, do you think you would have altered your behaviour to protect against going deaf?	
Yes	51%
No	13%
Not sure	21%
Some people with no experience of deafness might assume that this is burdensome for a person who has lost their hearing. Please can you say whether you feel, in reality, an actual burden of having a hearing loss?	
My hearing loss causes no burden to me	3%
My hearing loss causes very little burden	58%
The burden is moderately great, but I can cope with it	34%
The burden is very great, but I can cope with it	3%
The burden is too great and I have difficulty coping with it	1%
I'm not sure	1%
How successfully do you and your partner/significant other communicate with each other?	
Very successfully/Successfully	89%
OK (communicate on a basic level, but are not able to talk about complex issues due to problems with communication)	4%
Poorly	1%
Do you feel you are advantaged/disadvantaged in any way because of your hearing loss?	
Advantaged	3%
Disadvantaged	54%
Neither advantaged nor disadvantaged	39%
Both advantaged and disadvantaged	4%
Some people feel they need extra emotional support with coping with their hearing loss. Do you feel you receive enough support from family, friends and hearing professionals?	
Enough support received from family and friends	76%
Not enough support received from family and friends	1%
Enough support received from health professionals	59%
Not enough support received from health professionals	1%
Would you appreciate more specific emotional support from health professionals?	
Yes	34%
No	24%
Not sure	42%

Percentages for each question may not always add up to 100% due to missing numbers

RESULTS

All sociodemographic data as well as other variables were analysed according to whether patients had a family history or not. There was *no significant difference* between the responses from participants with a family history and without a family history of otosclerosis to any of the questions so the results have been presented as one group (Table 16.2).

DISCUSSION

The majority of participants in the study were female, married and aged 40–59, had a family history of otosclerosis and had a moderate level of hearing loss. This could be considered a typical representation of people with this condition (House & Cunningham, 2005).

The vast majority of the group said that they would want a cure or treatment for their deafness, the assumption from this being that this was a condition that was irritating to live with and they would rather they did not have it. The majority of participants in the present study will be assessed at some point to see if surgery is appropriate. It could be assumed that most of them would be keen to proceed with surgery; however, 25% of the group said they did not want to be treated or were not sure if they would want a cure for their deafness. This indicates that although surgery may be offered to them, perhaps not all would wish to pursue this. It is possible that, if there were alternatives to surgery, these would be preferable. Other research which considered the impact of having surgery on people with otosclerosis has shown that there are differences in 'temperament' and 'optimism – pessimism' scale pre- and post-operatively, in that before surgery people feel more negatively about their condition than after surgery (Gildston & Gildston, 1972). This would suggest that even though there may be fear and uncertainty about the surgical procedure prior to having it, afterwards there is psychological benefit. Larger and new studies looking at the psychological benefits of having surgery for otosclerosis would be useful.

The majority (75%) of the group said that, if it had been possible to predict when they were younger whether they were likely to develop a hearing loss when they were older, they would have wanted such a test. But, only half of the group said that they would have altered their behaviour to protect against going deaf. This indicates that people like to be forewarned as to what may befall them in the future, but that this is mainly for information's sake. It may also indicate that otosclerosis is not perceived as a condition to be avoided at all costs. This attitude was reflected in other questions assessing the perceived burden of the condition. More than 60% of the group said that their hearing loss caused no or little burden to them and 89% said they managed to have very successful or successful communication with their partner or significant other.

However, sadly, one member of the group said that the burden associated with their hearing loss was too great to cope with. It is hoped that this expression of despair has been discussed with the health professionals involved and appropriate support put in place. It also suggests that the psychological impact of otosclerosis should not be underestimated for some people affected with it.

The results of this study can be compared to other research that has documented attitudes towards the same issues, but using different population groups. Deaf and hearing parents of deaf children were asked to comment on the perceived level of burden of deafness for their children (Middleton, 2005). The results from this showed that deaf parents were less likely to perceive a burden of deafness in the children than hearing parents, the assumption being that deafness is perceived as more burdensome by hearing people, who do not have personal experience of deafness in themselves. Most people participating in that research had a severe – profound level of deafness, either in themselves or in their children and so this is a somewhat different situation to the participants in the present study with otosclerosis. However, it would be interesting to ask hearing people, with no knowledge or experience of otosclerosis, for their opinions on the perceived level of burden attached to this condition. One could hypothesise, like in the research already mentioned above, that they might perceive the level of burden to be higher than reported by people actually with the condition.

The majority of participants felt that they had received enough support from family, friends and health professionals in coping with their hearing loss, but 34% said they would have appreciated more specific emotional support from health professionals. This is an interesting finding as, even though most in this study felt that the condition was not too burdensome to deal with, more than a third of them still would have appreciated more emotional support from health professionals. This may be in relation to dealing with a health professional who is empathic to their situation or else spends a little time asking about and listening to the impact of the condition.

When asked about whether participants felt they were advantaged or disadvantaged because of their hearing loss, just over half said that they felt disadvantaged. This indicates that otosclerosis is disabling to some, but not for all people who have it.

Interestingly, 3% said that they felt advantages associated with their hearing loss; all these people had a family history of the condition. This could possibly indicate that having a family history of the same condition offers support and a connection that links people. This has been reported before within numerous other contexts. For example, an anecdotal study by Lemkens (2005) indicated that those with severe otosclerosis that warranted treatment with a cochlear implant, felt that having a family history of otosclerosis was an advantage to them as they felt more prepared for their situation. They also found their problems could be easily discussed in the family and they gained support from this.

Other work done on congenital deafness has shown that having a family history of deafness can help with how people cope with this, in particular in relation to schooling (Stephens, 2005) and whether parents feel there is a burden attached to their child's deafness or not (Middleton, 2005). Many different pieces of research across the world have shown that deaf children of deaf parents are less likely to have emotional and behavioural problems than deaf children of hearing parents (e.g. Meadow, 1980; Satapathy & Singhal, 2001; Polat, 2003). Other work presented elsewhere within this book has shown that those with a family history of late onset deafness or hearing impairment (i.e. different from the congenitally deaf) also have a more positive experience of deafness than those without a family history (Kramer et al., this volume, Chapter 6). Therefore, in the present study, although there was no significant difference in the responses from participants with respect to each question and whether they had a family history or not, those who did have a family history may have been more likely to feel there were advantages of sharing the 'family condition'. It is possible that this offered a connection to their family unit – a shared experience, from which they gained psychological benefit.

In summary, otosclerosis is a condition that the participants in this study found to be bearable. The vast majority felt that the burden associated with the condition was something they could cope with and most felt that their communication with their partners was not affected by the condition. However, there was enough of a burden attached to the condition to feel that a treatment or cure was warranted and most felt that they would have liked to have been forewarned of this before they developed signs of the condition.

REFERENCES

Declau F, Van Spaendonck M, Timmermans JP, Michaels L, Liang J, Qiu JP et al. (2001) Prevalence of otosclerosis in an unselected series of temporal bones. *Otology and Neurotology* 22: 596–602.

Gildston H, Gildston P (1972) Personality changes associated with surgically corrected hypoacusis. *Audiology* 11: 354–67.

House JW, Cunningham CD (2005) Otosclerosis. In CW Cummings, PW Flint, BH Haughey, KT Robbins, JR Thomas, KA Harker et al. (eds) *Otolaryngology Head and Neck Surgery*, 4th edn. Los Angeles: Mosby.

Lemkens N (2005) The effects of otosclerosis. In D Stephens, L Jones (eds) *The Impact of Genetic Hearing Impairment*. London: Whurr, pp. 195–200.

Meadow KP (1980) *Deafness and Child Development*. London: Arnold.

Middleton A (1999) Attitudes of deaf and hearing individuals towards issues surrounding genetic testing for deafness. PhD thesis, University of Leeds.

Middleton A (2005) Parents' attitudes towards genetic testing and the impact of deafness in the family. In D Stephens, L Jones (eds) *The Impact of Genetic Hearing Impairment*. London: Whurr, pp. 11–53.

Polat F (2003) Factors affecting psychosocial adjustment of deaf students. *Journal of Deaf Studies and Deaf Education* 8: 325–39.

Satapathy S, Singhal S (2001) Predicting social-emotional adjustment of the sensory impaired adolescents. *Journal of Personality and Clinical Studies* 17: 85–93.

Stephens D (2005) The impact of hearing impairment in children. In D Stephens, L Jones (eds) *The Impact of Genetic Hearing Impairment*. London: Whurr, pp. 73–105.

17 People's Reaction to Having a Family History of Otosclerosis

DAFYDD STEPHENS AND NELE LEMKENS

INTRODUCTION

Otosclerosis represents an interesting condition from the standpoint of psychosocial aspects of hearing impairment. It is a common condition, affecting some 2% of the British adult population (Browning & Gatehouse, 1992). Between 50% and 70% of all cases have a family history (Gordon, 1989) and the condition results in a conductive hearing impairment which may be amenable to surgical intervention. So far four genes which may result in the condition have been localiscd (Van Camp & Smith, 2005).

Despite this, and a plethora of papers which have been written on the surgical aspects of the condition, studies of its impact on those affected are sparse, and have recently been reviewed by Lemkens (2005). Within her review, she found a small number of studies beginning with the work of Gildston and Gildston (1972). Those authors found that a range of personality traits were significantly impaired in individuals with the condition, and that most of these improved after a successful stapedectomy.

Eriksson-Mangold et al. (1996) have argued, on the basis of in-depth interviews and associated questionnaires, that this was a somewhat simplistic approach, and that any changes in emotional adaptation were, in reality, more complex. Neither study considered specifically individuals who had a family history of the condition.

In the present brief account we shall present some results on the attitudes and reactions of individuals with otosclerosis and a family history of such a condition extending the pilot findings reported by Lemkens (2005).

METHOD

SUBJECTS

Thirteen consecutive subjects seen in the Welsh Hearing Institute, Cardiff, Wales, and nine consecutive subjects seen in the ENT department of the

The Effects of Genetic Hearing Impairment in the Family. Edited by D. Stephens and L. Jones.

Table 17.1 Demographics of subjects

	Mean age (years)	SD	Males (n)	Females (n)
Belgium	56.2	12.7	4	4
Wales	52.6	15.3	3	10
Total	54.1	14.5	7	14

Table 17.2 Hearing levels of subjects

	Air conduction				Bone conduction		Air – bone gap (dB)			
	BEHL		WEHL		Better ear		Right ear		Left ear	
	Mean (dB)	SD	Mean (dB)	SD	Mean (dB)	SD	Mean	SD	Mean	SD
Belgium	67.9	37.0	82.8	36.8	49.9	22.3	22.4	20.6	21.9	19.6
Wales	46.2	21.2	63.9	27.7	29.9	10.4	17.9	6.8	21.9	13.6
Total	55.5	34.7	72.0	32.5	40.5	20.1	20.0	14.7	21.9	16.4

BEHL = Better Ear Hearing Level; WEHL = Worse Ear Hearing Level (averaged over 0.5, 1, 2 and 4 KHz)

University of Antwerp, Belgium, comprised the subjects of this study. All had been diagnosed clinically as having otosclerosis. Their age, gender and hearing level distribution are shown in Tables 17.1 and 17.2.

QUESTIONNAIRE

Two different questionnaire formats were used in the present study. The Belgium arm of the study used the questionnaire described by Middleton in the next chapter but included key questions on the individual's reaction to having a family history of tinnitus. The Welsh arm had the latter questions but also two open-ended questions. Only the five overlapping questions will be considered in the present brief report.

These questions are shown in Appendix 17.1.

Question 1 may be discounted from the present analyses as it taps the subject's knowledge of having affected family members. Only subjects who responded affirmatively were included in the study.

Question 2 (attitudes towards discoveries in genetics) was included to provide comparison with the other studies on attitudes of deaf people (Middleton, 2005) and of other patients with otosclerosis (Middleton, this volume, Chapter 18).

Question 3 taps the patient's view as to whether the family history affected their own reaction to their hearing impairment and Question 4 examines the broad type of effect (positive or negative) that such a reaction had.

Finally the open-ended question, Question 5, taps into the specific effects that the patients had noticed.

RESULTS

The two groups of subjects (Belgian and Welsh) did not differ significantly from each other in age and gender distribution. Analysis of the hearing levels showed a wide difference of hearing levels among the respondents. The air conduction thresholds did not differ significantly between the Belgian and Welsh groups or either the better or worse hearing levels (averaged over 500 Hz and 1, 2 and 4 kHz). However, the better ear bone conduction thresholds were more sensitive in the Welsh population (z = 2.70; p = 0.008). There was no significant difference between the two population in terms of the air – bone gaps found. These results are shown in Table 17.2.

The responses to Question 2 on attitudes towards discoveries in genetics are shown in Figure 17.1. It may be seen that the three most commonly reported attitudes are all very positive (Hopeful = 14/22, Enthusiastic = 12/22, and Optimistic = 10/22). However, a small minority did report more negative attitudes with 3/20 reporting feeling pessimistic and a similar number feeling concerned. These responses were not significantly related to the country of origin, gender, age or any of the hearing level measures.

Interestingly the Welsh subjects marked more descriptors than did the Belgian subjects, with a median of 3 responses from the Welsh compared with a median of 1.5 by the Belgians (z = 2.70; p = 0.008).

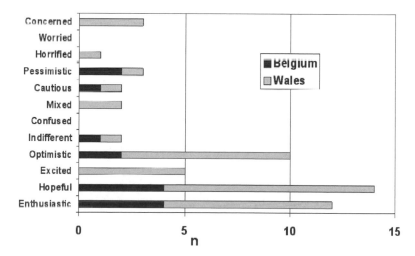

Figure 17.1 Number of times various descriptors were listed.

The responses to Question 3 on whether or not having a family history of hearing loss had any effect on their own reaction to their hearing loss are shown in Figure 17.2. This shows that 70% of the respondents indicated they felt that their family history had affected their reaction either definitely (7/20) or maybe (7/20).

There was no significant difference in the response to this question between the subjects from the two countries, nor did gender, age or hearing levels have any significant effect.

The responses to Question 4 on the type of effect such knowledge of a family history had on them (positive or negative) are shown in Figure 17.3. It may be seen that two-thirds of the respondents (12/18) indicated a positive effect with only two reporting a negative effect.

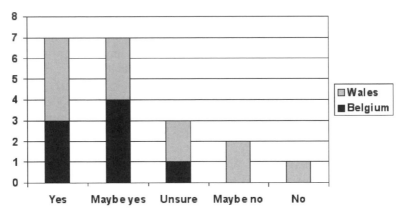

Figure 17.2 Influence of family history.

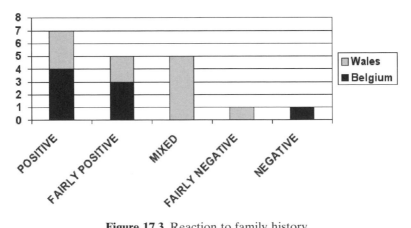

Figure 17.3 Reaction to family history.

The type of response given to this question did not depend significantly on the source of the subjects, their gender, their age or their hearing levels. However, it did relate to whether or not they felt that a family history had had an effect on them (χ^2 = 32.8; 12 df; p = 0.001). Thus those indicating a definite effect were also more likely to indicate that this was definitely a positive effect.

Twelve respondents specified ways in which their family history had affected them, listing between them 27 responses. Of these responses, ten were positive, five were negative and in five it was impossible to define the nature of the response or they did not seem to be related to the family history.

The positive responses are shown in Table 17.3.

The five negative responses are shown in Table 17.4, the three neutral responses in Table 17.5, and ten 'general' responses in Table 17.6. The last group are responses basically related to their hearing loss alone, independent of whether or not it is familial.

Table 17.3 Positive responses

S1	The problems of being hard of hearing is shared by many and therefore can be discussed.
S2	It is easier to speak about the problem because someone whose hearing is OK can hardly understand the difficulties associated with it.
S3	Because there are other people with hearing problems in my family, I was better prepared when my hearing worsened.
S3	You can react earlier concerning your future work situation etc.
S4	Finally understand reason behind hearing loss.
S4	Comparison with my mother as she had the same problem.
S5	General atmosphere within the family is one of understanding and tolerance, allowing us to anticipate and approach most problems with humour.
S5	Learnt from family members who have had a negative approach to their problem – we strive to overcome social isolation and an inferiority complex.
S6	Understand how they felt and being able to offer ways of coping and strategies for overcoming the difficulties which arise

Table 17.4 Negative responses

S4	Could my child have the same – her children etc?
S4	How will it affect my quality of life – i.e. will it affect my job, me driving?
S5	Concern for transmission to next generation.
S7	When my father and mother were alive they both suffered hearing loss and we had to talk louder.
S12	Concerned about children of the family.

Table 17.5 Neutral responses

S7	My mother had a hearing aid late in life but did not like to use it.
S12	Hope that treatment will be available for any children diagnosed.
S12	Parents were aware that the condition existed in the family.

Table 17.6 General responses

S4	Constantly say pardon/what did you say? Are you speaking to me?
S4	Unable to hear loud snoring.
S8	Communication, including my social life greatly diminished over the years.
S9	My marriage, job, social life.
S10	Having to talk loud.
S10	Playing in a band, found it hard to listen to low notes.
S11	I don't socialise much.
S11	Will make excuses when invited out to a formal dinner.
S11	Often feel embarrassed.
S11	Affects my job.
S11	Dislike meetings, attending new courses etc.

DISCUSSION

The results of this study show that patients with a family history of otosclerosis were broadly positive about their family history and about genetics as a whole. These general views about genetics are reflected in Question 2 in which the subjects have the option to mark as many descriptors of how they feel about genetics as they wish. Broadly speaking, four response options indicated very positive feelings about genetics, four rather neutral feelings and four reflected negative feelings.

It is difficult to explain why the Welsh respondents marked more descriptors than did the Belgian subjects, particularly as the breakdown of the responses did not differ significantly between the two groups. It could be that there were nuances in the translation.

That said, the most remarkable point about the results is that over 80% of the responses reflected enthusiasm for genetics, with only 8% being negative. In a group of Deaf people asked the same questions by Middleton (Middleton et al., 2001; Middleton, 2006) only 28% of the responses were positive and 32% negative. The differences in her hard of hearing/deafened group were less marked, but were still 44% positive and 22% negative, and those of her subjects who were hearing but had either a deaf parent or a deaf child gave figures of 56% positive and 17% negative. These results, together with those for the 'neutral' responses are shown in Figure 17.4.

Interestingly, the adjective most commonly endorsed by the patients with otosclerosis (64%) was 'hopeful', which was also the most commonly indicated by Middleton's 'hearing' subjects (51%). Thirty-seven per cent of her 'hard of hearing' subjects also reported being hopeful, but only 18% of her 'Deaf' subjects. However, while 54% of otosclerotics expressed 'enthusiasm' for developments in genetics, only 27%, 22% and 10% of Middleton's groups expressed similar feelings.

Only 14% of the present respondents expressed concern about such developments, whereas among Middleton's groups, those feeling concerned ranged from 23% in her hearing group to 33% among the Deaf.

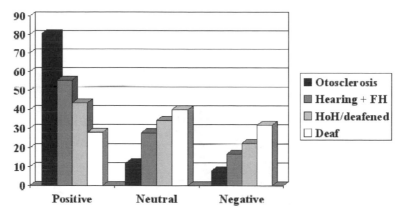

Figure 17.4 Percentages of responses to positive, neutral and negative descriptors of development in genetics.

All these indicate a strong positive attitude to genetics in the group of patients with otosclerosis compared to those who are associated with what is often a congenital hearing loss, and in particular in comparison with members of the Deaf community. This is presumably because they do not feel threatened by genetic developments and feel that such developments would be likely to help their own descendants. It is also interesting to note that Middleton (this volume, Chapter 18) found no difference between patients with otosclerosis and a family history and those without a family history in their attitudes to a range of specific genetic developments.

Figure 17.2 indicates that some 70% of respondents indicated that having affected family members affected their own response to their otosclerosis. This compares with 57% of patients with non-specific late onset hearing impairment and a family history, seen by Stephens and Kramer (2005). However, if we take only the results in otosclerotic subjects from Wales, whose data were collected in the same way in the two studies, the percentage reporting such an effect is 58%, almost identical to the non-otosclerotic subjects.

It may be seen in Figure 17.3 that 12/19 responding about the effect of a family history reported a positive effect, compared with only 2/19 reporting a purely negative effect. This may be interpreted as reflecting the generally positive effects of having a role model, and will be discussed further in the context of the specific effects below.

When we subdivided the specific responses, as shown in Tables 17.3 to 17.6, we found that 11 of the responses could be defined as 'General' responses (Table 17.6), independent of any family history and comparable with those reported in a number of studies from Barcham and Stephens (1980) onwards as consequences of their hearing impairment *per se*. Of the other 17 listed, nine could be regarded as positive (Table 17.3), five as negative (Table 17.4) and three as 'neutral' in that it was impossible to tell whether the respondent was indicating a positive or negative effect (Table 17.5).

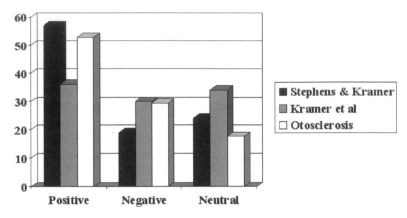

Figure 17.5 Percentages of positive, negative and neutral effects specified in response to having a family history.

Table 17.7 The total number of reported meaning units per theme and
the distribution of positive, negative and neutral responses
(based on Kramer et al., Chapter 6, Table 6.3)

Theme	Distribution of the number of positive, negative and neutral meaning units		
	Positive	Negative	Neutral
Role modelling	3		
Expectation/anticipation	1		1
Acceptance	1	2	1
Help-seeking	1		
Sharing knowledge	3		
Offspring / worry about future		4	1

Such a breakdown of responses has been discussed by Kramer et al. (this volume, Chapter 6) on the basis of their study and that of Stephens and Kramer (2005), and Figure 17.5 is an amalgam of their results and the present data. It may be seen that the results of this study fall within the bounds of the two studies on non-specific acquired familial hearing impairment.

Two different approaches to the classification of the responses, using the analysis approach of Graneheim and Lundman (2004) were used in the studies by Stephens and Kramer and by Kramer et al. and the present results fit quite well with both. Kramer et al. (this volume, Chapter 6, Table 6.2) defined six themes encompassing positive, negative and neutral elements within each. We have examined our results using the same approach and these are shown in Table 17.7, based on their Table 6.3.

While the number of responses being considered in this study is small, it is interesting to note that the breakdown of themes by positive, negative and neutral responses follows the same general pattern as that described by Kramer et al. Thus 'Role modelling' and 'Sharing knowledge' attracted positive responses, 'Acceptance' and 'Offspring / worry about the future' attracted predominantly negative responses.

CONCLUSIONS

It would seem, therefore, that the perceived and reported effects of having a family history in individuals with otosclerosis very much mirrors that of other patients with later onset hearing impairment and a family history. It is interesting to note that, despite the fact that surgery was discussed with all patients and that the Belgian centre is one of the leading centres in the world for such surgery, not a single patient referred to surgery in their responses in positive or negative ways. This contrasts markedly with the results of Eriksson-Mangold et al. (1996), in which surgery was highlighted repeatedly by their respondents.

REFERENCES

Barcham LJ, Stephens SDG (1980) The use of an open-ended problems questionnaire in auditory rehabilitation. *British Journal of Audiology* 14: 49–54.

Browning GG, Gatehouse S (1992) The prevalence of middle ear disease in the adult British population. *Clinical Otolaryngology* 17: 317–21.

Eriksson-Mangold M, Erlandsson SI, Jansson G (1996) The subjective meaning of illness in severe otosclerosis: a descriptive study in three steps based on focus group interviews and written questionnaire. *Scandinavian Audiology* 25 (suppl. 43): 34–44.

Gildston H, Gildston P (1972) Personality changes associated with surgically corrected hypoacusis. *Audiology* 11: 354–67.

Gordon MA (1989) The genetics of otosclerosis: a review. *American Journal of Otology* 10: 426–38.

Graneheim UH, Lundman B (2004) Qualitative content analysis in nursing research: concepts, procedures and measures to achieve trustworthiness. *Nurse Education Today* 24: 105–12.

Lemkens N (2005) The effects of otosclerosis. In D Stephens, L Jones (eds) *The Impact of Genetic Hearing Impairment*. London: Whurr, pp. 195–200.

Middleton A (2005) Parents' attitudes towards genetic testing and the impact of deafness in the family. In D Stephens, L Jones (eds) *The Impact of Genetic Hearing Impairment*. London: Whurr, pp. 11–53.

Middleton A (2006) Review of the attitudes of Deaf people and their families towards issues surrounding deafness. In A Martini, D Stephens, A Read (eds) *Genes, Hearing and Deafness*. London: Dunitz (in press).

Middleton A, Hewison J, Mueller RF (2001) Prenatal diagnosis for inherited deafness – what is the potential demand? *Journal of Genetic Counselling* 10: 121–31.

Stephens D, Kramer SE (2005). The impact of having a family history of hearing problems on those with hearing difficulties themselves: an exploratory study. *International Journal of Audiology* 44: 206–12.

Van Camp G, Smith R (2005) Hereditary Hearing Loss Homepage. Antwerp: University of Antwerp. http://webhost.ua.ac.be/hhh/

APPENDIX 17.1

1. Do or did you have other family members with the same type of hearing loss?

   Yes   No

2. Which of the given words best describe how you feel about new discoveries in genetics, in the light of your own hearing difficulties? (tick as many as you like)

Enthusiastic	Hopeful	Excited	Optimistic
Indifferent	Confused	Mixed feeling	Cautious
Pessimistic	Horrified	Worried	Concerned

If you answered yes to question no. 1 please also answer the following questions

3. Does the fact that you have other family members with the same type of hearing loss have any effect on your reaction to your own hearing difficulties?

   Definitely yes   Maybe yes   Unsure   Maybe no   Definitely no

4. If you think there is an effect of your family history, do you think this effect on your reaction to your own hearing difficulties is in general a positive or a negative effect?

Definitely positive	More positive	Both positive and negative effects	More negative	Definitely negative

5. We are interested in the particular ways in which this family history has affected you. Please write down as many effects as you can think of, you can use the back of this page as well. Continue overleaf if necessary.

IV Genetic Counselling and Family Reactions

18 Genetic Counselling and the d/Deaf Community

ANNA MIDDLETON

OVERVIEW

This chapter discusses the practicalities of seeing d/Deaf[1] clients within a clinical setting in the UK. This is considered within the context of issues surrounding genetic counselling, psychology of deafness and Deaf culture.

There have been numerous excellent reviews of how to conduct an evaluation of the genetic/inherited basis of hearing loss within genetic counselling (e.g. see Israel, 1989, 1995; Arnos et al., 1991, 1992, 1996; Israel & Arnos, 1995; Gorlin et al., 1995, Mueller, 1996; Arnos & Pandya, 2003; Smith et al., 2004) and so these will be considered the background to this chapter and will not be addressed in any specific detail here.

The culturally Deaf client may have a different perspective on genetics issues and also different communication needs from those who identify with the hearing world. So there may be particular considerations pertinent to a clinical service involving such clients. Therefore, this chapter gives attention to

---

[1] **Terminology**
Within this chapter the terms 'deaf' and 'deafness' refer to people with an audiological loss within severe/profound levels, 'hearing loss' is an all-inclusive term that refers to any level or type of audiological hearing loss. 'Deaf' written with an uppercase 'D' refers to a deaf person who is culturally Deaf, i.e. uses sign language (e.g. British or a National Sign Language) as their first or preferred language and has a positive identity attached to being deaf. The term d/Deaf refers to deaf people who identify with both the Deaf community and the hearing world; this term is generally used in relation to adults rather than children. The term 'hearing-impaired' is avoided as many Deaf people would not view themselves as 'impaired' in any way; however, it is acknowledged that this term is widely used among health professionals as a generic term instead of 'deafness' used in this context. The deaf community is an inclusive term to refer to all people with any level and perception of hearing loss. The Deaf community or culture is a specific term that refers to culturally Deaf people only. NSL (National Sign Language) is used as a general term to refer to the main signed language from any country (e.g. British Sign Language or French Sign Language). SSSL (Signed Supported Spoken Language) refers to the sign language, which is a literal translation of spoken language for any country (e.g. Signed Supported English).

The Effects of Genetic Hearing Impairment in the Family. Edited by D. Stephens and L. Jones.
Copyright © 2006 by John Wiley & Sons, Ltd.

these issues and offers information to help provide a Deaf-friendly genetic counselling service.

The author does not make the assumption that all d/Deaf people *should* participate in genetic counselling – potential clients are free to decide themselves as to whether they wish to access such services. There is also no underlying agenda to reduce deafness in society as an outcome of genetic counselling.

Firstly, an overview of the frequency of deafness is given, with reference to Deaf culture and how genetic counselling is relevant to d/Deaf people. Secondly, a historical picture is offered which gives a background to some of the attitudes of culturally Deaf people towards genetics. Thirdly, practical ideas suggest methods for effective communication with d/Deaf people in a clinic consultation. Finally, counselling issues relevant to d/Deaf people are discussed depending on the context of the family background.

The attitudes of those hearing people who have lost their hearing later on in life, due to genetic or inherited causes (the 'hard of hearing' or 'deafened'), as well as people who have specific needs due to syndromal deafness, are a different group that are not referred to specifically in any detail in this chapter, although some of the issues discussed will be relevant.

This chapter is introduced with a short account of the experience of working with Deaf people. A researcher or clinician from the genetics community may experience certain difficulties working with members of the Deaf community if this is not handled with insight and preparation. The following describes the author's initiation into such work.

INTRODUCTION

As culturally Deaf adults are often from large d/Deaf families, i.e. people with an inherited or genetic deafness, there is a huge resource here for understanding the molecular genetic basis of hearing loss as well as the psychological dynamics between members of a Deaf family (i.e. research that genetic counsellors might be interested in). However, given some of the strongly negative attitudes towards the perceived misuse of genetic technology (see later), it is unlikely that many culturally Deaf adults would seek out participation in molecular or psychological genetic research studies. Yet, when asked, d/Deaf families are often interested to know what the genetic basis is of their deafness and are also keen to be asked their views about genetics issues. Through transparent and sensitive explanation, and acknowledgement of the historical context within which the genetic services are placed, it is possible to work well as a genetic researcher in the Deaf community looking at either molecular genetic work or psychological studies.

When I originally started working in research with d/Deaf people the word 'genetic' in my job title seemed to be the codeword that closed doors to me. I was interested in documenting the views of d/Deaf and hearing parents of deaf children towards genetic technology, and yet just asking people's opinions about genetics issues was enough for Deaf people to be suspicious of me – the assumption being that if I worked in the field of genetics then I would view d/Deaf people from the 'medical model' and would advocate the demise of the Deaf community, e.g. via genetic testing in pregnancy and selective abortion of deaf foetuses. As a practising genetic counsellor I subscribe to a nondirective model which means I work with the values and direction of the client, so the idea that I would advocate the 'demise' of any community was alien to me.

I worked hard to gain trust and offer accurate information about what modern-day genetics services offer and by doing this carefully and sensitively I was gradually able to establish myself as less of a threat. By enrolling in British Sign Language classes and through this making an attempt to be linguistically and culturally adept I tried to engage with the Deaf community by visiting Deaf clubs, support groups, charities, schools and universities as well as seeing d/Deaf people in their homes.

I approached people who could be considered 'Deaf community leaders' – key policy-makers and advocates with levels of influence in the community. These people were invited to contribute to my research and were offered an opportunity to express their views to the medical profession. They helped me with my questionnaire design and gave their approval. Without this the process would have been much more difficult, also it would have been very easy to discredit my research as the Deaf community is very small and so expressed disapproval from an influential member would have been devastating to me personally (but also practically for the study). It is imperative that different d/Deaf people are involved in the design and creative stages at the beginning as well as participating in any study so that the process is transparent and culturally sensitive. It is also advisable that researchers learn the National Sign Language (NSL) for their country so that they can respectfully initiate conversations with Deaf people, even if an interpreter is used too.

There are many academics doing interesting work within the Deaf community. Those who are d/Deaf themselves have the advantage of being able to communicate on so many different levels, both in terms of language and culture, with the Deaf study participant. I had the 'disadvantage' of being both hearing and also working in genetics (a perceived threat!) and so I had to give much consideration as to how I conducted my research.

Work with the Deaf community can be enormously rewarding and I have felt privileged to be able to meet and learn from Deaf people across the world. I am indebted to the hundreds of d/Deaf people who have taken the time and commitment to offer their opinions. This has helped me to think through how genetic counselling services could be improved and how we, as health professionals, have an obligation to do this well. The present chapter offers a brief summary of some of the knowledge and experience I have been fortunate enough to gather.

EPIDEMIOLOGY OF DEAFNESS

There are many different causes of deafness; these include environmental and genetic factors. Out of the approximately 1 in 1000 children born with a severe – profound, congenital or early-onset deafness (Davis, 1993) more than 50% have a genetic cause (Parving, 1996; Smith et al., 2004). There are over 400 genetic syndromes that involve deafness as part of the phenotype (Gorlin et al., 1995). Approximately, 30% of pre-lingual hearing loss consists of syndromal deafness, the remaining 70% consists of non-syndromal deafness (Smith et al., 2004). Most people affected by syndromal and more than half with non-syndromal deafness would be eligible for referral to genetic counselling services. Therefore, within the UK alone there are likely to be several hundred thousand people for whom genetic counselling is relevant; within the world this number could reach millions.

People with an inherited form of deafness may have numerous similarly affected relatives within their family and may use a National Sign Language (NSL) (e.g. BSL) as their preferred language. They may also choose to mix and socialise with other d/Deaf people and as such may choose to have a partner who is d/Deaf. Some researchers have suggested that approximately 90% of Deaf individuals marry another d/Deaf person (not including individuals with late onset deafness) (Schein, 1989, in Prezioso, 1995). It is thought that 70% of d/Deaf couples who have only deaf children are thought to have their deafness because of alterations in the Connexin 26 gene (Nance et al., 2000).

MEDICAL OR CULTURAL MODEL?

The 'pathological' or 'medical' model perceives deafness as a medical defect to be treated, corrected or cured. For example, an ENT surgeon would advocate the use of cochlear implants and an audiologist prescribes hearing aids, both taking the perspective that to be hearing, or as close to this as possible, is the preferred option for the client. However, this perspective starkly contrasts the way deafness is perceived via the 'cultural' or 'linguistic' model. Here deafness is not viewed as a disability, but rather a way of life, often identified via communication using sign language. People who consider themselves 'culturally Deaf' do not feel disabled or 'impaired' with respect to this. They feel empowered by their language, they have a positive identity attached to their deafness and they tend to mix and socialise with many other Deaf people (Padden, 1980; Arnos et al., 1991; Christiansen, 1991). Deaf identity is something that evolves over time, the process of establishing an identity is influenced by the interactions deaf people have with other deaf people and also their hearing peers (Ohna, 2004).

Although exact figures are not known it is thought that there are at least 50,000 deaf people in the UK who use British Sign Language (BSL) as their first or preferred language (RNID, 2006a), and therefore may consider themselves 'culturally Deaf'. It is likely that many of these people come from families where there are numerous relatives with an inherited deafness. There is a large and vibrant 'Deaf culture' in many countries across the world, e.g. in the UK, USA, Netherlands, Sweden, Norway, Germany, Australia etc.

Being a member of the Deaf community is not determined by audiological level of hearing loss (Woll & Ladd, 2003). Although most people will have a congenital or early onset, profound level of deafness, there are many people with this audiological assessment who would consider themselves more associated to the hearing world. Conversely there are culturally Deaf people who have a relatively mild level of hearing loss and residual hearing.

Ninety per cent of deaf children are born to hearing parents (Cohen & Gorlin, 1995). Such deaf children may not have easy access to Deaf role models if they do not automatically have similarly affected relatives. This means that they may not develop their Deaf identity until they start school and begin to mix with other d/Deaf children through groups and clubs. If they are brought up in a mainstream school and an oral environment then they may not have an affinity with the Deaf community at all, or not until adulthood. However, studies have shown that those d/Deaf people who are able to accept, mix and work with the values of both the hearing world and the Deaf community appear to have the highest levels of self-esteem (Bat-Chava, 1994, in Calderon & Greenberg, 2003). Calderon and Greenberg (2003) argue that Deaf role models are vital throughout the education of deaf children, whether they are part of a hearing or deaf education system.

NEWBORN HEARING SCREENING PROGRAMME

As the majority of deaf children are born into hearing families a diagnosis of deafness may be delayed – due to parents and health professionals neither anticipating nor specifically looking out for it. The Newborn Hearing Screening Programme offers the opportunity to screen all newborn babies audiologically for deafness and, as such, means that deafness can be diagnosed much earlier than ever before (Cone-Wesson, 2003). The hope of this is that appropriate communication and educational tools can be implemented as early as possible thereby giving the deaf child the best possible chance of 'normal' development (Sass-Lehrer & Bodner-Johnson, 2003). By delaying a diagnosis, this may delay the acquisition of effective language. The knock-on effect of this on emotional and cognitive development can be enormous.

There is discussion as to whether genetic testing, e.g. for Connexin 26, should be an automatic part of the Newborn Hearing Screening Programme, so that both the audiological hearing loss and also the genetic cause are identified (Arnos & Pandya, 2003). There is some slight resistance to this, however, due to concern that such testing, although useful for parents to know what caused their child's deafness, may give the impression that pre-natal genetic testing for the next pregnancy should be utilised (Middleton, 2002a) and there is much resistance to the use of this from both deaf and hearing people (Middleton et al., 2001).

GENETIC COUNSELLING

Deaf individuals are often interested to know if and how they have inherited their deafness and what the chances are of passing this on to children (Arnos et al., 1992). These are questions that can be addressed by the clinical service of genetic counselling. Such a service is provided by genetic counsellors and clinical geneticists working in the Clinical Genetics department, found in most major teaching hospitals across many areas in the UK and elsewhere throughout the world.

Genetic counselling in general is 'the process by which patients or relatives at risk of a disorder that may be hereditary are [informed] of the consequences of the disorder, [and] the probability of developing or transmitting it' (Harper, 1993). Genetic counselling not only offers information about issues relating to genetics and inheritance, it also offers a supportive and non-judgemental environment, following a 'non-directive' code, where clients are neither advised nor coerced with regards to decisions.

Both geneticists and genetic counsellors undertake a genetic evaluation. It is usual for there to be overlap between the work that both these health professionals do. However, broadly speaking, one of the main differences between the roles is that any physical or diagnostic examination would be done by the doctor (geneticist) and, once a diagnosis is established, longer-term follow-up and support as well as information giving can be provided by the genetic counsellor. A medical history is taken and also a physical examination is carried out on the client to evaluate whether there could be a syndromal cause to the deafness. Medical records for relatives may also be collected for comparison and the obstetric history of the client's mother is documented. Genetic testing via a blood sample may be offered, which may confirm the clinical investigations.

Several hundred genes are known to be involved with deafness (Van Camp & Smith, 2006). Alterations in the Connexin 26 gene, are thought to account for up to 50% of genetic cases of childhood deafness, with 1 in 31 people carrying this gene in certain populations (Estivill et al., 1998; Kelley et al., 1998). Deafness resulting from Connexin 26 gene alterations is typically severe – profound and congenital (Mueller et al., 1999); however, there are also reports of people with mild – moderate loss too (Cohn et al., 1999). A result of the molecular genetic research means that, for certain families, it is possible to define whether a specific gene alteration has caused a person's deafness and subsequently, what the chances are of passing this on to children. Such testing and information relating to this is provided within the genetic counselling service.

Some people request genetic counselling with the aim of preventing genetic disorders from being passed on in their family, others simply want information so that they are better informed of the chances of passing on a specific genetic condition. Families may be interested in finding out the medical basis to their hearing loss, just for information's sake to 'piece together the jigsaw' or because they want to make specific decisions relating to having children.

Pre-natal genetic testing for deafness is not a service that is routinely available within genetic counselling and requests for this are few and far between. Most families are just interested to know if their deafness is genetic and what the chances are (for preparation) of passing this on to children (Middleton et al., 2001). However, pre-implantation genetic diagnosis for Connexin 26 deafness has been requested, where two hearing parents wanted to avoid having deaf children (Australasian Bioethics Information, 2002; Kelly, 2002).

There are often myths surrounding why deafness is present in a family. Many people make reproductive decisions based on assumption rather than medical information. The following case studies are examples of this.

CASE STUDY 1

One deaf couple known to the author through her work as a genetic counsellor were so frightened of having deaf children that they had decided not to have children. The burden that they attached to their own deafness meant that they felt a heavy responsibility to not 'inflict' this on their children. However, through genetic testing it was revealed that their chances of having deaf children were minimal. They were delighted with this news.

CASE STUDY 2

Another Deaf couple had assumed that their deafness was not inherited because they both came from hearing families; they were then surprised when their two children were born deaf. Genetic testing revealed that they were both deaf due to an alteration in the Connexin 26 gene and as a consequence all their children would be born deaf, they were also delighted with this news. They had a strong Deaf identity and, although their hearing families hoped that deafness would not be inherited, as a couple, they were really pleased to pass on their deafness, their language and culture to their children.

Both couples welcomed the opportunity to discuss their concerns about family planning and the process of genetic counselling and testing meant that they were better informed about their genetic heritage. This in turn meant that they were better able to psychologically engage in their future. They also had the opportunity to confidentially express the burden and responsibility they felt with respect to passing (or not) deafness on to their children. This was provided within a sensitive environment away from the perceived 'pressure' from their family and community.

The process of genetic counselling for deafness is therefore of direct relevance to the millions of d/Deaf people across the world with inherited deafness. However, generally the uptake for genetic counselling from such d/Deaf clients in the UK is very low. There are many possible reasons why this might be: d/Deaf people may just not be interested in knowing why they are deaf or what the chances of having deaf children are, although clinicians working with d/Deaf adults would indicate otherwise (Arnos et al., 1992). Other reasons may relate to fear of genetic services; this issue is addressed below.

DEAFNESS, EUGENICS, GENETICS AND ATTITUDES

Culturally Deaf people may often have quite negative attitudes towards genetic technology (Middleton, 2002b). The views of a collective group of culturally Deaf people attending a conference called the 'Deaf Nation' at the University of Central Lancashire, UK, in 1997 were studied to ascertain attitudes towards genetics (Middleton et al., 1998a, 1998b). Delegates were asked to complete a questionnaire which documented their views about genetic technology and how they felt about its use with respect to deafness (e.g. genetic testing in pregnancy for deafness). Of the 87 delegates who completed questionnaires, 55% thought that genetic testing for deafness would 'do more harm than good'; 46% thought that its potential use 'devalued d/Deaf people', and 49% were concerned about new discoveries in genetics (Middleton et al., 1998a, 1998b). This group indicated that they felt really threatened by the perceived 'misuse' of genetic technology, the biggest fear relating to pre-natal genetic testing for deafness followed by selective termination of pregnancy if the foetus was deaf. If this fear were realised then the net result of such actions could be the demise of the Deaf community.

A much larger study has since been completed (n = 1314), which replicated many of the above views. Here the attitudes of d/Deaf, hard of hearing and deafened adults as well as hearing parents of deaf children were documented (Middleton et al., 2001). This study indicated that Deaf people have quite different attitudes from those who do not identify with the Deaf culture including hard of hearing/deafened adults and hearing parents of deaf children. Those who mix more in the hearing world tend to have quite positive attitudes towards genetic technology. The majority of all participant groups indicated that not many people would actually be interested in using pre-natal genetic testing for deafness with selective termination of pregnancy involving a deaf foetus, which is a fear of the Deaf community. This work was completed in the

UK and has also been replicated in the US (Stern et al., 2002), with similar findings. Therefore, it is very unlikely at the moment that the Deaf community would diminish through the use of genetic technology. Nevertheless the perceived fear in relation to this is enormous.

HISTORICAL CONTEXT

Throughout history there have been numerous attempts to suppress and even deliberately destroy the Deaf community. Alexander Graham Bell (inventor of the telephone and leader of the eugenics movement) delivered a paper in 1883 called 'Memoir Upon the Formation of a Deaf Variety of the Human Race' to the National Academy of Sciences. In this he advocated that deaf people should marry hearing people (as opposed to other deaf people) so that they could reduce the chances of passing on deafness to their children (Bell, 1883). Despite his great respect for d/Deaf people (his own mother was deaf and so too was his wife) he took the view that deafness was a great disability and should be avoided if at all possible. Hitler during the Second World War advocated that d/Deaf children and adults should be sterilised so that they could not pass on deafness to their children; indeed 16,000–17,000 deaf people suffered sterilisation. In addition to this, other d/Deaf people were killed as part of 'Operation T4' the Nazi programme designed to destroy disabled citizens – all part of the eugenic pursuit of the perfect Aryan race (Biesold, 1999, in Schuchman, 2004).

Given the evidence above and many other attempts throughout history to prevent d/Deaf people from having children – all with the (often incorrect) assumption that deafness is always inherited, it is not surprising that d/Deaf people are often suspicious of modern-day genetics services. The very fact that pre-natal genetic testing for deafness with selective termination of pregnancy for a deaf foetus is even possible is enough for Deaf people to feel that there is another eugenic agenda being impressed upon them. There is a feeling that, historically, genetics services (and 'why should modern-day services be any different!') have devalued the role of Deaf people in society. It is therefore imperative that genetic counsellors and geneticists are mindful of the context within which they practise.

It is important to offer a 'culturally neutral' genetic counselling service (Arnos & Pandya, 2004), where Deaf clients are neither judged nor stereotyped. Assumptions should not be made about preferences for having deaf or hearing children and genetic counsellors should be aware of the historical sensitivity of such issues.

DEAF PEOPLE'S CLINICAL SERVICE REQUIREMENTS

The following sections consider the requirements of a clinical service for d/Deaf people. The UK Disability Discrimination Act (1995) gives some guidance on specific issues to consider in relation to communication and access to services.

THE DISABILITY DISCRIMINATION ACT (DDA)

The Disability Discrimination Act (DDA) 1995 in the UK prevents d/Deaf people from being discriminated against by any service providers, including the Health Service and hospitals (RNID, 2006b). This means that the health profession needs to ensure that communication issues are addressed, for example through the installation of text-based and video-based information and telephone systems as well as providing access to qualified interpreters supporting the preferred language of deaf clients. In an ideal world all health professionals would have Deaf awareness training and those working regularly with deaf clients would be proficient in signed language and lipspeaking.

The following sections give consideration to the different forms of communication tool that d/Deaf people may use.

COMMUNICATION

Deaf and hard of hearing individuals use a variety of different forms of communication: speech, National Signed Language (NSL), Signed Supported Spoken Language (SSSL), which refers to the sign language which can be a literal translation of spoken language for any country, lip-reading, writing, reading, cued speech, use of non-verbal cues through gesturing and facial expressions. Particularly within a counselling context, effective communication does not always have to mean fluency in language – the use of non-verbal cues, facial expressions and body language all offer a form of communication that can express what a person is feeling sometimes more than a language can. NSL has its own grammatical structure and is different from SSSL which usually follows the pattern of speech.

Lip-reading

It is important to give clear lip-patterns when speaking to a d/Deaf person, without obstructing these features (e.g. by chewing gum, eating food, or covering the mouth with hair or a hand or even a beard or moustache). It is also important to maintain eye contact and not repeatedly look away, for example, at a computer or set of patient records.

Speech

Profoundly d/Deaf people may not always be able to effectively communicate using speech. Individuals from large culturally Deaf families may use very little speech, if any. This means that conversations in a clinic setting that are totally focused around speech can be difficult. Deaf people will often have very good voice control and their speech may be quite clear. However, this can some- times be rather misleading to the hearing person, who wrongly assumes that all they are saying is being understood. As with any conversation, where one person is communicating in a different language, it is important not to make assumptions about the level of understanding. Checking this out throughout the conversation can help. The focus of good communication not only applies to the consultation, it needs to be in place right from the moment the indi vidual or family are referred, through to when they walk through the door of the genetics clinic, including the interaction with receptionist. The staff in the genetics clinic should know how to use IT that Deaf people use (e.g. by being famililar with TypeTalk or similar telephone relay services or having a mobile phone texting or video-phone service to inform about changes to clinic times). The receptionist needs to make sure they approach the Deaf person sitting in the waiting room to let them know visually of their consultation. Simple things like not calling out the client's name in the waiting room are easily overlooked yet so easy to put right.

Reading/writing skills

It has sometimes been the case that deaf children fall behind their hearing counterparts in reading and writing skills (Holt et al., 1992, in Ralston & Israel, 1995). Some older research has indicated that the average reading age of an 18 19-year-old deaf student fits that of an 8–9-year-old hearing student (Paul, 1998, 2003; Traxler, 2000). This may be due to the learning environment within which the deaf person was taught, or may be because English is the second language (with signed language as the preferred language thus using a differ- ent grammar and sentence construction). It is possible therefore that some deaf adults have difficulty in reading forms or questionnaires and written instruction. It is important not to assume that these difficulties are due to any problems with intellect. More recent research from Europe has suggested that deaf children who have deaf parents are more likely to have better educa- tional achievement than deaf children with hearing parents (Kramer, 2005). The assumption here is that having a positive role model in the family who understands how to solve communication issues leads to better academic achievement. However, aside from this it is still worth making sure that any written instruction from the clinic is clear, brief (short sentences) and Deaf- friendly (by checking with someone fluent in sign language).

The genetic counselling teams can produce information in NSL for delivery via DVD and video. The information can be given in NSL and also voice over in spoken language with subtitles (Belk & Middleton, 2004). This is a very useful tool for providing equal access to services and also complies with the Disability Discrimination Act (1995).

Communication over the telephone

Deaf people often have high levels of technological literacy. This may involve the routine use of the computer, text messaging and videophones, as well as more traditional text telephones (see Harkins & Bakke, 2003, for an overview). This technology can be incorporated into clinical practice.

Relay telephone systems also exist in the UK with information relayed to the deaf person via their text telephone through an operator.

Communication in a clinic setting

When choosing a sign language interpreter it is important to first check what sort of language is to be used. Interpretation of NSL is different from SSSL, which is different again from lipspeaking. It is also important to double-check whether the client would rather bring their own interpreter. As the local Deaf community may be small, confidentiality may be difficult to maintain and so clients may prefer to choose someone they know already. Alternatively they may prefer to use someone completely unconnected and not part of their local community (hearing interpreters are often involved in the Deaf community, and may be hearing children of Deaf parents themselves).

Whatever the situation, it is important to check whether the interpreter has interpreted genetic or even medical consultations before. If not, then it would be important to speak or meet with them beforehand to check their understanding and discuss ways that they intend to use when interpreting terms that they may not have encountered before. It is not sufficient to assume that the medical consultation will be interpreted word for word or even concept for concept with the inflection and tone of speech. There will almost certainly be differences, which unless specifically asked about, and checked, the hearing clinician will be unaware of.

Most hospitals in the UK use an agency of registered interpreters, or alternatively local freelance interpreters (agencies charge a booking fee, all interpreters charge travel costs and a minimum call-out charge on top of their fee). Interpreting is demanding and breaks are needed every half-an-hour or so (RNID, 2006d). Although ideally two interpreters should be booked, if a whole afternoon of interpreting is needed, this is not always possible. It is useful to discuss with the interpreter and the Deaf client the seating arrangements and the lighting before the consultation. It is important to talk directly to the Deaf person and maintain eye contact with them at all times. It is important not to ask the interpreter for opinions as they are meant to be neutral rather than an advocate for the Deaf person. Afterwards, as part of the feedback process, check with the Deaf person as to whether the interpreting arrangements were satisfactory (BDA fact sheet, 2005b)

Interpreters take recognised qualifications after many years of approved training (RNID, 2006d). They are highly qualified professionals and will often specialise in specific types of work, e.g. medical, theatre, law courts etc. It is important to use someone who is registered through a national agency or has an accreditation for interpreters in the chosen NSL. There is usually a directory of qualified interpreters in each country.

Lipspeakers

'Lipspeakers' are interpreters who help d/Deaf people use speech and lipreading. The lipspeaker sits next to the hearing person who is speaking, they repeat what is being said (without using their voice) using clear lip patterns that the lip-reader may find easier to follow. They can also use fingerspelling, gesture and facial expression as well as other cues that show the phrasing and emphasis of the spoken work. Normal speech uses up to 200 words a minute. It may be very difficult for a person lip-reading to compute this many words, so a lipspeaker can use less words without losing the intended meaning. Lipspeaking is skilful and involves detailed training (RNID, 2006e).

Electronic notetakers

There are different forms of note taking, all very similar. An electronic notetaker uses a laptop to type up a summary of spoken language, not every word is typed, the notetaker summarises what is being said. The d/Deaf person could network their computer to the notetaker's so that they can also communicate to each other. As a notetaker is summarising the spoken conversation the written interpretation is delayed and does not happen in real time.

Speech-to-text (STT) reporters use a specially designed keyboard that enables every spoken word to be phonetically transcribed by a software programme into text. This makes it quicker and easier to keep up with the pace of spoken language and requires the d/Deaf person to be able to read at high speed. STT reporters use Palantype® or Stenograph® in the UK (RNID, 2006f, 2006g).

GENETIC COUNSELLING CONSULTATIONS

Timing of consultations

Most genetic counselling consultations in the UK last between 45 minutes and an hour. As there is often much technical and clinical information to explain as well as emotional issues to address, it is usual for a post-clinic letter or leaflet to be sent afterwards that summarises the consultation. However, as mentioned above, if reading and writing skills are different from those of hearing counterparts, then this method for summarising information may not be very helpful. In addition to this, within the clinic consultation if memory-processing skills are being employed in the interpretation of language, then these will not immediately be so readily available to reinforce the technical information. Therefore, in these sorts of consultations, it is important to keep them shorter than normal and more frequent. So, instead of having a 1-hour consultation, it might be more useful to have two half-hour sessions instead. It would also be helpful to revisit the same concepts several times and rephrase them in different ways to help them embed in the d/Deaf client's memory.

Use of language

If a genetics professional is aware that a d/Deaf client does not view having a deaf child as a problem, then it would be insensitive to talk to them in terms of there being a 'risk' of having a deaf child or else referring to deafness as 'abnormal' and hearing as 'normal' within the genetic counselling process. Instead the geneticist or genetic counsellor would talk about the 'chance' of having a deaf child and use the terms 'deafness' and 'hearing' as they are without saying either is 'abnormal'. In addition to this, terms like 'mutation' and 'gene fault' also have negative connotations attached to them and so could be replaced with gene 'alteration' or 'change' instead.

Taking a pedigree

In order to make a genetic evaluation for a d/Deaf client the first piece of information collected is the family tree or pedigree; this should cover at least three generations. The hearing status and health of each individual is documented. For clients who are not aware of the details of their relatives, genetic evaluation is still possible as other data is collected too. The ethnic background of the family is relevant and so too is whether there is consanguinity (cousin or intermarriage in the family).

The experience of delayed or difficult communication between a deaf child and his/her hearing parents may lead to a feeling of exclusion in the home, a consequence of this is that there could be less knowledge about the family history (Israel & Arnos, 1995). Therefore, d/Deaf adults from hearing families may have less information about family relations to offer within pedigree taking than one might expect. It is not unusual for the genetic counsellor to be asked to telephone the hearing family on behalf of the d/Deaf client, to find out details for the pedigree. But d/Deaf adults from deaf families, who have grown up with a closeness to their relatives via a shared language, are more likely to have easier access to personal information about their family pedigree.

COUNSELLING ISSUES

Hearing children learn to express their emotions through voice and language; they are also taught to label their feelings via spoken interaction with their parents. However, sometimes deaf children born to a hearing family may have a delay in acquiring their communication skills and therefore may have a delay in emotional and cognitive processes (Henderson & Hendershott, 1991, in Ralston & Israel, 1995). This means that as d/Deaf adults they may find it more difficult to express and describe emotions (although it is important not to over-generalise this issue). Describing and expressing emotion can be a part of the genetic counselling consultation and so it is important to be aware that d/Deaf adults may do this differently from hearing adults.

There is much written about the social and emotional development of deaf children (e.g. Greenberg & Kusche, 1989, in Calderon & Greenberg 2003). Calderon and Greenberg (2003) summarise some of this work: 'deaf children are often delayed in language development, tend to show . . . poorer emotional regulation, and often have an impoverished vocabulary or emotion language'. Not everyone agrees with this negative labelling and can provide many examples of positive emotional expression amongst deaf children. The literature on the emotional development of d/Deaf people is somewhat controversial and there is much research to demonstrate that d/Deaf adults are resilient and able to overcome negative influences – the deafness may not impact negatively if the family environment is supportive, if the parents adapt and cope with the deafness and if there are adequate community and education resources available (Calderon, 2000; Stinson & Foster, 2000, in Calderon & Greenberg, 2003).

With regards to the emotional engagement within a clinical setting, d/Deaf adults may have a different emotional language and expression from hearing clients, depending on their life experience. However, this difference should not be viewed as deficient in any way.

Genetic counselling for deafness is of relevance to all sorts of people with differing backgrounds, many of whom will have different perspectives and experiences of deafness. The following groups and the specific nuances relating to each group are all considered in turn in the following sections.

Hearing parents of deaf children

The birth of a deaf child to hearing parents with no experience or understanding of deafness can be perceived as devastating to the parents and their extended family (Luterman & Ross, 1991, in Israel, 1995). There are many factors that may influence the grieving process as parents try to make sense of their situation. Eventual acceptance of the child as deaf may be influenced by these factors: prior perceptions of deafness, expectations and attitudes of friends and relatives, economic issues, stress factors in the family, previous coping strategies and relationships with health professionals and education network (Calderon & Greenberg, 1993, in Israel, 1995).

Hearing parents of deaf children are often very keen to understand what has caused their child's deafness, they may blame themselves and look to the pregnancy to see what could have gone wrong. Some research has suggested that the unexpected birth of a deaf child may cause parents to feel they are being punished in some way (Vernon & Andrews, 1990, in Israel, 1995). It is therefore very important that accurate and sensitive information is given about the causes of deafness, and this can be done via genetic counselling: 'parents must know, when possible, the cause of the child's deafness to realistically face issues about which they would otherwise fantasize' (Mindel & Feldman, 1987, in Israel, 1995).

With respect to genetics issues, hearing parents of deaf children generally have positive views. In a study looking at the attitudes of a group of 527 hearing adults with a family history of deafness (most of whom were parents of deaf children), the majority chose positive as opposed to neutral or negative words to describe their feelings about new discoveries in genetics, the most frequently chosen word was 'hopeful' (Middleton et al., 2001).

Four hundred and thirty-two parents of deaf children were asked specific questions about their family and children and attitudes towards testing in pregnancy for deafness; 69% said they preferred to have hearing children (as opposed to not minding the hearing status of future children); 53% said they would be interested to find out whether a baby is deaf or hearing before it was born (i.e. have a pre-natal genetic test); most of these said they would just want this information for preparation purposes rather than so that they could have an abortion if the foetus was deaf; however, 16% said they would consider this. The majority (67%) felt their deaf children were disadvantaged because of their hearing loss (which was not the case for many d/Deaf parents), and most felt there was some to great 'burden' for them attached to having a child who is deaf. More than 80% said, if it were possible, they would want a cure for their child's deafness. When asked about support at the time of the deafness diagnosis more than half the group (52%) said they felt they did not receive enough support from the health professionals. However, most said they received the required support from family and friends (Middleton, 2005).

Therefore, for this group of clients, attending a genetic counselling consultation, there tends to be quite a lot of interest as to why the deafness is present which is coupled with negative emotions surrounding the deafness. This group is most commonly referred for genetic counselling.

Deaf adults with hearing parents

The experience of growing up in a hearing family may be daunting for deaf children if the parents and extended family are unsure how to cope and adapt to the specific needs associated with deafness. If parents struggle to communicate with their child and the child never really feels understood by their parents then this can lead to a very difficult experience that could conceivably impact on the d/Deaf person as an adult. This could also mould their own attitudes towards having deaf children. However, if hearing parents make every attempt to establish communication channels (e.g. by learning sign language or helping children to lip-read and encourage their speech) and so too does the extended family, then this will help in all aspects of the child's development.

The perceived success of communication between parents and their deaf children has been documented. A study of 108 deaf/hard of hearing parents of deaf children reported that 67% felt that they communicated 'very successfully' with their deaf children, whereas only 33% of the 432 hearing parents of deaf children felt this was true. The vast majority of hearing parents felt the communication with their deaf child was less than perfect. Indeed 18% of this latter group said they felt communication issues were only OK or even poor (Middleton, 2005). Deaf adults who have hearing parents may feel an emotional distance between themselves and their parents, particularly if the hearing parents struggled to communicate with them when they were children.

Given the issues documented in the previous section about hearing parents' attitudes towards the impact of deafness on their children, it is easy to see how deaf children may develop low self-esteem as they grow into d/Deaf adults. Deaf and hearing researchers have suggested this can be overcome by developing positive interactions with deaf and hearing peers at school (Antia & Kriemeyer, 2003) and also through the provision of specific education systems and the incorporation of Deaf role models (Calderon & Greenberg, 2003).

Some deaf parents have said that they would choose not to have deaf children if it could be avoided (Middleton, 2005). One participant in this research said they 'would not wish deafness on [their] worst enemy'. This highlighted the negative personal experience they had while growing up with a hearing loss and struggle they had within a mainstream hearing society. But other Deaf parents of deaf children felt the experience was positive – they were lucky to have the opportunity to pass on their language, history and culture, as well as deafness, to their children and they were proud of this (Middleton, 2005).

Deaf parents of deaf children

Ten per cent of d/Deaf couples have deaf children (Cohen & Gorlin, 1995). The process of genetic counselling for deafness can be complicated as Deaf people often marry and have children with other Deaf people. As there are so many different genetic causes behind deafness, two people within a couple (particularly when there have been multiple d/Deaf relationships within the same family) may have complex and multiple genetic predispositions. This means the calculation of 'genetic risk' and the inheritance pattern may not be straightforward. A study of the frequency of Connexin 26 gene changes showed that families where there was deafness in both the parents and their children (n = 43), 42% had this due to Connexin 26 (Pandya et al., 2003).

The birth of a deaf child to d/Deaf parents may not be a total surprise but may still elicit a mixed response. Much depends on the d/Deaf parents' own values and beliefs about their deafness and the place of deafness in society.

Deaf parents of deaf children are much more likely than hearing parents of deaf children to feel that their deaf children do not place a burden on the family (Middleton, 2005). They are also more likely to feel that the deafness in their children is more of an advantage than disadvantage: one deaf parent (who did not identity with the Deaf community) said she felt an advantage in having deaf children as '*I could share my skills and knowledge of deafness. I could understand her needs better*'. Another deaf parent of deaf children said: '*being deaf myself, the children were advantaged as I knew what the problems were and knew what to do*'. Finally, one culturally Deaf parent of deaf children said: '*at home we're all deaf so [the children] never felt left out. It's society without "deaf awareness" that made them feel disadvantaged! Otherwise we are all happy and [a] close-knit family with [the] same rich language [and] culture*' (Middleton, 2005).

Hearing children and adults with deaf parents

Approximately 90% of d/Deaf couples have hearing children (Israel, 1995). The birth of a hearing child to d/Deaf parents can often lead to a feeling of confusion (Hoffmeister, 1985, in Israel, 1995). In a family that only uses sign language it is much easier for a hearing child to learn sign language first and spoken language second. Research has shown that normal speech and language can develop in a hearing child from a d/Deaf family if that child has contact with hearing speakers approximately 5–10 hours per week (Schiff-Myers, 1988, in Israel, 1995).

A hearing child born to d/Deaf parents may be used by their d/Deaf parents as the link between the Deaf and hearing world. Hearing children may be used as interpreters for their Deaf parents and this may be inappropriate as well as appropriate in different situations. Hearing children within d/Deaf families may be perceived as having the 'best of both worlds' – they can participate in the Deaf culture with their family, but also have access to the hearing world too. However, in order to develop a 'healthy psychosocial perspective' hearing children/adults of d/Deaf parents need to maintain a balance in the relationship between these cultures (Myers & Marcus, 1993, in Israel, 1995).

ETHICAL CONSIDERATIONS: CHOOSING TO HAVE DEAF CHILDREN

For culturally Deaf families, where there are many relatives in the family who are d/Deaf, there may be a preference for having deaf children. This concept is not new and has been well documented in the past (Hoffmeister, 1985; Dolnick, 1993; Erting, 1994; Israel, 1995; Middleton et al., 1998a). Research from the author has indicated that a very small number of d/Deaf people may consider the application of pre-natal genetic testing for deafness with selective termination of pregnancy if the foetus was likely to be hearing. One participant in this study indicated that she wanted to avoid having hearing children as she worried they would not learn speech and be taken away from her by social services (UK) (Middleton et al., 2001; Middleton, 2004).

Deaf adults may be interested to use genetic counselling so that they can find out their genetic heritage and use this to choose a suitable d/Deaf partner with whom they can have deaf children. At Gallaudet University, Washington, DC, the author met many d/Deaf students who were interested in the process of genetic counselling. One student said that she knew her deafness was due to having two gene alterations in the Connexin 26 gene; she said she would be interested to know if any future partners also had their deafness due to Connexin 26 as she wanted to ensure that her children would be deaf.

At the time of publication no readily available, published medical evidence indicates whether any d/Deaf parents have chosen to actually use pre-natal genetic testing with selective termination of pregnancy for a hearing foetus. However, there are unsubstantiated suggestions within the genetics field to suggest that this may have been done. Given the worldwide negative press that Deaf people have received in relation to this issue, it is not surprising that neither d/Deaf parents nor the genetics professionals seeing them would advertise such an issue openly.

In 2002 a Deaf, lesbian couple from the US decided that they wanted to have another deaf child. Their deliberate choice to have a deaf child caused great debate across the world (e.g. Anstey, 2002; Fletcher, 2002; Levy, 2002; McLellan, 2002; Savulescu, 2002; Spriggs, 2002). The following are some comments from these articles:

Couples who select disabled rather than non-disabled offspring should be allowed to make those choices, even though they may be having a child with worse life prospects. (Savulescu, 2002)

Deaf people are behaving like hearing people. They feel good about themselves and want to have babies like them. Why should they be morally blamed? (Fletcher, 2002)

Cultures are simply the kind of things to which we are born, and therefore to which the children of deaf parents, hearing or deaf, normally belong. Thus these parents are making a mistake in choosing deafness for their children. Given their own experience of isolation as children, however, it is a mistake which is understandable, and our reaction to them ought to be compassion, not condemnation. (Levy, 2002)

VIEWS OF GENETICISTS AND GENETIC COUNSELLORS

It is not clear to what extent parents should be allowed to externally control the genetic makeup of their own children (American Medical Association, 1994). Within genetic counselling practice it is considered best practice to offer a 'non-directive' service where clients are not told what to do nor directed to make certain decisions. Therefore, it should be possible for a d/Deaf couple to have a pre-natal genetic test with selective termination of pregnancy for the absence of the gene faults for deafness (i.e. if the foetus is likely to be hearing). Offering preimplantation genetic diagnosis with active selection for embryos that have the gene faults for deafness, could also be possible. However, it is debatable whether hearing geneticists and genetic counsellors would feel comfortable with such a use of genetic technology.

Wertz and Fletcher (1999) asked genetics professionals across the world to comment on whether they would offer pre-natal genetic diagnosis to a d/Deaf couple wanting to have deaf children. Of those who said they would offer pre-natal genetic diagnosis with selective termination of pregnancy, 43% were from Cuba, 35% were from the US, 18% were from Canada, 9% were from the UK and 0% were from Norway. Those who were in favour of this used the 'autonomy' argument – i.e. if this is what the parent chose, and they were able to make a fully informed autonomous decision, then this was acceptable to the genetics professional.

THE HUMAN RIGHTS ACT

The Human Rights Act 1998 brings the European Convention on Human Rights into UK law (RNID, 2006c). This is particularly relevant to d/Deaf parents. The Act protects the rights of d/Deaf parents not to be discriminated against. For example, a d/Deaf couple should not be told they couldn't have children because they might pass deafness on. They must also not be told to end a pregnancy if there is a chance their baby might be deaf. Deaf couples also obviously have a right to fertility treatment. In terms of whether they could use the Act to gain support for actively creating a deaf child, via implementation of genetic technology, it is not clear whether this would be covered.

THE BRITISH DEAF ASSOCIATION POLICY ON GENETICS

The 'Sign Community' or British Deaf Association (BDA) is 'the UK's largest national organisation run by Deaf people for Deaf people' (SignCommunity website) It does stress concern over the use of pre-natal genetic testing with the selective termination of 'deaf' pregnancies and *demands* that: 'all genetic counsellors should receive Deaf awareness training to ensure a clear understanding of the Deaf community and Deaf culture . . . [and that] . . . parents are not formally or informally pressured to take pre-natal tests or to undergo termination where it is discovered that the foetus is deaf' (BDA, 2005a).

Therefore, the BDA believe that d/Deaf and hearing parents attending a genetic counselling consultation in the UK currently do not receive adequate information to enable them to make informed decisions about deafness and intend to rectify this by implementing more Deaf awareness training among genetics professionals.

THE UK NATIONAL DEAF CHILDREN'S SOCIETY POLICY ON GENETICS

The National Deaf Children's Society also has a Policy on Genetics. In it they advocate choice and information:

> The Society . . . recognises the rights of potential parents from families who have a history of deafness to take advantage of genetic testing and ante-natal diagnosis and to use the results of such tests in a way that suits the individual family. If asked for advice, the Society will ensure that the family receives positive information about deafness in order to enable them to make an informed choice. (NDCS, 2005)

To date there is no consensus across the world on whether deliberately choosing to have deaf children should be endorsed by medical science. It is of interest and useful to know that Deaf parents may prefer to have Deaf children so that, within a clinical setting, there is awareness of and preparation for such attitudes. However, it is not useful to focus entirely on this view; only a very small number of Deaf people may ever consider this option.

CONCLUSIONS

Genetic counselling services for d/Deaf people and their relatives require a specialist knowledge of deafness, Deaf culture and the role that genetics has played within history for d/Deaf people. It is imperative that communication and language differences are embraced as well as attitudinal differences. Training in Deaf Awareness would be valuable for any health professional wanting to start working in this area.

Deaf people and their families are often very interested in the services offered by genetic counselling. With prior consideration of the nuances specific to the Deaf culture it is possible for genetics professionals to offer a culturally sensitive service.

Working with deaf people who use sign language as their first language is both interesting and rewarding. All health professionals who engage in this work enjoy learning from their clients. Hopefully this chapter has offered some ideas for health professionals thinking of entering this field as well as providing an overview for existing practitioners.

REFERENCES

American Medical Association (1994) Ethical issues related to prenatal genetic testing. *Archives of Family Medicine* 3: 633–42.

Anstey KW (2002) Are attempts to have impaired children justifiable? *Journal of Medical Ethics* 28: 286–8.

Antia SD, Kriemeyer KH (2003) Peer interaction of deaf and hard of hearing children. In M Marschark, PE Spencer (eds) *Oxford Handbook of Deaf Studies, Language and Education.* Oxford: Oxford University Press, pp. 164–76.

Arnos KS, Israel J, Cunningham M (1991) Genetic counselling of the deaf. Medical and cultural considerations. *Annals of the New York Academy of Science* 630: 212–22.

Arnos KS, Israel J, Devlin L, Wilson MP (1992) Genetic Counselling for the Deaf. *Otolaryngologic Clinics of North America* 25: 953–71.

Arnos KS, Israel J, Devlin L, Wilson M (1996) Genetic aspects of hearing loss in children. In J Clark, F Martin (eds) *Hearing Care in Children.* Needham Heights, MA: Allyn & Bacon, pp. 20–44.

Arnos KS, Pandya A (2003) Advances in the genetics of deafness. In M Marschark, PE Spencer (eds) *Oxford Handbook of Deaf Studies, Language and Education.* Oxford: Oxford University Press, pp. 392–405.

Arnos KS, Pandya A (2004) Genes for deafness and the genetics program at Gallaudet University. In JV Van Cleve (ed) *Genetics, Disability, and Deafness.* Washington, DC: Gallaudet University Press, pp. 111–27.

Australasian Bioethics Information (2002) Designer babies/go ahead to screen out deafness. *Australasian Bioethics Information Newsletter* [serial on the Internet]. 27 Sept. Available from: http://www.australasianbioethics.org/Newsletters/047-2002-09-27.html.

Bat-Chava Y (1994) Group identification and self esteem in deaf adults. *Personality and Social Psychology Bulletin* 20: 494–502.

Belk RA, Middleton A (2004) Seeing chromosomes – translating genetic information into British Sign Language. European Psychosocial Aspects of Genetics Conference, Munich, 12–15 June. Joint spoken presentation EWSO6. *European Journal of Human Genetics* 12 (Suppl 1): 355.

Bell AG (1883) Upon the formation of a deaf variety of the human race. *National Academy of Sciences Memoirs* 2: 177–262.

Biesold H (1999) *Crying Hands: Eugenics and Deaf People in Nazi Germany.* Washington, DC: Gallaudet University Press.

BDA (British Deaf Association) (2005a) Genetics policy statement. In-house publication, London.

BDA (British Deaf Association) (2005b) Factsheet on using a sing language interpreter. In-house publication, London.

Calderon R (2000) Parent involvement in deaf children's education programs as a predictor of child's language, reading, and social-emotional development. *Journal of Deaf Studies and Deaf Education* 5: 140–55.

Calderon R, Greenberg M (1993) Considerations in the adaptation of families with school-aged deaf children. In M Marschark, MD Clark (eds) *Psychological Perspectives on Deafness*. Hillsdale, NJ: Lawrence Erlbaum Associates, pp. 27–47.

Calderon R, Greenberg M (2003) Social and emotional development of deaf children. In M Marschark, PE Spencer (eds) *Oxford Handbook of Deaf Studies, Language and Education*. Oxford: Oxford University Press, pp. 177–89.

Christiansen JB (1991) Sociological implications of hearing loss. *Annals of the New York Academy of Sciences* 639: 230–5.

Cohen MM, Gorlin RJ (1995) Epidemiology, etiology and genetic patterns. In RJ Gorlin, H Toriello, MM Cohen (eds) *Hereditary Hearing Loss and Its Syndromes*. New York: Oxford University Press, pp. 9–21.

Cohn ES, Kelley PM, Fowler TW, Gorga MP, Lefkowitz DM, Kuehn HJ et al. (1999) Clinical studies of families with hearing loss attributable to mutations in the connexin 26 gene (GJB2/DFNB1). *Pediatrics* 103: 546–50.

Conc-Wesson B (2003) Screening assessment of hearing loss in infants. In M Marschark, PE Spencer (eds) *Oxford Handbook of Deaf Studies, Language and Education*. Oxford: Oxford University Press, pp. 420–33.

Davis A (1993) A public health perspective on childhood hearing impairment. In B McCormick (ed) *Practical Aspects of Audiology, Pediatric Audiology 0–5 Years*, 2nd edn. London: Whurr, pp. 1–41.

Disability Discrimination Act (1995) Code of Practice: rights of access – goods, facilities, services and premises. London: HMSO, 1999.

Dolnick E (1993) Deafness as culture. *Atlantic Monthly* 272(3): 37–53.

Ellis NC, Hennelley RA (1980) A bilingual word-length effect: implications for intelligence testing and the relative ease of mental calculation in Welsh and English. *British Journal of Psychology* 50: 449–58.

Erting C (1994) *Deafness, Communication, Social Identity: Ethnography in a Pre-school for Deaf Children*. Burtonsville, MD: Linstock Press.

Estivill X, Fortina P et al. (1998) Connexin-26 mutations in sporadic and inherited sensorineural deafness. *Lancet* 351: 394–8.

Fischer SD, van der Hulst H (2003) Sign language structures. In M Marschark, PE Spencer (eds) *Oxford Handbook of Deaf Studies, Language and Education*. Oxford: Oxford University Press, pp. 319–31.

Fletcher JC (2002) Deaf like us: The Duchesneau-McCullough case. *L'Observatoire de la genetique – Cadrages*. July/Aug (5).

Gibson I (2004) Summary: teaching strategies used to develop short-term memory in deaf children. *Deafness and Education International* 6: 171–2.

Gorlin RJ, Toriello HV, Cohen MM (eds) (1995) *Hereditary Hearing Loss and its Syndromes*. New York: Oxford University Press.

Greenberg M, Kusche C (1989) Cognitive, personal and social development of deaf children and adolescents. In MC Wang, MC Reynolds, HJ Walberg (eds) *Handbook of Special Education: Research and Practice (Vol. 1)*. Oxford: Pergamon Press, pp. 95–129.

Harkins JE, Bakke M (2003) Technologies for communication. In M Marschark, PE Spencer (eds) *Oxford Handbook of Deaf Studies, Language and Education*. Oxford, Oxford University Press, pp. 406–19.

Harper P (1993) *Practical Genetic Counselling*. Oxford: Butterworth-Heinemann.

Henderson D, Hendershott A (1991) ASL and the family system. *American Annals of the Deaf* 136: 325–9.

Hoffmeister RJ (1985) Families with deaf parents: a functional perspective. In KS Thurman (ed) *Children of Handicapped Parents: Research and Clinical Perspectives*. London: Academic Press, pp. 111–30.

Holt JA, Traxler CV, Allen TE (1992) *Interpreting the Scores: A User's Guide to the 8th Edition Stanford Achievement Test for Educators of Deaf and Hard of Hearing Students*. Washington, DC: Gallaudet Research Institute.

Israel J (1989) Counseling in deaf/hearing-impaired adult populations. *Perspectives in Genetic Counseling* 22: 1–4.

Israel J (1995) Psychosocial aspects of deafness: perspectives. In J Israel (ed) *An Introduction to Deafness: A Manual for Genetic Counsellors*. Washington, DC: Genetic Services Center, Gallaudet University, pp. 147–80.

Israel J, Arnos K (1995) Genetic evaluation and counselling strategies: the genetic services center experience. In J Israel (ed) *An Introduction to Deafness: A Manual for Genetic Counsellors*. Washington, DC: Genetic Services Center, Gallaudet University, pp. 181–208.

Kaplan H, Bally SJ, Garreston C (1987) *Speechreading: A Way to Improve Understanding*, 2nd edn. Washington, DC: Gallaudet University Press.

Kaplan H, Gladstone VS, Lloyd LL (1993) *Audiometric Interpretation: A Manual of Basic Audiometry*, 2nd edn. Boston: Allyn & Bacon.

Kelley PM, Harris DJ, Comer BC et al. (1998) Novel mutations in the connexin 26 gene (GJB2) that cause autosomal recessive (DFNB1) hearing loss. *American Journal of Human Genetics* 62: 792–9.

Kelly J (2002) Designer baby to have perfect hearing. *Herald Sun*, Sept 21.

Kramer S (2005) The impact of having a family history of hearing problems on those with hearing difficulties themselves: an open-ended and a structured questionnaire. Verbal presentation at the 'Genes, Hearing and Deafness' Conference, 17–19 March 2005, Caserta, Italy.

Levy N (2002) Deafness, culture and choice. *Journal Medical Ethics* 28(5): 284–5.

Luterman DM, Ross M (1991) *When Your Child Is Deaf: A Guide for Parents*. Parkton, MD: York Press.

McLellan F (2002) Controversy over deliberate conception of deaf child. *Lancet* 359(9314): 1315.

Marschark M (2003) Cognitive functioning in deaf adults and children. In M Marschark, PE Spencer (eds) *Oxford Handbook of Deaf Studies, Language and Education*. Oxford: Oxford University Press, pp. 464–77.

Middleton A, Hewison J, Mueller RF (1998a) Attitudes of deaf adults towards genetic testing for hereditary deafness. *American Journal of Human Genetics* 63: 1175–80.

Middleton A, Hewison J, Mueller RF (1998b) Attitudes of deaf adults towards testing in pregnancy for hereditary deafness. *Deaf Worlds* 14(3): 8.

Middleton A, Hewison J, Mueller RF (2001) Prenatal diagnosis for inherited deafness – what is the potential demand? *Journal of Genetic Counselling* 10: 121–31.

Middleton A (2002a) Pre-natal testing for deafness – attitudes and ethics. Department of Health Steering Group Conference on the Newborn Hearing Screening Programme, London, 3 Sept. 2002.

Middleton A (2002b) Genetics and the culturally Deaf. In *Nature Encyclopaedia of the Human Genome*. London: Macmillan Reference Ltd, Nature Publishing, Vol. 1. pp. 1062–64.

Middleton A (2004) Deaf and hearing adults' attitudes towards genetic testing for deafness. In JV Van Cleve (ed) *Genetics, Disability, and Deafness*. Washington, DC: Gallaudet University Press, pp. 127–47.

Middleton A (2005) Parents' attitudes towards genetic testing and the impact of deafness in the family. In D Stephens, L Jones (eds) *The Impact of Genetic Hearing Impairment*. London: Whurr, pp. 11–53.

Mindel ED, Feldman V (1987) The impact of deaf children on their families In ED Mindel, M Vernon (eds) *They Grow in Silence: Understanding Deaf Children and Adults*, 2nd edn. Boston: Little, Brown, pp. 1–29.

Mueller RF (1996) Genetic counselling for hearing impairment. In A Martini, A Read, D Stephens (eds) *Genetics and Hearing Impairment*. London: Whurr, pp. 255–64.

Mueller RF, Nehammer A, Middleton A et al. (1999) Congenital non-syndromal sensorineural hearing impairment due to connexin 26 gene mutations – molecular and audiological findings. *International Journal of Pediatric Otolaryngology* 50: 3–13.

Murray JJ (2004) 'True love and sympathy': the Deaf–Deaf marriages debate in transatlantic perspective. In J Vickery Van Cleve (ed) *Genetics, Disability and Deafness*. Washington, DC: Gallaudet University Press, pp. 42–71.

Myers R, Marcus A (1993) Hearing mother, father deaf: issues of identity and mediation in culture and communication. In *Deaf Studies III: Bridging Cultures in the 21st Century*. Washington, DC: College for Continuing Education, Gallaudet University, pp. 171–84.

Nance WE, Liu XZ, Pandya A (2000) Relation between choice of partner and high frequency of connexin 26 deafness. *Lancet* 356: 500–1.

NDCS (National Deaf Children's Society) (2005) Genetics and deafness – policy statement. London, accessed through http://www.ndcs.org.uk, last updated 2003.

Ohna SE (2004) Deaf in my own way: identity, learning and narratives. *Deafness and Education International* 6: 20–38.

Padden C (1980) The Deaf community and the culture of Deaf people. In S Wilcox (ed) *American Deaf Culture*. Silver Spring, MD: Linstock Press, pp. 1–16.

Pandya A, Arnos KS, Xia XJ, Welch KO, Blanton SH, Friedman TB et al. (2003) Frequency and distribution of GJB2 (Connexin 26) and GJB6 (Connexin 30) mutations in a large North American repository of deaf probands. *Genetics in Medicine* 5: 295–303.

Parving A (1996) Epidemiology of genetic hearing impairment. In A Martini, A Read, D Stephens (eds) *Genetics and Hearing Impairment*. London: Whurr, pp. 73–81.

Paul P (1998) *Literacy and Deafness: The Development of Reading, Writing, and Literate Thought*. Needham Heights, MA: Allyn & Bacon.

Paul PV (2003) Processes and components of reading. In M Marschark, PE Spencer (eds) *Oxford Handbook of Deaf Studies, Language and Education*. Oxford, Oxford University Press, pp. 97–109.

Prezioso CR (1995) Cultural aspects of deafness (the Deaf community). In J Israel (ed) *An Introduction to Deafness: A Manual for Genetic Counsellors*. Washington, DC: Genetic Services Center, Gallaudet University, pp. 131–46.

Ralston F, Israel J (1995) Language and communication. In J Israel (ed) *An Introduction to Deafness: A Manual for Genetic Counsellors*. Washington, DC: Genetic Services Center, Gallaudet University, pp. 63–84.

RNID (Royal National Institute for the Deaf) (2005a) Facts and figures on deafness and tinnitus. In-house publication. London, http://www.rnid.org.uk.

RNID (Royal National Institute for the Deaf) (2005b) The Disability Discrimination Act 1995 (DDA) – a guide for providers of goods, facilities and services. In-house publication. London, http://www.rnid.org.uk.

RNID (Royal National Institute for the Deaf) (2005c) The Human Rights Act 1998 – information for deaf and hard of hearing people. In-house publication. London, http://www.rnid.org.uk.

RNID (Royal National Institute for the Deaf) (2005d) Working with a BSL/English interpreter. In-house publication. London, http://www.rnid.org.uk.

RNID (Royal National Institute for the Deaf) (2005e) Lip-reading and lipspeaking. In-house publication. London, http://www.rnid.org.uk.

RNID (Royal National Institute for the Deaf) (2005f) Working with an electronic note-taker. In-house publication. London, http://www.rnid.org.uk.

RNID (Royal National Institute for the Deaf) (2005g) Working with a speech-to-text reporter. In-house publication. London, http://www.rnid.org.uk.

Sass-Lehrer M, Bodner-Johnson B (2003) Early intervention: current approaches to family-centred programming. In M Marschark, PE Spencer (eds) *Oxford Handbook of Deaf Studies, Language and Education*. Oxford: Oxford University Press, pp. 65–81.

Savulescu J (2002) Deaf lesbians, 'designer disability,' and the future of medicine. *British Medical Journal* 325: 771–3.

Schein DJ (1989) Family life. In *At Home with Strangers*. Washington, DC: Gallaudet University Press, pp. 106–34.

Schiff-Myers N (1988) Hearing children of deaf parents. In D Bishop, K Mogford (eds) *Language Development in Exceptional Circumstances*. New York: Churchill Livingstone, pp. 47–61.

Schuchman JS (2004) Deafness and eugenics in the Nazi era. In J Vickrey Van Cleve (ed) *Genetics, Disability and Deafness*. Washington, DC: Gallaudet University Press, pp. 72–8.

Smith RJH, Green GE, Van Camp G (2004) *Deafness and Hereditary Hearing Loss Overview*. Seattle: University of Washington. Last Revision: 15 July 2004. www.genereviews.org.

Spriggs M (2002) Lesbian couple create a child who is deaf like them. *Journal of Medical Genetics* 28: 283.

Stern SJ, Arnos KS, Murrelle L, Welch KO, Nance WE, Pandya A (2002) Attitudes of deaf and hard of hearing subjects toward genetic testing and prenatal diagnosis of hearing loss. *Journal of Medical Genetics* 39: 449–53.

Stinson MS, Foster S (2000) Socialization of deaf children and youths in school. In PE Spencer, CJ Erting, M Marschark (eds) *The Deaf Child in the Family and at School: Essays in Honor of Kathryn P Meadow-Orlans*. Hillsdale, NJ: Lawrence Erlbaum Associates, pp. 191–209.

Traxler C (2000) The Stanford Achievement Test, 9th edn: National norming and performance standards for deaf and hard of hearing students. *Journal of Deaf Studies and Deaf Education* 5: 337–48.

TypeTalk (2005) website: http://www.rnid-typetalk.org.uk/frame.html.

Van Camp G, Smith R (2006) Hereditary Hearing Loss Homepage. Antwerp: University of Antwerp [cited March 2006]. http://www.uia.ac.be/dnalab/hhh/.

Vernon M, Andrews J (eds) (1990) Psychodynamics surrounding the diagnosis of deafness. In *Psychology of Deafness – Understanding Deaf and Hard of Hearing People*, New York: Longman, pp. 119–36.

Wertz D, Fletcher J (1999) Ethics and genetics: in global perspective. Personal correspondence.

Woll B, Ladd P (2003) Deaf communities. In M Marschark, PE Spencer (eds) *Oxford Handbook of Deaf Studies, Language and Education*. Oxford: Oxford University Press, pp. 151–63.

19 Seeing Chromosomes: Improving Access to Culturally Sensitive Genetic Counselling through the Provision of Genetic Information in British Sign Language

RACHEL BELK

This chapter looks at one area of work undertaken over the last two years within a specialist genetic counselling post aiming to develop the service for d/Deaf people in a Regional Genetics Service in the UK. The post has particularly focused on identifying barriers to access and communication and ways in which these can be removed.

INTRODUCTION

The two central tenets of genetic counselling are that it should be provided from a non-judgemental standpoint and that it should work towards maximising the autonomy of the person(s) attending for genetic counselling by giving complete information in a non-directive manner. This emphasis on individual autonomy is the direction in which medicine has been moving since the latter part of the twentieth century, but clinical genetics has been debating and promoting this ethical stance for longer than most specialities. In no small part, this is because of the reaction against the legacy of the eugenics movement, which espoused explicit prejudice against individuals by emphasising the 'improvement' of the genetic health of the population through the non-reproduction of those individuals or families perceived to be at genetic disadvantage (Walker, 1998).

However, practitioners have debated at length whether totally non-directive genetic counselling can be achieved (Clarke, 1991; Clarke, 1997). One thread of the argument is that making an individual aware of the very existence of genetic tests for an inherited condition may give an implicit recommendation of their use. This may be regardless of the professional's own

The Effects of Genetic Hearing Impairment in the Family. Edited by D. Stephens and L. Jones.
Copyright © 2006 by John Wiley & Sons, Ltd.

views and the way in which the information is given. This is a particular concern in genetic counselling for deafness where the availability of tests could further emphasise the 'medicalisation' of deafness, highlighting the difference between this and the Deaf Community's perspective of deaf sign language users as a linguistic minority (Ridgeway, 2002; Middleton, 2005).

The discovery of genes causing syndromal and non-syndromal deafness, particularly Connexin 26 (Denoyelle et al., 1997; Lench et al., 1998), has caused concern within the Deaf Community that it could lead to prenatal testing and termination of pregnancy for deafness. A discussion of this debate and the research into attitudes towards genetic testing is not part of this chapter, but has been addressed elsewhere in this book and beyond (Middleton et al., 1998, 2001; Brunger et al., 2000; Stern et al., 2002; Taneja et al., 2004; Dennis, 2004). Middleton discusses the broader issues relating to equitable provision of genetic counselling in Chapter 18, while I will address the specific area of making genetic information available in British Sign Language (BSL) as an important part of this process.

I mention the debate around genetic testing here as an understanding of this is essential to the provision of culturally-sensitive and non-directive genetic counselling for deafness. Despite the concerns raised by the Deaf Community towards genetic developments, it is recognised that Deaf individuals or couples may find genetic counselling of benefit in many ways. Arnos et al. (1991), in a paper from the Genetics Services Centre based at Gallaudet University, stated that

> deaf individuals have a deep curiosity about the cause of their own deafness and the implications for future generations. When genetic information is presented in a manner that is sensitive to their cultural and linguistic differences, deaf people are very enthusiastic about participation in the genetic counseling process.

Anecdotally, I have also found this to be the case. During discussions with Deaf individuals outside the genetics clinic, I have found that, once we have moved past their common, though not universal, mistrust of my motives and understood what we offer through genetic counselling, they have been very keen to bring up their own family history and explain their own understanding of the cause of their deafness.

A discussion of the possible causes of the familial condition, leading to greater understanding on the part of the genetic counselling client is therefore an aim in itself. One Deaf couple who came for genetic counselling told me at the home visit that they would be just as happy to have deaf or hearing children. However, they were keen to know about the chances of this prior to trying for a family as it would affect their plans as to where they would live – if they were likely to have a deaf child they would move so that they were living in the catchment area for a school with a strong total communication policy where BSL would be the first language rather than in an adjoining area where the school had a predominantly oral tradition.

We believe that a lack of knowledge about the nature of genetic counselling is likely to be a factor affecting the number of Deaf individuals who are seen in the genetic counselling clinic. There is evidence to show that those seen are a very small proportion of all those for whom it may be applicable. In our Regional Genetics Service, 586 people were referred in the six years between 1998 and 2003 where the primary reason for referral was hearing loss. However, only a very small proportion of these are adults identifying themselves as part of the Deaf community as a BSL interpreter is booked for a genetic counselling consultation on average less than 10 times a year. Figures from the RNID suggest that, from the North-West population of 4.6 million people, there are likely to be as many as 5000 BSL users (RNID, 2005). Arnos et al. (1991) found in one study that, of 175 families contacted with likely hereditary deafness, 58% had a clear family history of deafness or a clear syndromal cause, but only 16% had been referred for genetic counselling. This group were parents of deaf children so they comment that the proportions are likely to be smaller for deaf adults where there may be additional cultural and linguistic differences.

Lack of knowledge about genetic counselling is by no means confined to this group. Many members of the population are unaware of what genetic counselling is unless they come into contact with it personally. However, the Deaf community have similarities with other cultural minority groups in that they often encounter prejudices that limit opportunities, they rarely encounter a doctor from their own cultural group and their language differences and health knowledge limitations often create barriers to appropriate health care. They also have limited access to English language-based information and have, on average, lower education and literacy levels and socioeconomic status than the general population (Barnett, 1999). All of these factors make it more difficult for a Deaf individual to have access to information incidentally about genetic counselling through, for example, a chance mention by their GP during a consultation about another issue.

IMPROVING ACCESS TO INFORMATION AND COUNSELLING

Within our Regional Genetics Service, we have been working on improving access to the information and counselling provided for all people referred with deafness or hearing loss. In the context of the factors above, however, I am focusing in this chapter on the Deaf community in particular.

This focus on improving access is being debated in wider fora than just the genetic counselling community. For example, the UK Council on Deafness, the national umbrella organisation for charities and professional bodies working in the field of deafness (UKCoD, 2005), hosted a seminar on 'Access to the NHS' in March 2004 at which RNID reported back on a recent survey of deaf and hard of hearing people. This found that, for example, a third of patients were unsure about the correct amount of medication to take because of mis-understood communication with their doctor and a quarter of patients had missed appointments in the past due to poor communication (Adams-Spink, 2004). An essential part of identifying where improvements are needed is therefore to consult with both service users and Deaf professionals. For this reason, consultation groups with Deaf and hearing professionals working in this area are planned for autumn 2005.

Some of the changes already instigated are straightforward and aimed at avoiding the types of miscommunication above. A one-page pre-clinic com-munication questionnaire is completed by the counsellee or with the genetic counsellor so that the need for an interpreter is recorded clearly in the notes. This is not so much for the initial appointment as the nature of the service's pre-clinic contact means that this would be asked about routinely by a genetic counsellor – it is so that there is an easy reference for future review appoint-ments and referral letters to other professionals involved.

A dedicated clinic for people attending because of hearing loss has been established so that one clinical geneticist and one genetic counsellor can focus expertise. This means that links are being developed with audiologists, ENT specialists and community paediatricians around the region to improve liaison in areas such as aetiological investigations carried out before referral. The clin-ical geneticist and genetic counsellor working in this area are also an easy source of information for other colleagues who, for example, need to contact a BSL interpreter.

PRODUCING INFORMATION ON GENETIC COUNSELLING

We have recently been working on the development of 'video leaflets' in BSL. There are dual aims to this project: both to improve knowledge levels about the nature of genetic counselling and to produce high-quality information to supplement clinic discussions and personalised post-clinic summary letters. This has grown from a departmental and, to some extent, a national move to produce a greater number of high-quality written information leaflets. Genetic information is highly complex and this complexity can clearly make it more difficult for a person to understand and therefore assimilate the material being presented (Andrews et al., 1994). As a result, it is seen as imperative that patients receive a detailed summary of the information discussed in clinic (Hallowell & Murton, 1998). This has been found to serve as a good reference in the future, sometimes years ahead (Stayner & Kerzin-Storrar, 2004).

For many years in our department, we have made use of leaflets to support verbal and written information giving. The Regional Genetics Service based at Guy's and St Thomas' Hospital in London developed a range of excellent leaflets within the last couple of years and made these freely available to the

Clinical Genetics community (BSHG, 2005). We have adapted some of these leaflets and updated existing departmental leaflets to expand our range of printed information. Leaflets also have the advantage of being able to include the diagrams and pictorial representations sometimes used in clinic.

However, the use of these written leaflets depends on the reading ability of the user.

English is the second language for most culturally Deaf people and the average reading age of a BSL user is between seven and a half and ten years (Conrad, 1979; Solomon, 1994; RNID, 1996; UK disability forum, 2005). While guidelines suggest that written leaflets should be pitched at a maximum reading age of 12 (Kent, 1996; Nicholls, 2003) and this has been achieved where possible, it is usually impossible to simplify complicated genetic information to this lower level.

As I highlighted earlier, Deaf people may have extra difficulty in accessing accurate facts about genetic conditions and genetic counselling from other sources and therefore the information supplied through their contact with us is potentially even more important than for most people. In addition, the implementation in October 2004 of the final section of the Disability Discrimination Act in the UK (Great Britain, 1999) means that there is now a legal obligation for organisations to provide information in a form that is accessible to all its service users.

PRODUCING VIDEO-RECORDED INFORMATION ON GENETIC COUNSELLING

Because BSL cannot be clearly represented on paper, the necessary format was a video, DVD or CD-ROM with the leaflets signed by an interpreter in BSL. The five leaflets chosen for translation were ones that were likely to be of the greatest value to Deaf people attending the department. They are:

- Introduction to genetic counselling
- The genetics of sensorineural deafness
- Autosomal recessive inheritance
- Autosomal dominant inheritance
- X-linked inheritance

While working on the written leaflets, we were discussing the best means of producing the translations with local (hearing) BSL interpreters and a group of culturally-Deaf interpreters based in the West Midlands. The Deaf BSL interpreters were just reaching the end of their training and we benefited from them being able to work on the project as a group to share ideas about the most accurate and understandable way to translate the genetic concepts. There was the additional benefit for them of being able to add this to their training portfolios. We agreed that it was far preferable for Deaf people to record the translation. The producer of *See Hear*, a Deaf magazine programme on British television, wrote in a piece about Deaf people interpreting on television that:

> even the best hearing interpreter, native signer or no, will not achieve the same audience appreciation as the best Deaf interpreters. And for a complete cultural translation, geared to the minds of Deaf viewers, Deaf interpreters will nearly always do it better. (Duncan, 1997)

The National Deaf Children's Society (NDCS, 2005) agreed to fund the project. We collaborated with the Faculty of Media at Trinity and All Saints (an accredited college of the University of Leeds, UK – TASC, 2005), who specialise in television and radio production at degree level. A group of undergraduate students took on the leaflet production as part of their professional placement, working in a professional standard television studio with autocue and computer editing facilities. There was a pleasing symmetry in being able to involve two groups of students from diverse fields in a joint project. It also meant, importantly, that we were able to keep down the production costs significantly.

During the course of several meetings between the interpreters and me, we had wide-ranging discussions about the genetic concepts underpinning the leaflet content. Genetic counsellors always aim to be aware of neutral language, but it was even more important in this setting. Terms like 'risk', 'disorder', 'mutation' or 'normal' were not acceptable, whereas 'chance', 'condition', 'gene change' and 'deaf' or 'hearing' were fine. As in English, the terms 'gene', 'chromosome', 'genetic' and 'DNA' do not mean very much to a lay person without further explanation so the fact that these terms tend to be signed in BSL with the same hand shape (the fingertips of the first two fingers on each hand touching and then separating while twisting to give the impression of the double helix) combined with the lip pattern for each word is not, in itself, a problem: it would not be enough in either English or BSL to just use the word in order to transmit the meaning.

Once the interpreters had more background knowledge about the relationship between the cell, chromosome, gene, DNA etc., they were able to agree on a definition of these terms in BSL. As a visual language, BSL has the advantage of being able to make the relationship between different genetic definitions more explicit by using three-dimensional 'placement' without adding extra 'words'. I also explained and expanded on an analogy I sometimes use in the clinic setting to explain the terms above: that each cell is rather like a library, where the shelves are chromosomes, the books are genes, a mutation is a spelling mistake or a missing page and the DNA is the paper and ink. The interpreters felt that viewers would find this a very helpful and visual image and reminded me that Deaf people like specific examples. We decided that to avoid repetition during the signing of each leaflet and to define the genetic terms used, we would draw up a glossary. This was signed independently and added to the end of each leaflet. The advantage of the DVD format is that this can be particularly easily accessed as an 'extra'. However, the terms were still reiterated and set in context within each leaflet.

Prior to the start of recording, consensus was reached on small but important issues such as clothing. The media team asked the interpreters to avoid wearing some colours that do not show up well on television. As the interpreters were all Caucasian, they also chose darker colours so that there was a better contrast between their hands and their background clothing. They also avoided patterned tops which could be too 'busy' and detract from the signing. For similar reasons, a plain dark blue background was chosen. The camera was positioned so that the interpreter was framed from their head down to just above the knee: this meant that the whole 'signing frame' could be seen while leaving enough space for the subtitles without them obscuring the hands.

The illustrations from the leaflets, contact addresses and credits were added during editing. When the interpreter is referring to a picture from the leaflet, the main shot of the interpreter is brought down to a small screen in the bottom corner while the picture fills most of the screen. The interpreters were aware of this prior to recording so they could indicate over their left shoulder when referring to the picture. Two of the five Deaf interpreters plus their hearing tutor met following the editing to reach a consensus on the back-translation for voiceover and subtitles. The final master copy can be produced on video, CD-ROM and DVD at a minimal cost of less than a pound per copy.

DISSEMINATION

Master copies of the leaflets will be freely available to other clinical genetics departments around Great Britain. The recording has been left deliberately 'unaffiliated' so that it can be used in any region of the country, although the addresses of all the Regional Genetics Services in the UK are included in the contact details at the end. Local contact details can be added to either the insert for the casing or, even more simply, as a sticker on the outside. The leaflets on modes of inheritance and genetics of sensorineural deafness should be used following genetic counselling rather than as a substitute, so it is felt that they should not be made widely available outside the clinical genetics setting.

The leaflet on 'What is Genetic Counselling?' could potentially be made available through selected deaf/Deaf organisations and through GP surgeries and audiology/ENT departments. This was something that the Deaf interpreters felt strongly about as d/Deaf people are often not able to discuss options like genetic counselling face-to-face with their GP or other doctor, as mentioned previously. We hope that this leaflet, particularly, will also address the second aim of the project: to increase knowledge about the non-directive nature of genetic counselling and, by doing so, allay the fears of some from the deaf community.

We will monitor demand for the leaflets in our department and will ask other genetics departments to do the same. A simple user questionnaire will be included with each 'video leaflet', along with a stamped addressed envelope for return to the department. This comprises very short questions in written English with responses given pictorially wherever possible, e.g. a scale of five faces with broad smile through to frown. In collaboration with Nowgen, The North-West Genetics Knowledge Park (Nowgen, 2005), we are assessing the acceptability of the video leaflets to Deaf people and professionals.

We are also involving other experts in the quality assessment of the translations so that we can learn from this for future projects. Although much preparatory work was done prior to translation, an independent view will be able to highlight any terms which have been particularly difficult or ambiguous and therefore may cause problems for BSL interpreters when translating for genetic counselling appointments. It is hoped that the development of high-quality translations of genetic information is informing a discussion of genetic terminology in BSL. There have been precedents in other areas such as mental health and sex education around discussions of vocabulary and cultural equivalence of terminology (Coleville, 1985; Deaf Professionals in Mental Health, 2000). The lessons learned are being incorporated in a study day for BSL interpreters interested in genetic counselling and other areas of medical interpreting. This is scheduled for autumn 2005 in collaboration with ASLI, the Association of Sign Language Interpreters (ASLI, 2005), and Nowgen.

There has been an interesting debate within the Deaf and the interpreting community reflecting the evolution of thinking about the role of the interpreter (Cragg, 2002; Hull, 2002; Turner & Harrington, 2002). Historically, it is accepted that the interpreter is there to translate the conversation taking place as transparently as possible, adding none of their own judgements nor missing out any asides not directed towards the Deaf person, but which a hearing person would have heard. However, over time it has been recognised that the maturing interpreting profession has developed the view of interpreter as 'machine' where one language goes in and another comes out with identical meaning to a point where the interpreter is seen to 'generate action, make choices and exercise decisive power' (Tate & Turner, 1997). This recognition of working in the 'real world', where a completely disinterested and neutral perspective is difficult if not impossible to achieve, strikes me as having interesting parallels with the developing debate about non-directiveness in genetic counselling that was discussed earlier. Both groups suggest that this may be a necessary stage for the respective emerging professions to go through.

CONCLUSION

The work described in this chapter is a small development in trying to provide equal access to genetic information and is only one aspect of the wider access issues relating to genetic counselling (UKCoD, 2001a). The Deaf Community's views on improving access continue to be sought through discussion with individual professional representatives and through wider consultation, as mentioned earlier, in line with published guidelines (UKCoD, 2001b).

I do not feel myself to be any type of expert in the provision of services for the Deaf Community, but aim to facilitate discussion between this group and the genetic counselling professions. In a piece about the concept of the Deaf Nation, Turner writes about the relationship of hearing people to the Deaf Community:

> The role of [hearing] academics as allies in this context, it seems to me, have to do not with presuming to provide answers – despite the fact that this is what students expect! – but more with trying to ask revealing questions, to generate opportunities for dialogue, to be aware of and feed in ideas from other sources, to offer reasoned and constructive critique, to help direct attention to insights that might otherwise be overlooked and generally to facilitate the development of a thoughtful environment. (Turner, 2002)

As genetic counsellors with a commitment to equal access for the Deaf community and aiming to provide culturally-sensitive services, I hope that we can have a similar role.

REFERENCES

Adams-Spink G (2004) NHS 'failing' deaf patients. BBC News website http://news.bbc.co.uk/1/hi/health/3527099.stm 03.03.04.

Andrews LA, Fullarton JE, Holtzman NA, Motulsky AG (1994) *Assessing Genetic Risks: Implications for Health and Social Policy*. Committee on Assessing Genetic Risks, Institute of Medicine. Washington, DC: National Academy Press.

Arnos KS, Israel J, Cunningham M (1991) Genetic counseling of the Deaf: medical and cultural considerations. *Annals of the New York Academy of Sciences* 212–22.

Association of Sign Language Interpreters website (2005) http://www.asli.org.uk/.

Barnett S (1999) Clinical and cultural issues in caring for Deaf people. *Family Medicine* 31: 17–22.

British Society for Human Genetics website leaflet forum (2005) http://www.bshg.org.uk/leaflets_forum/leaflets.htm.

Brunger JW, Matthews AL, Smith RH, Robin NH (2000) Parental attitudes toward genetic testing for pediatric deafness. *American Journal of Human Genetics* 67: 1621–5.

Clarke A (1991) Is non-directive genetic counselling possible? *Lancet* 338: 998–1001.

Clarke AJ (1997) The process of genetic counselling: beyond non-directiveness. In PS Harper, AJ Clarke (eds) *Genetics, Society and Clinical Practice*. Oxford: Bios, pp. 179–200.

Coleville M (1985) *Signs of a Sexual Nature*. Coleford: Forest Books.

Conrad R (1979) *The Deaf School Child: Language and Cognitive Function*. London: Harper & Row.

Cragg S (2002) Peeling back the skins of an onion. *Deaf Worlds* 18(2): 56–61.

Deaf Professionals in Mental Health (2000) *Sign Language in Mental Health*. Coleford: Forest Books.

Dennis C (2004) Deaf by design. *Nature* 431: 894–6.

Denoyelle F, Weil D, Maw MA et al. (1997) Prelingual deafness: high prevalence of a 30delG mutation in the connexin 26 gene. *Human Molecular Genetics* 6: 2173–7.

Duncan B (1997) Deaf people interpreting on television. *Deaf Worlds* 3(13): 35–9.

Great Britain (1999) *Disability Discrimination Act 1995. Code of Practice: rights of access – goods, facilities, services and premises*. London: HMSO.

Hallowell N, Murton F (1998) The value of written summaries of genetic consultations. *Patient Education and Counselling* 35: 27–34.

Hull S (2002) To interpret or not to interpret. *Deaf Worlds* 18(2): 50–5.

Kent G (1996) Shared understandings for informed consent: the relevance of psychological research on the provision of information. *Social Science and Medicine* 43: 1517–23.

Lench N, Houseman M, Newton V, Van Camp G, Mueller R (1998) Connexin-26 mutations in sporadic non-syndromal sensorineural deafness. *Lancet* 351: 415.

Middleton A (2005) Parents' attitudes towards genetic testing and the impact of deafness in the family. In D Stephens, L Jones (eds) *The Impact of Genetic Hearing Impairment*. London and Philadelphia: Whurr, pp. 11–53.

Middleton A, Hewison J, Mueller RF (1998) Attitudes of Deaf adults toward genetic testing for hereditary deafness. *American Journal of Human Genetics* 63: 1175–80.

Middleton A, Hewison J, Mueller RF (2001) Prenatal diagnosis for inherited deafness – what is the potential demand? *Journal of Genetic Counselling* 10: 121–31.

National Deaf Children's Society website (2005) http://www.ndcs.org.uk/index.html.

Nicholls S (2003) *A Clear Writing Resource*. Manchester: Nowgen.

North-west Genetics Knowledge Park website (2005) www.nowgen.org.uk.

Ridgeway S (2002) I'm happy my child is deaf. *Guardian*, Manchester 09.04.02 and Guardian Unlimited website http://www.guardian.co.uk/women/story/0,,681109,00.html.

Royal National Institute for the Deaf (1996) *Factsheet on Deafness Statistics*. London: RNID.

Royal National Institute for the Deaf website (2005) http://www.rnid.org.uk/information_resources/aboutdeafness/statistics/.

Solomon A (1994) Defiantly Deaf. *New York Times* magazine, 40–5.

Stayner B, Kerzin-Storrar L (2004) Genetic counselling summary letters: patients' views and uses. Poster presentation at European Meeting on Psychosocial Aspects of Genetics (EMPAG), Munich, Germany.

Stern SJ, Arnos KS, Murrelle L, Welch KO, Nance WE, Pandya A (2002) Attitudes of deaf and hard of hearing subjects towards genetic testing and prenatal diagnosis of hearing loss. *Journal of Medical Genetics* 39: 449–53.

Taneja PR, Pandya A, Foley DL, Nicely LV, Arnos KS (2004) Attitudes of Deaf individuals towards genetic testing. *American Journal of Medical Genetics* 130A: 17–21.

Tate G, Turner GH (1997) The code and the culture: sign language interpreting – in search of the new breed's ethics. *Deaf Worlds* 3(13): 27–34.

Trinity and All Saints Department of Media website (2005) http://www.tasc.ac.uk/depart/media/index.htm.

Turner GH (2002) The Deaf Nation notion: citizenship, control and courage. *Deaf Worlds* 18(2): 74–8.

Turner GH, Harrington FJ (2002) The campaign for real interpreting. *Deaf Worlds* 18(2): 69–72.

UK Council on Deafness (2001a) *Good Practice Guide: Providing Access to Public Services for Deaf People*. Colchester, UKCoD.

UK Council on Deafness (2001b) *Setting up a Deaf Users' Forum*. Colchester, UKCoD.

UK Council on Deafness website (2005) www.deafcouncil.org.uk.

UK disability forum website (2005) www.ukdisabilityforum.org.uk.

Walker AP (1998) The practice of genetic counselling. In DL Baker, JL Schuette, WR Uhlmann (eds) *A Guide to Genetic Counseling*. New York: Wiley-Liss, pp. 1–20.

20 Ethnicity, Spirituality and Genetics Services

LESLEY JONES, GHAZALLA MIR AND REHANA KHAN

Issues about ethnicity and spirituality do not apply to the study of genetic deafness alone. Much of what we will be discussing in this chapter applies to other areas of healthcare, such as palliative care and end of life issues as well as those surrounding childbirth and pregnancy itself. Genetic counselling raises particular concerns as discussed with reference to deafness by Middleton and Belk in this volume and by authors such Ahmed, Green and Hewison (2005) and Ahmad and Atkin (2000) in the context of thalassaemia.

There is a core of central beliefs about health care provision which rests on the appropriate and sensitive delivery of healthcare within a system based on equity and quality. Inequalities in health extend to other areas besides ethnicity and the picture is a complex one if age, education, gender, income, disability and sexuality are taken into consideration. Ethnicity does not rest on nationalism alone or colour of skin. The very notions of 'race' and ethnicity are challenged and endlessly redefined (as discussed later on). Spirituality too extends beyond the boundaries of organised religion to include people's faith and beliefs when challenged by difficulties such as receiving the news of a genetic history affecting the potential birth of a child. The sense that we make of the problems we encounter is influenced by the beliefs we have about the meaning (or otherwise) of life.

This chapter is based on research on the relevance of spirituality to management of chronic conditions within the Pakistani community Mir (2005), and on health care delivery to deaf children and adults from minority ethnic communities (Chamba et al., 1998; Ahmad et al., 1998) as well as on the practice of genetic counselling in a large northern town in the UK (Khan). It highlights the importance of understanding ethnicity and faith (both aspects of culture) in the policy, practice and study of genetic counselling in deafness. To do this we look at genetic counselling in deafness and ways of changing practice to encompass ethnic, religious and cultural difference and at a study of Pakistani Muslims in the UK as a specific example. Although this chapter is based largely on the experience of South Asian people in the UK, it can also be used as a

The Effects of Genetic Hearing Impairment in the Family. Edited by D. Stephens and L. Jones.
Copyright © 2006 by John Wiley & Sons, Ltd.

basis for providing appropriate care for other groups of healthcare users in other countries with diverse populations . . .

This chapter looks at some of these issues raised in genetic counselling about deafness raised by the above research and practice, as in Table 20.1.

Table 20.1 Issues of ethnicity and religion affecting genetic counselling

Ethnicity and marginalisation of religion
Access
Interpreting
Link workers
Assumptions and stereotypes
Perceived judgement and blame
Training
The concept of change
Implementing equitable practice

We begin by looking at the relationship between faith and ethnicity, then at genetic counselling and practice in that context, followed by a detailed look at one population within the UK in order to see what lessons can be learnt from close analysis of one group of people's views of the situation.

ETHNICITY AND MINORITY ETHNIC COMMUNITIES

PAKISTANI MUSLIM COMMUNITIES IN THE UK

Studies on health and healthcare within communities have most often adopted the framework of ethnicity as a basis for research, while excluding or marginalising consideration of the religious identity of respondents. This has reflected a more general trend within studies of health and social care (Selway & Ashman, 1998). Studies about the impact of religion on the health of minority ethnic communities is limited by both these factors and the available literature is consequently sparse.

Studies of ethnicity and health, group identities based on shared physical features, ancestry, geographical origins and social and political heritage have been used to define ethnic communities (Bhopal, 1997). Such studies have been instrumental in highlighting the experiences of service provision and the healthcare needs that exist within minority ethnic groups. The value of studying ethnic variations has also been highlighted as a tool in aetiology.

Despite the widespread use of this framework, however, the use of ethnic groupings has been criticised by a number of writers. As a concept, ethnicity is recognised as underdeveloped in its ability to recognise diversity (Ahmad, 1999). There are many views of how ethnicity or the contested term 'race' can be used. Stephen Rose talks of the term 'biogeographic ancestry' as a more accurate one. It does at least cover all the options!

The construction and use of ethnic categories, though often adopted by people from minority ethnic groups, have also been described as racist and imposed by the dominant ethnic group, which has led to the possible racialisation of health research (Barot, 1993; Dyson, 1998). Specific ethnic categories, such as those developed for the Census, may not be the same as terms used by social groups to describe themselves (Rankin & Bhopal, 1999). Confusion surrounding ethnic categories can result in inconsistency and inaccuracy in the terms used to describe these groups (Bhopal & Rankin, 2002). Contemporary definitions of ethnicity emphasise the need to unpack categories such as 'Asian' which imply homogeneity across wide geographical areas and to break the concept down into its different dimensions (Karlsen & Nazroo, 2002). Irish became a category of ethnicity in the 2002 Census, for example, which indicates the fluidity of the use of such terms.

Attempts have been made to include religion as a part of ethnicity (Modood et al., 1997; Nazroo, 1997; Aspinall & Jackson, 2004; Audit Commission, 2004); however, the relationship between ethnicity and religion is not straightforward. Ethnic group categories (such as those used in the Census) focus on nationality, which, in the case of Muslims and some other faith groups, can hide religious identity. In areas such as diet and dress there is an overlap in the influence of ethnicity and religion – for example, Muslims from Malaysia and Bangladesh are likely to eat different kinds of food influenced by regional availability and traditions. Nevertheless, they will still share with each other and with Muslims in all other ethnic groups the principles of a halal diet. In this respect, their food and drink will differ significantly from others within the same ethnic category who do not share their faith. Such variations in diet and regional traditions are clearly of relevance to healthcare and to health workers in providing accessible and appropriate services.

There is evidence that health inequalities within South Asian communities, for example, may be revealed more accurately using faith identity than ethnic groupings: greater socio-economic and health inequalities exist between the different faith groups within the Indian population, for example, than between Indians and other ethnic groups. This is likely to be because Indian Muslims have more in common with the lifestyles, beliefs, customs and historical perspectives of Pakistani Muslims than with those of Indian Sikhs and Hindus (Ahmad, 1999). This suggests that religion should be recognised as an aspect of identity that may at times overlap with ethnicity but cannot be subsumed by it. Both aspects of identity are important in terms of belonging and social relations and therefore both are likely to have a bearing on health and well-being. Ignoring the influence of religion in research means that only a partial picture will emerge of the issues affecting a particular social group. The same is true of Afro-Caribbean people and those from different parts of Africa such as Nigeria or Somalia. They may all be classified as Black or Afro-Caribbean (even when born in this country) yet may have nothing in common. The differences between the Rastafarian religion and Islam are numerous and include dietary as well as religious beliefs and observance.

The British Medical Association has recognised that shared ideas about health and illness affect health beliefs and ideas about causation (British Medical Association, 1995). There is also evidence that shared beliefs influence willingness to give and receive care and the perception of appropriate roles for those who are ill or disabled (Selway & Ashman, 1998). Shared beliefs are implied rather than explicitly included in the definitions of ethnicity mentioned at the beginning of this section. However, common beliefs are the explicit and essential foundation on which faith communities are formed; the values and principles of a faith will necessarily permeate such communities at various levels. Within communities in which faith is an important aspect of identity, interventions that fail to address religious beliefs are, therefore, unlikely to comply with BMA guidelines about incorporating relevant health beliefs into treatment methods.

Within the wider literature on health and social care there is little to be found on the need to address religious beliefs in service provision. For example, little work has been done on families with a history of deafness and the impact of religion and beliefs (Chamba et al., 1998). Indeed, attempts to introduce attention to this aspect of identity into service frameworks may meet with hostility and resistance (Hatton et al., 2004). Interestingly, provision relating to palliative care and bereavement counselling appears to be an exception, though consideration of religious beliefs may be subsumed within the concept of spirituality (Speck et al., 2004). As highlighted earlier, this concept is in some ways significantly different to religion.

Faith beliefs are likely to affect lifestyle, communication patterns and decision-making as well as social networks and relations. Failing to analyse findings in relation to religious groupings may therefore mean that important issues in all these areas are not identified.

Studies that focus on ethnicity may result in findings that relate to faith only because participants raise the significance of their religious practice, rather than as a result of deliberate exploration and inclusion in the design of a study (see, for example, Cinnirella & Loewenthal, 1999). Consequently findings of inequity are unlikely to differentiate between religious and ethnic discrimination. Yet, this important distinction is applied in practice within UK society. Indeed racism within the UK has historically focused on religious practices, particularly those related to Islam (Runnymede Trust, 1997; Commission for Racial Equality, 1998). The concept of Islamophobia has arisen in recent years to represent a particular form of racism experienced by Muslims and targeting their faith identity. This is particularly highlighted in the present political climate within Europe at the time of writing.

If needs are identified only within the conceptual framework of ethnicity, while minimising the significance of religious identity, recommendations for service development may fail to increase access to and take-up of services. In this case, ethnicity becomes an imposed framework that can result in misrepresentation or only partial acknowledgement of the kinds of needs that exist.

Minority groups have traditionally been obliged to accept such imposed categories and have packaged themselves according to state-created identities in order to secure resources and have needs met (Ahmad, 1996). This has often meant hiding or compromising their prime identity (Barot, 1993). Faith identity may not only be undermined in this way but the ability of religious values to make sense of the world and to be a valid foundation for self-organisation is simultaneously called into question. In order to apply for funding groups may 'market' themselves as a homogeneous population. For example a group of older people requiring day care may describe themselves as Asian in order to comply with funding criteria. They may encompass Sikhs, Hindus and Muslims, each with different dietary, religious and linguistic needs. Carib Care in London is another example of elder care, which includes people from different islands in the Caribbean and with different languages and cultures.

Failure to acknowledge religious identity also means that the influence it can have on interaction is not addressed in professional training programmes. Professionals may consequently feel ill equipped to understand value frameworks other than their own (Hatton et al., 2004). Many feel constrained to avoid referring to faith at all.

A disparity in expectations and an emotional distance between patients and professionals, and between professionals with different religious backgrounds, may result from this lack of engagement with alternative beliefs and values (Bhopal, 1997). The quality of these relationships may subsequently suffer through mutual criticism (Bowler, 1993; Murphy & Clark, 1993). Studies show that such inability to form a holistic relationship may lie at the root of suboptimal care, poor take-up of services and other types of discrimination such as stereotyping (Auluck & Iles, 1991; Bowler, 1993; Vangen et al., 1996).

There is evidence that health professionals have successfully used knowledge of beliefs that affect social action in various ways. For example, a campaign to reduce smoking after the end of Ramadan, was based on knowledge that Muslims would have reduced or finished their smoking habit completely during the month (Kelleher & Islam, 1996). Knowledge of the links between religious beliefs and diet has also been used to aid the aetiology of stomach cancer, which has different rates of incidence in different ethnic communities (Bhopal, 1997).

Ethnicity and religion are thus both important aspects of identity that need to be acknowledged in any study of minority ethnic communities alongside other influences such as age, gender and social class, which are also known to impact on communication and decision-making in people with chronic illness (Chamaz & Olesen, 1997). A conceptual framework is needed therefore that encompasses all these elements and that can take account of the complex relationship between them.

INFLUENCE OF RELIGION ON INDIVIDUAL, FAMILY AND COMMUNITY

INFLUENCE ON THE INDIVIDUAL

Faith beliefs exist within cultural and social contexts, which also influence relationships and interactions and, as already highlighted, there is considerable overlap between age, gender, social class, ethnic and religious influences (Modood et al., 1997). Although these may be considered separately, within everyday experience they are essentially interconnected.

Religion may define a condition, such as deafness, positively, giving the experience meaning and purpose and providing knowledge of how to respond in such circumstances. These teachings can act as a source of energy to patients (Ahmed, 2000). Alternatively, religious beliefs may encourage negative interpretations, for example, of illness as a punishment. Such punitive interpretations have been found to damage patients' ability to negotiate their condition and to have a harmful influence on the self-concept of people with chronic illness and disability (Selway & Ashman, 1998).

There is evidence that the meaning and thus the implications of illness or disability may differ considerably between professionals and individuals from minority ethnic backgrounds and faith values are presented as one reason for this disparity (Hill, 1994). The difficulty of communicating concepts based on faith to health professionals who focus primarily on physical health is clear.

Medical explanations about the cause of a condition may be differentiated from explanations about why (in terms of meaning) a condition exists. These explanations may be formulated in the light of personal biographies and other sources of knowledge, including religious beliefs and family or community norms (Popay & Williams, 1996). Individually or socially held beliefs may at times conflict with medical explanations: professional attitudes towards mental illness and towards consanguineous marriages are good examples of conflicting medical and social interpretations. It has been suggested that such conflicts may lead to confusion as people struggle to make sense of their situation (Popay & Williams, 1996).

Understandings of the relationship between the individual and society may also be an area in which belief frameworks differ. The Islamic view that individuals are responsible for their behaviour is held alongside the recognition that societies and individuals have equal co-existence and that individuals influence and are influenced by each other. The well-being of an individual is thus closely related to the well-being of society (Al-A'ali, 1993). This understanding is not supported by a professional culture, which may emphasise the role of the individual in decision-making, without addressing social influences on action and choice (Dyson, 1999).

INFLUENCE ON FAMILY

The influence of family members on health-seeking behaviour among Pakistani people living in the UK, and the way in which this is exercised, is an under-researched area. Studies which do explore these dynamics often focus on gender roles and particularly women's position within the family. These have been shown to affect access to information and contact with healthcare providers. Pakistani men, for example, in both urban and rural settings in Pakistan are more likely than their wives to know how to obtain healthcare (Mahmood & Ringheim, 1997). A number of studies show that this situation is mirrored in the UK with men taking a lead role in contact with health and social care practitioners (Ahmad, 2000; Mir & Tovey, 2003). However, this may be an enforced position arising from greater fluency in English among men (Mir et al., 2003). There is some evidence that women's decision-making on health issues may be influenced by men: the attitude of husbands, for example, may significantly affect South Asian women's decisions about whether or not to consult a male general practitioner (Bowes & Domokos, 1996). The prospect of dishonouring the family and being ostracised can also be a powerful constraint on women's choices in this community (Wheeler, 1998). However, research is limited as to whether such constraints are gender-specific and whether they reflect religious or other influences. Family dynamics have a powerful effect in genetic counselling and decisions are usually guided by beliefs and values upheld a family unit. Engaging with these values lies at the heart of providing counselling support.

INFLUENCE ON COMMUNITY

The consequences of being part of a faith community have, for some groups, been shown to influence access to healthcare. A study of information networks relating to contraception and reproduction found that adherents of well-established large urban churches had more intensive and diverse channels of information, both inside and outside their congregations, than women who were excluded from such networks. As a result, they participated more actively in the exchange of information about choices open to them.

In terms of health promotion, it has been suggested that use might be made, for example, of Islamic teachings on the body as a trust from God to promote the idea of personal responsibility, preventive healthcare and an active approach to seeking out advice for health problems (Ahmed, 2000).

Although some religious communities have been shown to provide practical support to families within their congregation (Selway & Ashman, 1998; Walsh, 1998), this has not been demonstrated at a practical level for South Asian communities. There is evidence of moral support, however, and religious communities may serve as a primary means through which individuals adapt to illness (Cinnirella & Loewenthal, 1999; Mir et al., 2000). Narratives from religious scriptures, passed among members of a faith community, have been shown to help promote positive examples of others who model resilience within families and communities (Mir & Tovey, 2003; Walsh, 1998). They may also serve to transmit cultural and family beliefs that guide personal expectations and actions. Anecdotes about the experience of other people may serve a similar function. A study of South Asian carers found that such anecdotes could reinforce carers' fears about the quality of care in hospital settings as well a moral obligation not to 'give away' the person cared for (Bhakta et al., 2000).

Although, as mentioned earlier, religious beliefs may become harmful if rigid and punitive, they more often act as a resource for families and may be integral to the well-being of patients and carers. A number of studies have shown that religious orientation plays an important role as a coping strategy in the lives of carers from many ethnic groups (Atkin & Ahmad, 1998; Mir et al., 2000; Mir & Tovey, 2003). In addition, religious factors are associated with beneficial effects on health and well-being in patients with blood pressure and those needing long-term haemodialysis (Selway & Ashman, 1998). Faith, prayer and spiritual rituals, especially at sites of high spiritual energy such as places of pilgrimage or worship, have also been shown to aid healing by triggering emotions that influence the immune and cardiovascular systems (Walsh, 1998).

INFLUENCE WITHIN THE WIDER SOCIETY

In contrast to the largely positive influence of religious beliefs at an individual, family and community level, there is evidence of a lack of understanding and deliberate discrimination in relation to Muslim communities within the wider UK society. A report on Islamophobia (Runnymede Trust/Commission on British Muslims and Islamophobia, 1997) highlighted that Muslims face a degree of discrimination, which does not appear to be mirrored in other social/ethnic groups, related to their beliefs. This makes the experience of Muslims different to that of other minority groups – as well as discrimination based on ethnic origin, their attempts to maintain beliefs and practices that differ from those dominant in the UK is a significant further source of prejudice which adversely affects their psychosocial well-being.

INFLUENCE ON INTERACTIONS WITH
HEALTHCARE PROVIDERS

There is considerable evidence that the needs of Pakistani communities in the UK are often not addressed by health and social welfare services, resulting in inappropriate provision and consequently low take-up of services (Acheson, 1998; Chamba et al., 1998). Institutional racism has been a fundamental force in the difficulties faced by these communities and studies have highlighted both ethnic and religious discrimination. For example, stereotypes of South Asian families who 'look after their own' are sometimes used by service providers to explain low take-up (Atkin & Ahmad, 1998). There is little evidence that families are in fact able to be self-sufficient in providing care; however, studies within South Asian communities do reflect a perception of duty among carers towards those for whom they care. Institutional failure to encourage take-up of services may thus exploit and reinforce carer values and sustain inequalities in access to provision (Mir et al., 2000; Mir & Tovey, 2003).

These studies suggest that emotional engagement requires a degree of shared understanding and some shared values and that these form the basis of positive relationships between patients and professionals. It is not surprising, therefore, that some groups may hold a strong preference for professionals from their own community, emphasising the difficulties of 'difference' and believing that same 'race' professionals better understand the context in which they live (Cinnirella & Loewenthal, 1999). People may feel that such professionals have an awareness of patients' socio-cultural milieu and the pressures they face as well as an ability to understand the specific symptoms of mental illness that they experience. The use of religious practices as part of therapy, seen as a useful resource for treatment, was considered by Pakistani people in one study as only possible with professionals who shared the same faith background (Mir et al., 2000).

This section has demonstrated that religious beliefs can influence cognition and choice and that religious identity co-exists with, and is balanced against, other aspects of the self, each of which may be more or less significant in different contexts. The way research is conducted in the minority ethnic communities often blurs the distinction between religious and other influences. As a result of this, the relationship between religious identity, social action and health beliefs is unclear in most studies of these communities. The influence of religious teachings on caring, for example, may be bound in with economic and gender influences and experiences related to migration. Exploring each of these influences in its own right can prevent an approach that inappropriately privileges one influence and uses it to explain everything, while ignoring the diversity that may exist within a community. Attention to diversity is important also in highlighting the different ways in which religion may be practised and the different levels of religiosity within a faith group. Having considered the influence of religious beliefs, the following section considers how these and other aspects of culture may relate to genetic counselling.

GENETIC COUNSELLING

ETHNICITY AND SPIRITUALITY

In order to improve service provision, there is a purpose in studying families with a history of genetic deafness and for each family there will be a different set of circumstances surrounding their knowledge about genetic deafness. The next stage is to move on to their understanding of their situation as well as the way in which the information is transmitted and understood in a two-way process. There is implicit difficulty in translating concepts central to one culture into another where those concepts may be marginal. Language carries values over from one culture to another but may become distorted in the process.

COMMUNICATION

Genetic counselling is based on effective communication and one of the major problems raised in this area is still the language in which communication takes place.

Language emerges as significant in terms of interpreting, the use of link workers and the concept of informed consent. The provision of informed consent relies on the quality of information both provided and received by those being counselled. Access to that information is crucial in all of the ways applicable to interpreting in health settings as shown in Table 20.2.

Table 20.2 Access to information in health settings

Is it available?
Is it accessible?
Is it funded?
Is it appropriate?
Is it knowledgeable?
Is it confidential?

Competency in both the language and interpreting skills is a basic requirement for this work. The use of neighbours of family members, even children, as interpreters in consultations still exists and in this emotionally sensitive area this is not always appropriate and indeed is often adding pressure to an already fraught situation. Parents are often being asked to make a decision on the basis of incomplete information because the would-be interpreter has not understood the technical language, or sometimes the translations of words such as chromosome or gene or cell simply do not exist in the same way. For example, 'inherited condition' may be translated as 'condition you are born with', which has a fundamentally different meaning about what is happening. Concepts such as risk are complicated to explain in any language and can be difficult to grasp in an emotionally fraught atmosphere of a genetic consultation.

TRAINING NEEDS AND TIME CONSTRAINTS

Knowledge about genetic terms and concepts need to be taught in training courses for interpreters or link workers. Health professionals may also be unused to working with interpreters and may need to learn how to do this effectively. Health professionals also need to have the confidence to ask parents to wait for an appointment to be booked with a suitably qualified interpreter. Obviously this is not always possible and because of time constraints this inadequate provision, without interpreting support, can become the norm. Time exerts pressure on the clinicians, interpreters and link workers and prevents them from being able to prepare for interviews with the use of more than one spoken language.

The exchange between parents, health and language workers are usually under-resourced in time and training on all sides. For the genetic counsellor time spent with a link worker or interpreter before an interview can be valuable as terms are explained and complicated notions such as risk and uncertainty can be effectively translated and negotiated. In a packed clinic this may not always be easy to arrange. Interpreting concepts, which require some knowledge of the topic as well as some understanding of the ethical consideration requires an interpreter with high-level professional skills. Link workers may well not be trained as interpreters but be asked to fulfil that role as part of their work without any preparation or support. Access to trained professional interpreters specialising in the field of genetics is rare and often only available in areas of high population and well-resourced healthcare settings.

Problems may arise in all inadequately resourced consultation with one or more family members and poor language support. For the clinician there may be the frustration of listening to a long exchange and being given only a very short translation without having access to the full sense of the reply. For the parents there is similar frustration. Extra time is required for this process to work and for the use of pictures and illustrations to be explained properly before the process of reflection and decision-making can even begin. Without being given access to the tools for understanding this complexity it is very difficult for the process of informed consent to take place (Chamba & Ahmad, 2000; Ahmad et al., 2005).

To summarise this section the four main areas of concern in genetic counselling within more than one spoken language are given in Table 20.3. In order to provide this, resources are required to fund training and extra time to complete the process effectively.

Table 20.3 Necessary factors for effective genetic
counselling in a multilingual situation

Language competency
Knowledge of technical terms
Understanding of complex concepts
The appropriateness of the interpreter

A sensitive, confidential and knowledgeable interpreting service relies not only on full language support but cultural knowledge too. Interpreting support may be quite inappropriate if a family uses a different dialect from the interpreter, for example rural and urban areas may have entirely different languages and culture. Mirpuri speakers may not understand Urdu or Punjabi interpreters well.

LINK WORKERS

Link workers or specialist genetic counsellors can often be working outside their own language skills with people from other linguistic communities. An asylum seeker or refugee from rural Somalia speaking Somali, Italian or Arabic may have little in common with someone used to working within a Northern urban British/Pakistani context using Urdu or Punjabi. Islam might be a shared religion but the cultural and language differences could be considerable.

Together with other link workers in health and social care there is the shared experience of short-termism, marginalisation and a lack of career progression for this group of workers (Ahmad et al., 1998). Their posts are often funded through short-term contracts at the end of which there is little prospect of secure employment. The expertise about how to accommodate faith needs into a service accumulated during these contracts is sometimes undervalued and on the completion of the contract the worker moves on only to be replaced later on by an inexperienced worker as funding becomes available. This is a danger of 're-inventing the wheel' with each new appointment as further funding becomes available. Another problem for link workers who do manage to stay in post, is that there is no career structure and they often cannot move on to more demanding posts in the same area of work. They also report that white workers sometimes pass on all the problems concerning anyone who is non-white, whether or not the link worker has any knowledge about the patient's language or culture. White professionals' fear of causing offence may lead to reluctance to engage with families from non-Caucasian backgrounds. This can then lead to the passing on of those families to the link worker who might have knowledge about some groups but none at all about others (Ahmad et al., 1998; Chamba et al., 1998). Numerous studies highlight the wide distinctions between African Caribbean, Chinese and South Asian people, to consider only three definitions of ethnicity.

PATIENTS' PERSPECTIVES

From the patients' viewpoint genetic counselling and their response to what is offered may be influenced by their own beliefs but also by what they perceive as the expectations of the professionals. Some of these views taken from practice focus on perceived judgement and blame including:

- first cousin marriages (consanguinity)
- reluctance to terminate a pregnancy after screening or testing
- not understanding the implications of the results of tests.

The first area has been a focus of concern in the literature (Ahmad, 1999) for some time as the perceived racism of Caucasian clinicians is seen to concentrate on consanguinity as the main and only reason for the passing on of inherited conditions. This has led some parents to conceal their relationship to their spouses from counsellors on the grounds that that they do not wish to be discriminated against (Chamba et al., 1998). As a part of a complex causality consanguinity as a factor in genetic conditions is often seen by the parents as being 'their fault' if a child is born with an impairment.

The second area of concern for parents is that clinicians will disapprove if they do not accept termination after having undergone genetic testing or screening. They may feel that health professionals will think that a child born with a disability such as deafness will be a drain on resources. It may be perceived as a burden on the health, education and social services, particularly in a family with one or more children who are already deaf. The financial implication of the birth of a deaf child may well be different in the countries of the South with completely different economic systems, where services must be paid for. There the birth of a disabled child will have greater costs in terms of support services and employment prospects of a family member. However, within the present climate for genetic counselling in the UK, termination is a matter of personal choice and this is the context of decision-making for parents within the UK Health Service.

A clinician's view of a disabled child as a 'burden' may not be one shared by the family with clinicians. If there are existing deaf children, they may be seen as valued members of the family. These parents can feel that the child they already have is being diminished by this perceived pressure towards termination. As highlighted elsewhere in this volume (Middleton et al. Chapter 16; Middleton, Chapter 18; Belk, Chapter 19), where the parents are themselves deaf the birth of a deaf child may well be a source of unequivocal joy, in addition to that of the birth of any child. Parenting is a changing experience and it may be that, having brought up one child who is deaf, parents gain more confidence about how they will cope with another.

They may still want the right to find out before making their decision about whether or not to terminate the pregnancy. When clinicians are seen as disapproving of choices made, as in the case of thallassaemia (Atkin & Ahmad, 1998), parents may internalise this negativity and it may obscure their decision-making.

Parents report being aware that they are not fully informed about the implications of test results. Poor understanding of the full implications of these test results may well be a result of poor access to information. As seen earlier, this may be because the right access to understanding complicated concepts has not been given to the parents to enable them to make an informed decision.

ASSUMPTION AND STEREOTYPES

Assumptions made by professionals about attitudes to termination mean that sometimes parents feel uncomfortable about asking either for prenatal testing in the first instance or for a termination. This may mean that more individualised approaches need to be made to couples seeking genetic counselling. Caucasian clinicians may feel that in the current atmosphere of cultural sensitivity they will offend by saying the wrong thing to people from a different religion to themselves. This may prevent them from finding out what the needs of a parent are.

Cultural competence training may help develop the flexibility required to approach people as individuals within communities. Micro-cultures exist within minority ethnic communities just as they do within any other communities. Issues of nationality, religious observance, location, education and income all differentiate between groups of people, as discussed previously, moving away from training based on the 'They eat special foods' or 'Muslims don't have abortions' approach. This was characterised in the 1980s in the UK in multicultural education as the 'Samosas, Saris and Steel bands' approach. There is a move away from this prescriptive account of what each group of people are stereotyped as doing. At the start of a session of counselling, the visible features of a couple attending might be the first thing to strike the clinician; this might be, for example, style of dress, such as wearing the hijab. Perhaps we all need to train ourselves to step out of this stereotyping behaviour between and among groups. Treating people as individuals and always observing the basic rules of patient-centred care, such as checking out what a patient believes about their treatment, is something which benefits the wider community as well. This means that asking a patient how they feel about having a deaf child or about terminating a pregnancy can open up discussion rather than closing it down by assuming that they will react negatively to either of these options.

The other assumption made about Muslim patients particularly is that they will adopt a fatalistic stance about the birth of a deaf child. This is based on the idea that all Muslim will accept what is given to them as the will of Allah.

As with Roman Catholics there may be a range of beliefs, as discussed in Mir's 2005 study findings.

COMMUNICATION AND FAITH IDENTITY

A study of the impact of faith identity on chronic illness management in the Pakistani community (Mir, 2005) reveals that reference to faith is considered part of an appropriate response to the diagnosis of a chronic condition for Pakistani people. Religious beliefs provide a therapeutic resource and can offer individuals an emotional distance from the chronic condition by placing it in the wider context of human experience as a whole. The ability to distance oneself from a chronic condition in order to cope with its effects is a resource in European culture too (see Bury, 1982); however, for Pakistani people this feature of culture is strongly connected to faith beliefs.

Contemporary European healthcare treats faith as a private issue that has no place in the treatment of medical conditions. Even in the treatment of mental health conditions, where the use of belief frameworks in cognitive therapies might be considered more likely, faith beliefs do not appear to be positively exploited. The evidence suggests that such an approach to treatment appears to be far removed from what Pakistani patients can expect – adjustments to clinical practice for this population do not always offer even basic communication in the same language. The research supports the notion that most health professionals are not adapting clinical practice to the ethnic or religious identity of their patients and that they lack the skill or inclination to adequately distinguish between the two.

The study showed that Pakistani people with chronic illness most often take the lead from health practitioners about what to discuss, and that they often go along with the view that healthcare contexts are irrelevant to discussion of faith beliefs. It is clear from the findings that this perception is not, however, accurate; the religious identity of Pakistani people with chronic illness can affect their communication patterns in significant and distinct ways. Nevertheless, patients adapt to healthcare contexts by making this aspect of their identity almost invisible with adverse consequences for treatment and self-care. Religious identity cannot always be confined to the private sphere and there is a need for European secular contexts to engage with this identity (Cesari, 1998).

In cases where the issue of religious or ethnic identity is raised, practitioners may deny that these have the same impact on communication or self-care as other aspects of identity such as age, class or education. A vacuum exists in healthcare policies in respect of religion and, while ethnic health inequalities are acknowledged, there is little attempt to address these inequalities in policy or practice. The effect of this vacuum is to legitimise the position of those who deny ethnicity and religion as factors that can affect interaction between practitioners and patients. In addition, this may mean that professionals use their own, often negative, ideas about Pakistani or other groups of families, and particularly the position of women within them, to interpret family dynamics in relation to self-care.

These findings could be used to argue that deliberate attention is not paid to the religious and ethnic identity of any people with chronic illness in clinical settings. However, the idea that religious beliefs are a private aspect of identity and so not relevant to social communication is a cultural construct peculiar to the history of religion and science in Europe (Asad, 1993). Dominant patterns of behaviour and organisation in healthcare do reflect the prevailing culture in UK society. For example, routine appointments are unlikely to be offered over Christmas or Easter, whereas the festivals of Eid are unlikely to be taken into account when appointments are offered to Muslim patients. The same thing applies to Passover, Diwali or Chinese New Year. Showing a level of understanding and respect about important times for people from minority religious groups clearly has relevance to genetic counselling and appointments for families with deaf children.

Dismissiveness of religious and ethnic identity in the broad thinking about communication may explain why findings in Mir's 2005 study show that no action was being taken to address the specific needs of people's religion or ethnicity with chronic illness in some clinical settings. Service development can only take place after an initial acknowledgement that specific needs exist and that services are lacking in terms of meeting these needs.

DECISION-MAKING AND FAITH IDENTITY

Findings demonstrate that the personal judgement of Pakistani people with chronic illness is the most important influence on their decision-making and this judgement is affected by beliefs and values. This is of particular significance in genetic counselling where judgement is of the utmost importance. Religious beliefs contribute in varying degrees to decision-making about chronic illness but were influential for more than half the sample of this study and consequently cannot be ignored as a factor in the decision-making process. Religious beliefs could set the boundaries within which any decisions had to be taken and religious practices, such as fasting and prayers, could influence, for example, the way medication was taken.

The level of influence practitioners may have on decision-making in healthcare is linked to the quality of relationships between professionals and patients. The ability of physicians and other health professionals to engage with some patients in the management of impairment may well be limited. It suggests that it would be considerably enhanced if they were equipped with knowledge about the context in which these patients make decisions, of which religious beliefs and practices form an important part. Currently this knowledge appears to be almost absent from clinical settings. This results in a lack of confidence to engage in discussions about how religious beliefs and ethnic traditions influence management of a chronic condition or disability This lack of engagement is a barrier to the development of shared understanding between professionals and Pakistani patients as with other groups. Consequently, concordance is less likely to be achieved and poor management of chronic illness is less likely to be detected and addressed early.

As well as explicit beliefs, Mir (2005) found certain implicit values held by Pakistani people with chronic illness, which is relevant to our topic. For example, sincerity in putting patients' interests first is expected in the care provided by professionals. Expectations that family members should be supportive and feel responsible for a person who is ill are also embedded in respondent narratives. Explicit and implicit values contribute to the context in which Pakistani people with chronic illness make decisions about how to manage their condition. These values exist in families, in communities and in society, as do the shared understandings and values that exist in relation to Islam both within and outside the Pakistani community. The wider social context throws further light on the various ways in which religious identity affects the lived experience of people within the Pakistani community. This exploration also helps to link inequalities in healthcare to broader issues relating to inequalities in health and offers further reasons why religious identity needs to be specifically recognised in social policy.

UNDERSTANDING FATE AND FATALISM

Most respondents accepted their condition as part of their destiny and interpreted this experience as a test of their patience or (more rarely) a punishment for past misdeeds. However, this position risked misinterpretation by health professionals as discussed in the section on genetic counselling. Individuals sometimes expressed their belief in ways that could be interpreted as fatalism; when asked about his expectations for the future, one respondent in this study, for example, said that this was in God's hands, 'A person can't do anything'. Another similarly fasted in Ramadan saying, 'If my health is meant to become worse then let it, it doesn't matter'. At the same time, both respondents were taking regular medication, paid attention to any deterioration in their symptoms and respected the advice they had been given by health professionals. Such statements could, however, be taken at face value and out of context by health professionals. Religious justifications that were used to support an individual's decision on treatment could be understood in isolation and could prevent health practitioners from considering other reasons why a Pakistani person might resist certain forms of treatment. Religious views about destiny and accepting one's fate may be used as back-up reasons for decisions that are driven by other beliefs about health.

Developing a shared understanding at this level was far more complex than attributing decisions to an area such as religion or culture, which health professionals could treat as a personal arena. Pakistani patients who felt strongly that they did not wish to begin 'injections for life' may, indeed, be using this 'hands-off' approach to religion as a way of preventing health practitioners from attempting further persuasion. As with the example above, this line of argument might be used to head off a discussion where respondents had already made up their mind on a course of action and did not want to be dissuaded.

Poor understanding of the health beliefs of Pakistani and other minority ethnic patients appears to present a block to health professionals entering into any dialogue of negotiation. The absence of this dialogue was clearly detrimental to individuals with chronic illness who consequently had more limited input from professionals in decision-making than people from the ethnic majority.

A variety of reasons for lack of engagement in such decision-making appear to exist. Whereas with white patients efforts were being made to develop a shared understanding of health beliefs, practitioners did not feel confident about discussing the health beliefs of Pakistani patients if they had limited knowledge of their cultural context. This is likely to apply just as strongly to other cultures. Patients were often equally unwilling, sometimes assuming professionals who did not share these values would either undermine or dismiss their concerns or wouldn't understand the influence of religion on their experience. As one male patient with coronary heart disease commented:

> Fasting and prayer do not concern the doctors . . . They don't even know what it is.

This lack of confidence on both sides presented a block to shared understanding of how patient beliefs affected decisions about treatment. Given the significance of shared understanding, however, and the high influence religion had on decision-making, the findings suggest that these are precisely the areas in which practitioners need to develop dialogue and understanding with Pakistani patients. This type of engagement is in fact no different to discussing lay health beliefs with white patients.

Findings from this study support the argument that practitioners who are equipped to engage with patients' cultural context are more likely to develop relationships in which concordance can be developed and better health outcomes achieved. Given that religious beliefs influenced a significant number of respondents in this study and were very important for most of these individuals, exploring the impact of this particular sphere on the self-care of Pakistani individuals is likely to improve professional practice.

FAITH IDENTITY IN UK SOCIETY

Mir's research suggests that Pakistani individuals need social support to successfully incorporate faith beliefs into their daily routines and to draw on faith as a resource. Social policy support for faith identity can indirectly help Pakistani people with chronic illness by increasing the emotional and spiritual resources available to help them manage their condition. This kind of support is currently lacking within the Pakistani community and may be deliberately restricted by social policy. This has implications for work in this area about deafness.

There is diversity in the way in which faith is understood both within and outside the Pakistani Muslim community. In this respect they confirm the already well-established argument that representations of Islam as a fixed monolithic culture are mythical (Said, 1995). Islam is more than a series of Muslim identities. Shared understandings about the values and boundaries promoted by this religion show that it possesses its own culture, which can be, and has been, adapted to innumerable regional and local traditions. Furthermore, defining Islam as equal to the culture of a Muslim community could be seen as an extension of the idea, rooted in European culture, that religion is no more than a social construction and that understanding of Islam should be restricted to its human elements (Asad, 1993).

CONCLUSION

The evidence thus suggests that better levels of shared understanding are needed, not only between health practitioners and people from minority ethnic communities but between members of these communities and others in UK society. Differences in ethnic and religious background are not necessarily a barrier to achieving this understanding. Sincerity and willingness to offer practical support to others in need are considered key foundations for successful interaction by most people. For practitioners, knowledge of the faith and ethnicity of their patients which would enable them to ask sensible questions and to negotiate treatment without causing offence would help achieve the kind of understanding that is required. This chapter has also revealed the potential for finding common ground between different linguistic, cultural and faith groups in the UK. For most people in the desire to be understood and accepted as part of the wider community is balanced alongside other needs. There is evidence too that racism exacerbates an already difficult situation when stereotyped views of different ethnic and religious groups are allowed to dominate practice.

Examples of successful cross-cultural interaction provide evidence that common values can form a solid foundation for social cohesion as long as power relationships are simultaneously addressed. The current lack of power experienced by people from minority ethnic communities in their social relations with others in UK society, and lack of opportunities to engage, will need to be addressed in strategies to improve social cohesion within neighbourhoods, communities and society as a whole.

PRACTICAL IMPLICATIONS

Interpreting of a high quality and training for interpreters and health and link workers are all vital parts of this process – training that is continuous and at relevant points in time is required. Other practical steps are the provision of tape recording what was said in the consultation. Ideally this should be in the appropriate language or even audio, recorded for those whose language is spoken rather than written. Financially this is not always possible so it may be better to ensure that the clients understand what the contents of any written communication from the hospital may contain. This will enable them to make arrangements for their letter to be translated by an appropriate person with whom they do not mind sharing such confidential information.

Another practical step, which is being taken, is the provision of Race Equality Schemes in hospitals with a diversity officer employed to reflect on and monitor the schemes being put in place. The Genetic Interests Group within the UK also has an Ethnic Monitoring Team with a website for advice. This enables the identification of gaps in the service. A basic plan for providing an accessible and appropriate service for people from minority ethnic communities seeking genetic counselling might be the one shown in Table 20.4.

Table 20.4 Model for provision of genetic counselling for ethnic communities

1. Identifying the client group
2. Providing and funding adequate interpreters
3. Quality training for health and link workers continuously and at different points in time
4. Identifying a professional person chosen by the client who is accountable for ensuring that there is access to understanding the entire complex of issues necessary for making informed choices
5. Basing best-quality care on respect and an understanding of the individual – a synthesis of their upbringing, religion, education and life experience

The relationship between faith, ethnicity and genetic counselling raises many of the complex issues that contribute to inequalities in health such as access to services, cultural competence and power differentials. Understanding each others' views and sharing the basic universality of experience faced when making life-changing decisions is a good beginning to the delivery of healthcare in this context.

REFERENCES

Acheson Sir Donald (Chair) (1998) Independent Inquiry into Inequalities in Health. London: Stationery Office. http://www.archive.official-documents.co.uk/document/doh/ih/part2h.htm (accessed June 2004).

Ahmad W (1996) The trouble with culture. In D Kelleher, S Hillier (eds) *Researching Cultural Differences in Health*. London: Routledge, pp. 190–219.

Ahmad, W (1999) Ethnic statistics: better than nothing or worse than nothing. In *Statistics in Society*, D Dorling, S Simpson (eds). London: Arnold.

Ahmad W (ed) (2000) *Ethnicity, Disability and Chronic Illness*. Buckingham: Open University Press.

Ahmad W, Atkin K (2000) Pumping iron: compliance with chelation therapy among young people who have thalassaemia major. *Sociology of Health and Illness* 4: 500–24.

Ahmad W, Darr A, Jones L, Nisar G (1998) *Deafness and ethnicity: Services, Policy and Politics*. Bristol: Polity Press/JRF.

Ahmad W, Atkin K, Jones L (2002) Being deaf and being other things: young Asian people negotiating identities. *Social Science and Medicine* 55: 1757–69.

Ahmed A (2000) Health and disease, an Islamic framework. In *Caring for Muslim Patients*, A Sheikh, AR Gatrad (eds). Oxford.

Ahmed S, Green J, Hewison J (2005) Antenatal thalassemia carrier testing: woman's perception of information and consent. *Journal of Medical Screening* 12: 69–77.

Al A'ali (1993) Assumptions concerning the social sciences: a comparative perspective. *American Journal of Islamic Social Sciences* 10: 485–90.

Asad T (1993) *Genealogies of Religion, Discipline and Reason of Power in Christianity and Islam*. Baltimore. Johns Hopkins University.

Aspinall P, Jackson B (2004) *Ethnic Disparities in Health and Health Care: A Focused Review and Selected Examples of Good Practice*. London: Department of Health/London Health Observatory.

Atkin K, Ahmad W (1998) Genetic counselling and haemoglobinopathies: ethics, politics and practice. *Social Science and Medicine* 46. 445–8.

Atkin K, Ahmad WIU, Anionwu EW (2000) Service support to families caring for a child with a sickle cell disorder or beta thalassaemia major: parents' perspectives. In WIU Ahmad (ed) *Ethnicity, Disability and Chronic Illness*. Buckingham: Open University Press, pp. 103–22.

Audit Commission (2004) *Journey to Race Equality: Delivering Improved Services to Local Communities*. London: Audit Commission.

Auluck R, Iles P (1991) The referral process – a study of working relationships between antenatal clinic nursing staff and hospital social workers and their impact on Asian women. *British Journal of Social Work* 21: 41–61.

Barot R (ed) (1993) *Religion and Ethnicity: Minorities and Social Change in the Metropolis*. Kampen: Kok Pharos.

Bhakta P, Katbamna S, Parker G (2000) South Asian carer's experiences of primary health care teams. In W Ahmad (ed.) *Ethnicity, Disability and Chronic Illness*. Buckingham: Open University Press, pp. 123–39.

Bhopal R (1997) Is research in ethnicity and health racist, unsound, or important science? *British Medical Journal* 314: 1751.

Bhopal R, Rankin J (2002) Concept and terminology in ethnicity, race and health: be aware of the ongoing debate. *British Dental Journal* 186: 10.

Bowes A, Domokos T (1996) Pakistani women and Maternity Care: raising muted voices. *Sociology of Health and Illness* 18: 45–65.

Bowler I (1993) Stereotypes of women of Asian descent in midwifery: some evidence. *Midwifery* 9: 7–16.

British Medical Association (1995) *Multicultural Health Care: Current Practice and Future Policy in Medical Education*. London, BMA.

Bury M (1982) Chronic illness as biographical interruption. *Sociology of Health and Illness*, 4: 167–82.

Cesari J (1998) Muslim representation in a European political context. *Encounters* 42(149): 155.

Chamba R, Ahmad WIU (2000) Language, communication and information. In WIU Ahmad (ed) *Ethnicity, Disability and Chronic Illness*. Buckingham: Open University Press, pp. 85–102.

Chamba R, Ahmad W, Jones L (1998) *Improving Services for Asian Deaf Children*. Bristol: Polity Press.

Charmaz K, Olesen V (1997) Ethnographic research in medical sociology – its foci and distinctive contributions. *Sociological Methods and Research* 25: 452–94.

Cinnirella M, Loewenthal KM (1999) Religious and ethnic group influences on beliefs about mental illness: a qualitative interview study. *British Journal of Medical Psychology* 72: 505–24.

Commission for Racial Equality (1998) *Stereotyping and Racism: Findings from Two Attitude Surveys*. London: Commission for Racial Equality.

Dyson S (1998) Race, ethnicity and haemoglobin disorders. *Social Science and Medicine* 47: 121–31.

Dyson S (1999) Review of *Human Genetics, Choice and Responsibility*, BMA/Oxford University Press, 1998. *Social Science and Medicine*, 49: 1427–9.

Hatton C, Azmi S, Caine E, Emerson E (1998) Informal carers of adolescents and adults with learning disabilities from South Asian communities. *British Journal of Social Work* 28: 821–37.

Hatton C, Turner S, Shah R, Rahim N, Stansfield J (2004) Religious expression, a fundamental right. Report of 'Meeting the religious needs of people with learning disabilities'. London: Foundation for People with Learning Disabilities.

Hill SA (1994) *Managing Sickle Cell Disease in Low Income Families*. Philadelphia: Temple University Press.

Karlsen S, Nazroo J (2002) Agency and structure: the impact of ethnic identity and racism on the health of ethnic minority people. *Sociology of Health and Illness* 24: 1–20.

Kelleher D (1996) A defence of 'ethnicity' and 'culture'. In D Kelleher, S Hillier (eds) *Researching Cultural Differences in Health*, London: Routledge, pp. 69–90.

Kelleher, D Islam S (1996) "How should I live?" Bangladeshi people and insulin dependent diabetes. In *Researching Cultural Differences in Health*, D Kelleher, S Hillier (eds). London: Routledge.

Mahmood N, Ringheim K (1997) Knowledge, approval and communication about family planning as correlates of desired fertility among spouses in Pakistan. *International Family Planning Perspectives* 23: 122–9.

Mir G (2005) Social policy and health inequalities: the relevance of faith to chronic illness management in the Pakistani community PhD, University of Leeds School of Medicine.

Mir G, Nocon A, Ahmad W (2001) *Learning Difficulties and Ethnicity*. London: Department of Health.

Mir G, Tovey P (2003) Asian carers' experience of medical and social care: the case of cerebral palsy. *British Journal of Social Work* 33(465): 479.

Mir G, Tovey P, Ahmad W (2000) *Cerebral Palsy and South Asian Communities*. Leeds: Centre for Research in Primary Care, University of Leeds.

Mir G, Nocon A, Ahmad W (2001) *Learning Difficulties and Ethnicity*. London: Department of Health.

Modood T, Berthoud R, Lakey J, Nazroo J, Smith P, Virdee S et al. (1997) *Ethnic Minorities in Britain: Diversity and Disadvantage*. London: Policy Studies Institute.

Murphy K, Clark J (1993) Nurses' experiences of caring for ethnic minority clients. *Journal of Advanced Nursing* 18: 442–50.

Naeem Z, Newton V (1996) Prevalence of sensorineural hearing loss in Asian children. *British Journal of Audiology* 30: 332–9.

Nazroo J (1997) *The Health of Britain's Ethnic Minorities*. London: Policy Studies Institute.

Popay J, Williams G (1996) Public health research and lay knowledge. *Social Science and Medicine* 42: 755–68.

Rankin J, Bhopal R (1999) Current census categories are not a good match for identity. *British Medical Journal* 318(7199): 1696.

Runnymede Trust (Commission on British Muslims and Islamophobia) (1997) Islamophobia: a challenge for us all: report of the Runnymede Trust Commission on British Muslims and Islamophobia, London.

Said F. (1995) *Orientalism*. London: Penguin Books.

Selway D, Ashman A (1998) Disability, religion and health: a literature review in search of the spiritual dimensions of disability. *Disability and Society* 13: 429–39.

Speck P, Higginson I, Addington Hall J (2004) Spiritual needs in healthcare. *British Medical Journal* 2004: 123–4.

Vangen S, Stoltenberg C, Schei B (1996) Ethnicity and use of obstetrical analgesia: do Pakistani women receive inadequate pain relief in labour? *Ethnicity and Health* 1: 161–7.

Vanniasegaram I, Tungland OP, Bellman S (1992) A five-year review of children with deafness in a multiethnic community. *Journal of Audiological Medicine* 2: 9–19.

Walsh F (1998) *Strengthening Family Resilience*. New York: Guilford Press.

Wheeler E (1998) Mental illness and social stigma. *Gender and Development* 6: 37–43.

21 Living with NF2

PETER CRAWSHAW AND CYNTHIA CRAWSHAW

Peter Crawshaw was 25 and had just qualified in medicine when surgery for bilateral acoustic neuromas rendered him deafened. His wife Cynthia recently retired from a senior clinical nursing post. Their children, now in their twenties, have both obtained degrees and are developing their careers.

MY DEAFENED EXPERIENCE

Peter Crawshaw

INTRODUCTION

I was 22 and a fourth-year medical student working in wilderness Canada. Following a bad cold I lost significant hearing in one ear. Investigations in the UK a few weeks later (this was prior to the availability of CT scans), suggested viral deafness.

Three years later I awoke following my stag night party to find I was almost completely deaf. My new wife and I coped with the wedding and honeymoon prior to full investigation on one of the early CT scanners. I was diagnosed with NF2, having two large acoustic neuromas. Major neurosurgery followed. I then spent eight years training as a radiologist. For the past twenty years I have worked as a consultant in a busy general hospital in the north of England. During that time I have had neurosurgery three more times, once for tumour re-growth and twice to remove meningiomas.

IMPACT

The bald facts do not convey the stress, patience and effort it has taken, by my family, friends and colleagues at work to allow me to achieve such a normal life.

On becoming deaf the first thought was one of shock, quickly followed by irritation. I had so many plans for life and deafness threatened to disrupt them all. My wife, a nurse, seemed to take our problems in her stride, but not so my parents. Mother coped surprisingly well, but my father, from whom it emerged I had inherited the syndrome, was terribly upset. In his presence I spent my time consoling and counselling him rather than him me.

My biggest problem was to develop my lip-reading. It took years to become reasonably proficient, during which time most people had to write to communicate with me. My other serious problem was acute loss of confidence. I would cross the road to avoid friends, so I did not have to try and communicate. At work I just about coped with patients – they have always been very tolerant – but had much more difficulty with my older consultant colleagues. A small but significant number of the highly trained doctors I have worked with seem unable or unwilling to cope with disabled patients and colleagues.

I was very fortunate that my professor and his teaching staff found the time and patience over the years of training to teach and encourage me. Towards the end I failed my final viva numerous times. My fellow students took it upon themselves to give me mock teaching almost every day for three months. The only way to thank everyone was to succeed. Fortunately they had boosted my confidence sufficiently and I passed.

A year later I moved to a quiet country hospital for an easier life. Hectic modern medicine rapidly caught up with me. At work I was, and am, fortunate to have a superb secretary who looks out for me and aids communication considerably. At home my long-suffering wife has managed to work, raise two children and act as nurse, communications manager and friend to her husband.

Both my children have inherited NF2 and so life has turned full circle. Following their initial diagnosis I felt significant guilt and regret that they would have to suffer my disability. I had lived through a similar situation with my father, who became so guilt-ridden on my diagnosis (he had minimal signs of NF2) that he was unable to help me at the time I needed it most. I resolved to be optimistic and positive and help my children cope. We are a close-knit family so, while the children were growing up, we taught each other how to cope with problems and succeed in life.

My staff, colleagues and managers at work have always gone out of their way to help and support me.

For over 30 years one of my hobbies has been providing medical support for motor-sport, usually car rallies. This has introduced many good friends into my life.

Apart from loss of confidence, other problems I have encountered include irritability at the end of the day, which I tend to take out on my close relatives. This is exceedingly counterproductive, but difficult to eradicate. I also have a tendency to talk and not 'listen' – it is easier!

The deafened population fall between two stools. They do not usually want to join (and are rarely accepted by) the deaf society. Our mainstream society regards them as disabled; this can limit their ambitions and culture.

It is exceedingly traumatic to become totally deaf after years of normal hearing. The full implications of becoming suddenly deafened – with the inevitable isolation and exclusion from normal life, the impact on employment, learning, and personal life.

NOT BEING EASILY UNDERSTOOD BY PEOPLE WITH NORMAL HEARING

Most 'young' deafened people, and many older ones, want to continue with their normal life, i.e. job, social activities, friends etc. Much of this is possible but there are limitations and conditions which the deafened person has to come to terms with.

It is necessary to develop considerable self-confidence and a thick skin. This takes time and requires sympathetic friends, family and work colleagues who can boost confidence when the opportunity arises and can also pick up the pieces and lead the way to the pub, when difficulties occur. Most young people have a rapid turnover of friends and associates.

When I became deafened many of my friends melted away. Some lacked the patience to communicate. With some we no longer had a common interest, e.g. music. Others just moved on. Coupled with a massive loss of self-esteem this reduction in social life and contacts can be very hard to cope with especially if the deafened person does not have a partner.

A further problem can be physical appearance. After my initial operations I was left with gross unilateral facial palsy. The grafted nerve took almost two years to function adequately but I still have significant facial nerve and eye problems. This undoubtedly lowers confidence and hinders developing relationships.

HOW CAN THE NEWLY DEAFENED PERSON START TO REBUILD THEIR LIFE?

Provision for rehabilitation for deafened people is minimal. The National Association of Deafened People (NADP) and the LINK centre (which runs residential courses for deafened people and their partners) offer help, advice and a short rehabilitation course. They also introduce you to the deafened world. It is a huge relief to realise there are many thousands of people just like you.

Try to maintain a small circle of friends and associates who are prepared to help communication. Do not rely on one or two people: helping a newly deafened person is emotionally stressful and physically tiring. This also applies to one's partner. Developing different interests to allow breathing space can be vital for a relationship to succeed.

Use texting, and emails to communicate with distant friends. Text phones, using an operator to type out for you, are slow but can be a great help, particularly if the deafened person lives alone.

At work, at college and socially make everyone aware of your disability and gently explain the limitations and requirements of lipreading. Many people will be embarrassed to try and communicate but, given help and encouragement from you, they will persevere. Always carry a pen and some paper. A couple of written words can make a huge difference.

In lectures sit next to someone and ask if they will write down salient points not covered by the visual text. In meetings ask if you can sit next to the secretary and crib the minutes. This frequently enables you to follow meetings better than if you could hear!

Try to develop new sports, hobbies and interests that are not so hearing-dependent. These will give you an interest and help to generate new friends. Try not to become bitter: it is no one else's fault and bitterness drives friends away.

It is important to remain positive; with a certain amount of determination and some lateral thinking, it should be possible to overcome most problems and attain a high quality of life.

LIVING WITH A DEAFENED HUSBAND

Cynthia Crawshaw

I am writing this piece on our 29th wedding anniversary. I don't suppose anyone would say being married that long is easy. I will write about my experience but I hesitate to offer advice as no two people or their situations are alike.

I have long thought that I am the carthorse and my husband the racehorse. I am slow and patient, he is quick and impetuous. However, we are both determined. Our ability, or otherwise to cope with problems is no doubt largely determined by our personalities.

As the years have gone by we have changed our behaviour in the light of our evolving circumstances. When we were first married I was able to give my husband almost my sole attention and no doubt this helped to build up his lipreading and social skills. I learnt that people found it easier to communicate if I was present and could act as a go-between. This situation still exists, and can become trying at times.

We both wanted children. A visit to a geneticist 27 years ago suggested that the risk of inheritance was small. As the children grew we had some suspicions, seeing café au lait patches for example, but were not able to obtain genetic screening until they were about 9 and 11 years old. A CT scan at this time showed our son had small bilateral acoustic neuromas. The genetic screening merely confirmed his diagnosis but it was quite a blow to find our daughter was also genetically positive for NF2. I think our determination to help them as much as possible pulled us through.

They needed us to be positive optimistic and practical. There was no time for the sadness we felt, except occasionally at night when we were alone. This attitude was also important with our friends, family and colleagues. Most people were shocked enough. We have learned that being positive enables more support from other people who, most of the time, simply do not understand.

We have encouraged our children to be optimistic and adventurous and fortunately they are both as determined as their parents.

We only have one life; it seems a waste to spend time dwelling on ill-health and disability. We have concentrated on education, careers, sport and having fun. Between us we have managed to do most of the things we wanted.

The ongoing developments in the diagnosis and treatment of NF2 have been a significant boost. We feel the future can only get better. We both hope that our children can benefit from pre-implantation screening before having their own families but, if not, they say they want children anyway, suggesting their lives are well worth living.

Living with a deafened husband has made me more independent and self-sufficient than I would otherwise have been. My husband's work has become increasingly tough over the years, so that in the evenings he is frequently too tired to want to lip-read much. I found it hard when I developed cancer a few years ago. My husband who had always been used to help from me, found it difficult to reciprocate in the way I needed. On reflection it was probably due to habit and a fear of losing my support.

As I recovered I realised that I needed to concentrate on things important to me. This I am now doing with my husband's help and support.

We are now in an empty-nest situation and readjusting to our new found freedom and eventual retirement.

There are many terrible situations in this world. Our lives seem predominantly happy and successful by comparison.

My only advice: life is what you make it!

22 The Meaning of Hearing Loss in the Same Family over Nearly 200 Years

ANNA-CARIN REHNMAN

INTRODUCTION

This study started when I read a family story about a man born in 1816. His name was Pehr Hansson and he lived in a small parish in the north of Sweden. He was the youngest son in a family with two older brothers and one sister. At this time, before the introduction of elementary schools, only a few inhabitants of the parish had writing and counting skills. Pehr Hansson's father was a churchwarden and a member of the parish council and had at least a limited ability to write his name and to read handwritten material. Pehr Hansson and his brothers were able to read well, and were awarded the highest marks for reading in the church register. They also learnt to write and count in spite of the fact that they had no formal education.

Pehr Hansson grew up to become a physically strong and talented farmer, like his father and brothers. He was a member of the Parish Council, the Board of Education and the Tax Authority, and served as the banker of the parish. He also started a sawmill in the middle of the nineteenth century which gave him, his sons and other farmers in the village, jobs and income. But the family story also tells us that Pehr Hansson suffered from a severe degree of deafness. He had nine children from two marriages. Seven of them, five from his first marriage and two from his second, in all six men and one woman, developed deafness like their father, possibly already then recognised as a genetically dominant hereditary impairment. When I read about them I wondered what had happened to those children who inherited the deafness in the following generations.

AIM AND RESEARCH QUESTIONS

The central aim in this study is to describe and understand the meaning of hearing loss and its personal and environmental implications in the same

The Effects of Genetic Hearing Impairment in the Family. Edited by D. Stephens and L. Jones.
Copyright © 2006 by John Wiley & Sons, Ltd.

family spanning several generations, over nearly 200 years. It concerns how they interact with developments in society, and how different generations focus on possibilities for family life, education, health, gender and different strategies.

- How widespread was the hereditary hearing loss passed on by Pehr Hansson, born 1816, and his children?
- To what extent did the hearing loss have an impact on their life situation?
- In what way did the hearing loss have an effect on the following generations with regard to their education, family life and ability to make a living?

METHODS

TRACING RELATIVES

All members of families related to the progenitor Pehr Hansson, were traced in old parish registers and books, and the public population register.

QUESTIONNAIRES

About 100 relatives, living today and aged between 40 and 85 years who were descended from Pehr Hansson, were sent questionnaires in which they were asked if they knew anybody with a hearing impairment in their families. If so, who and where are they? More than 80 people replied.

INTERVIEWS

Thirty of those still alive today and 12 of their children had developed a hearing loss. Sixteen interviews of those 30 people were recorded. They told about themselves, their parents, the lives of their grandmothers or grandfathers and how the hearing loss had influenced their lives. I asked them for their audiograms or had their permission to obtain records from their medical files.

CASE STUDIES AND ANALYSIS

Thirty-four life stories of 18 women born between 1870 and 1963 and of 16 men born between 1877 and 1955 were constructed, including information from the interviews, examination of photographs, newspapers, letters and other sources. These life stories were collected and analysed by their time period in order to highlight any changes, with the aim of understanding the meaning of hearing loss over several generations.

RESULTS

RESULTS FROM THE QUESTIONNAIRES

More than 80 people answered the questionnaire. Only a few of them did not know anyone with a hearing impairment. Most of them knew a grandmother or a grandfather, an aunt or an uncle and described them as more or less deaf. Some had a parent, sisters or brothers. Thirty of those living today, and 12 of their children, had also developed a hearing loss themselves. The family tree was gradually created after checking that the different information sources tallied with the audiograms and other available information.

The hearing loss was widespread.

In three familes, the genetically dominant hearing loss came to an end after 3 generations. In four families it still continues after 5, 6 and 7 generations.

In the 2nd generation 6 men and 1 woman out of 9 with a likely genetic background, developed a hearing loss.

In the 3rd generation 9 men and 10 women out of 32 with a likely genetic background developed a hearing loss.

In the 4th generation 10 men and 11 women out of 60 with a likely genetic background developed a hearing loss.

In the 5th generation 13 men and 10 women out of 52 with a likely genetic background developed a hearing loss.

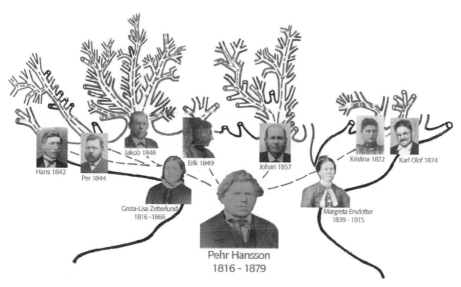

Figure 22.1 Family tree.

In the 6th generation 5 men and 10 women out of 28 with a likely genetic background developed a hearing loss.

In the 7th generation out of 6 children with a likely genetic background there are so far 2 girls who have developed a hearing loss.

RESULTS FROM THE INTERVIEWS

I started interviews with 16 people born between 1923 and 1963 who had a hereditary hearing loss, 7 women and 9 men. They told me about themselves, their parents, grandmothers or grandfathers and their lives. I learnt how they gradually lost their hearing and how it influenced their live. Here are some examples from the interviews.

The hearing loss started at different times for different people but has always become severe over time.

Everybody in the family had normal hearing as a child and developed normal speech and language. The progressive hearing loss varies as to at what age it starts and can also be different between different individuals in the same branch of the family. The first audiogram (Figure 22.2), which is my own, shows

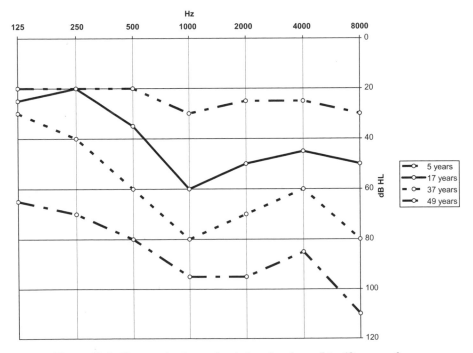

Figure 22.2 Changes in the author's hearing from 5 to 49 years of age.

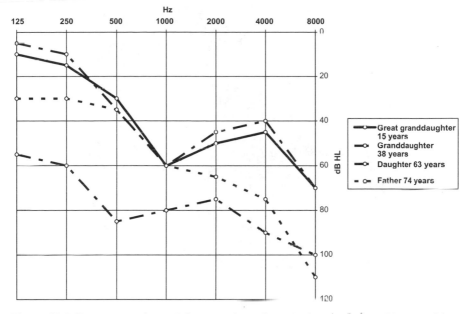

Figure 22.3 Four generations of the same branch of the family: father, 74 years old at the time of testing; daughter, 63 years old at the time of testing; granddaughter, 38 years old at the time of testing; great-granddaughter, 15 years old at the time of testing.

a progressive hearing loss from 5 to 49 years of age. The other example (Figure 22.3) shows four generations of the same branch of the family: a father, 74 years old when tested, his daughter, 63 years old, a granddaughter aged 38 years and a great-granddaughter aged 15 years. Independent of minor variations, the hearing loss has become severe over time for all of them.

HEARING LOSS – AN EVERYDAY ASPECT OF FAMILY LIFE

Hearing loss was an everyday aspect of family life. It was considered normal not to hear. To maintain functional communication they would touch each other before talking and talked loudly and clearly. The families lived in villages and their grandmother and grandfather lived in the same house or in their neighbourhood. As children, they had good contact with the older generation (Figure 22.4). Other family members, as well as neighbours, respected their talking rules and adapted themselves to those who heard least. Even in the village school, the teacher and their fellow pupils talked loudly and clearly. Those in the family, always one of the parents and some of the brothers or sisters with normal hearing, were considered exceptional because they heard perfectly.

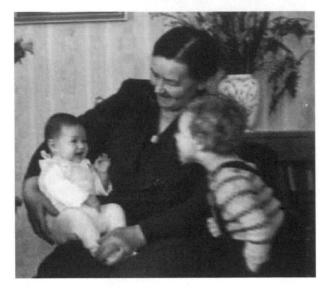

Figure 22.4 Deaf grandmother from family with her grandchildren.

My grandmother's brother was really stone deaf, and when he visited her, she lived upstairs, and was also deaf; downstairs, we could hardly bear the sound level when they were talking together. (Man, 2004)

Yes, the two eldest [sisters] couldn't hear well. But [my youngest sister] she heard perfectly well/.../ one knew that it was hereditary and that it came from mum, dad had perfect hearing and it was only my youngest sister who inherited from him as far as hearing is concerned. (Old man, 2004)

EDUCATION

The elementary school played a minor role for them in learning how to read, write and count because they had a strong tradition of home education that continued through the generations (Figure 22.5). In the second and third generations, they attended school for certain periods of the year or every other day. Even today there are strong reading habits in the families. Most of the people I interviewed had learned to read and write before starting school. Often it turned out to be their deaf grandfather who had taught them.

Grandfather taught me how to read and write before I went to school, even to write using my right hand. I was lefthanded which was not acceptable at that time. (Woman, 2004)

Throughout the generations all were avid readers of news and interested in social and political issues. Some of them took part in different social groups,

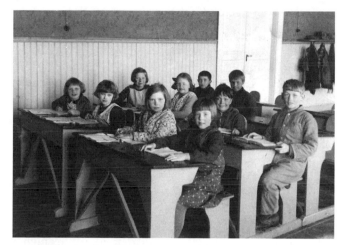

Figure 22.5 Elementary school with family members.

political, economical, religious and cultural, and in societies for the hard of hearing. In this way they could make use of their talents and skills.

Brothers and sisters without hearing loss were the first to receive higher education. Only one of those with a hearing loss received higher education before 1960. One reason was that their parents could not foresee hearing aids. When the first hearing-impaired ones started higher education, some failures occurred before they were fitted with hearing aids. They also tried, without success, to receive education from which people with handicaps were excluded.

IDENTIFICATION OF HEARING PROBLEMS

Those whom I interviewed, identified their hearing problems mostly in relation to sounds of nature and the perception of similar sounds that slowly faded away, i.e. sounds that man could not influence, rather than in communication with other people. They went to a school doctor or an ordinary doctor, but they did not like to receive a diagnosis.

> At the age of thirteen or fourteen I remember hearing crickets. Since then I never heard them again. At that moment I thought that this sound is something I shall never come close to hearing again. The others said they could hear it and, as I said before, I heard it once so in a way I know it exists. (Man, 2004)

> I went to the doctor when I was thirty, because I thought I had a lump of wax in the ear. I could no longer hear my watch ticking and was sent for a hearing test. Then the doctor told me to get a hearing aid because my hearing loss was so severe. (Woman, 2004)

CONSULTATIONS WITH DOCTORS AND DIAGNOSES

The first time I came across someone who had consulted a doctor, it was a young woman with a hearing loss, who worked in the office of a general practitioner in 1914. She writes in a letter that her 25-year-old sister has let her know about 'ear problems' and that she can hardly hear anything. The letter ends with the following words:

> It is a long time since I brought it up with the doctor [i.e., the hearing loss]. It is all in the hands of God.

An old man told me in an interview that he did his military service in 1943 during the Second World War.

> Had the recruitment rules then been the same as they are today, they would have rejected me.

A young boy [17 years old in 1952] who had to break off his higher education after some school failures because he could not hear, went to see a doctor and received the following prognosis:

> Then I was told that I would become deaf if . . . well, in a year's time or so. That doctor in the regional hospital really made me feel miserable. I really was hit badly . . .

Another man told me in an interview about his first consultation with a doctor around 1970:

> I was told by the doctor that I would have a decrease in my hearing capacity. That gave me a shock, because I was hearing rather well at the time. Nevertheless, I was told that the hearing nerve had permanent damage that would never heal. Oh no, I really felt let down and miserable after that consultation.

Some of them met the doctor at school and they knew that their hearing ability was poor but they did not take any notice of it. Only when some of them left the village elementary school and entered secondary school and started to learn foreign languages did they meet a school environment in which they could not cope.

CHANGES IN THE INTERACTION BETWEEN INDIVIDUALS AND THEIR ENVIRONMENT OVER TIME

Without any hearing aids a loud and uncontrolled voice always signalled that a person had a hearing loss [i.e. the level at which the individual can hear] to those talking to them. People in their environment who wanted to talk to them immediately adjusted their speech habits.

When some of them started to get hearing aids, their voices became more normal but they wanted to hide the hearing aid, because they were ashamed of their hearing loss. They did not want to talk about their hearing loss and some of them denied that the hearing loss was hereditary. People in their environment, not in the family, became insecure as to how to address them.

> My mother was deaf. For her, it meant a great handicap. She suffered a lot because of it and felt she was silly when she could not understand what people around her were talking about. She refused to use any hearing aid. Probably, because she was ashamed. (Woman in a questionnaire, 2003)

Now, when they use modern hearing aids and have a normal voice, they inform people around them about their hearing loss, in which situations they have a problem hearing and what they should do if a person does not hear. Often people meet them halfway and adjust their speech, but they soon tend to forget.

> I have always told everybody about my hearing impairment. I have let people know that if there is no reaction, they should give me a nudge. (Woman, 2004)

RELATIONSHIP BETWEEN SPEECHREADING AND HEARING AIDS

The only possible solution for communication for those in the family who lost their hearing in the past was speechreading. For a long time, through several generations, it was the best and safest way. No one learned sign language. In many situations they could not use a ear trumpet or early hearing aids and therefore their speechreading skill was very important. Later on, some talk about speechreading as an art, something they could not do, something which was too difficult and was meant only for those who were born deaf. When some

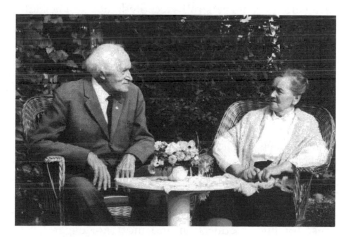

Figure 22.6 Family members speechreading.

of them had courses in speechreading they were surprised that they became good speechreaders. One among those I interviewed used only speechreading today. In his job he receives incoming orders by telephone and meets customers in a shop.

> I participated in a hearing test [at the hearing centre] and was asked if I had any job. I have been working all my life, I replied. The remaining time he serves behind the counter. I explained how I work. That is unbelievable, she said, that you have been able to keep the job. I know how to lip-read. I would be at a loss if customers turned around. (Man, 2004)

The others that I interviewed said that they can use both speechreading and hearing aids. They combine the best available hearing aids and speechreading skills to obtain the best possible communication.

> More ability than being able to see? But one can hear. I can hear some and the rest I can substitute with my eyes. Not everybody is hard to understand, some I can hear clearly. Some speak in a loud voice but with a slurred articulation. So speaking in a loud voice doesn't necessarily make for clarity. (Woman, 2004)

ATTITUDES TO HEARING AIDS CHANGE OVER TIME

It is impossible to know whether Pehr Hansson had a ear trumpet or not. There are notes indicating that at least two of his sons produced home-made trumpets which they used sometimes when talking to people and when attending church. Then, when early hearing aids came, some of them were afraid of losing what was left of their hearing ability if they used hearing aids. Those who had lived a long time without hearing aids often became irritated when they tried to use them and they could never reconcile themselves to using them.

When hearing aids became generally accepted, they still hesitated for a long time before getting one. When they finally went to see the doctor, their hearing loss had become severe. Those who really needed them concealed their hearing aid and were annoyed that they had to use them. At this time they received only one hearing aid per person, sometimes for the better ear, sometimes for the worse. They did not know the reason for choosing one ear or the other 'They took whatever they got.'

> However, when I look at the curve printed on the accompanying information sheet, there was nothing to indicate that it would not be possible to use two aids. Some people believe that the hearing capacity, would suffer in that case. (Man, 2004)

Attitudes to hearing aids have changed today. But they still hesitate for a long time before they get, usually, two hearing aids. For some, hearing aids have become a must for higher education and most are eager to learn how to use them and other hearing devices. Now many of them keep up with developments and use 'state-of-the-art' technical devices. They choose the most powerful hearing aids on the market and two of them have had cochlear implants.

FROM A WELL-KNOWN ENVIRONMENT TO A NEW, UNKNOWN ONE

I have not written much about how they made a living. From the beginning, the families were farmers. It was a privilege to inherit the farm and a sure way to support oneself. Even that has changed. When brothers and sisters with normal hearing had higher education, those relatives who were deaf and male often stayed at home and took care of the farm. Therefore it is interesting to see that it was women who left the familiar environment first. Often there were men involved who had plenty of resources to support them. In their new homes they tried to create a family environment where deafness was considered normal.

The life situation has changed a lot between those I interviewed and their parents. Apart from using hearing aids, most of them had moved from villages to towns, received higher education and were employed in different jobs. In addition, they try to establish relationships in their workplaces in order to reduce the impact of the hearing loss.

Another thing which has changed is their coping strategies. Their parents mostly took a personal responsibility to hear and prepare themselves and create a manageable situation before meeting other people. An old deaf woman came to see a doctor who wanted to interview her. Then the old lady said: 'Can we change seats?' and the doctor changed seats with her. Then she said: 'Now the light is falling on you so that I can speechread what you are saying'. This responsibility is still practised, but now they even share the responsibility of hearing with husbands, wives, colleagues and friends. A woman told me how her husband shared the responsibility with her when they attended big meetings.

> My husband and I are rather wrapped up in the work of the golf club, among other things. Now, we talk about large gatherings of about 100 people in big meeting in Stockholm. Then he chooses to sit with me in front, in order for me to be able to hear those people up front, but then somebody talks some place in the back, and then I get lost. Then he, of course will listen to them and retell it all to me. I pity him, of course I do. But it is a fact. Nevertheless he does his very best.

CONCLUDING REMARKS

Without describing the social changes that have taken place in society over time as far as family life, employment and attitudes towards impairment are concerned, I want to reflect upon the meaning of hearing loss given by different generations and their contemporaries.

Throughout the nineteenth century and in the beginning of the twentieth, hearing loss was considered to be part of natural variation and not a medical problem. The communication problems that arose were something to be resolved within the family and among close neighbours, where those involved shared the responsibility for finding a workable solution. The deaf did their part through speechreading and the others by adapting their speech habits to those who heard least. Children grew up in such circumstances and found it all normal.

People still lived in countryside villages between 1910 and 1960 but, perhaps because of their great interest in social matters and strong interest in reading, they knew at an early stage that people with some kind of deficiency were not regarded as full, worthy citizens. As a result, those children who had inherited the hearing loss, stopped short of going on to further education but kept in their home which provided, for them, a normal way to communicate. To remain in familiar surroundings, and at the same time trying to conceal the hearing loss in a new setting, must be considered a reasonable measure to cope with their hearing loss which even then had developed a medical implication. They tried to protect themselves from the medical aspect by avoiding seeing a doctor, because they knew that consulting a doctor would give them a definite diagnosis.

During this period of time new ideas came about as to the cause of the hearing impairment. To some, it was easier and less painful to blame it on noise rather than accepting it as a hereditary matter that might be transferred to their children. The first types of hearing aids could not provide satisfactory compensation, which, in fact, added uncertainty even to the speechreading skills. This might have been one reason why they hesitated so long before consulting doctors and starting to use hearing aids.

How is it that most of those whom I interviewed were able to turn the tide of these ongoing negative implications? Several factors should be considered, for example increased access to education, improved technical achievements and a change in attitudes towards people with an impairment. I have noticed that they have become aware of their speechreading skills in combination with hearing aids. They even dare to leave some responsibility for functional communication to others. They have reconciled themselves to their hearing loss and have a sense of belonging to the life of their ancestors which was valued more than a hereditary hearing loss.

Finally, I wonder what has happened to the hereditary aspect and the meaning of the hearing loss. One of my informants whose mother blamed his hearing loss on noise says it is an advantage to know the origin of the hearing loss. His son was diagnosed with a hearing loss at the age of three. As for himself, he feels part of a continuous flow across the generations. His son has high ambitions in life and does not consider his hearing loss as something dramatic as he knows where it comes from. The son looks up to his father as a good example to follow, confident that it is fully possible to live a rather normal life in spite of the hearing loss.

I want to quote a woman who comes from a family that never questioned the hereditary aspect of the hearing loss. She has now lost her hearing completely and is using a cochlear implant:

Today I feel in a way that I belong to the deaf. Yes I do. I know I do and it does not frighten me at all. Because the hearing loss is my life, a part of my life, it is part of my identity and it is hard to separate it from its context. That's why this connection to identity and confirmation becomes closely tied together for generations. And because I see both my dad and his mother, my grandmother, as good examples it is not a heavy burden to carry this deficiency. (Woman, 2004)

V Research Needs

23 Family History of Hearing Impairment and Its Psychological and Social Consequences – What Next?

BERTH DANERMARK
(WITH CONTRIBUTIONS FROM PER-INGE CARLSSON,
LESLEY JONES AND DAFYDD STEPHENS)

INTRODUCTION

One of the main conclusions in the review of literature on psychological and social consequences which we presented earlier (Stephens & Jones, 2005), was that the published literature does not provide us with any pointers regarding the different impacts of hearing impairment in adults with genetic and non-genetic aetiologies. This was an impetus to us to collect new data, from both retrospective and prospective studies, in order to take the first steps in creating an understanding of having a family history of hearing impairment (FHHI) and its psychological and social consequences. The underlying question is whether there is a difference between those hearing-impaired people with a family history and those without.

The studies we have collected in this book cannot give an unequivocal answer to this question. Some of the studies indicate that there is a difference, some that there is no difference. In some cases the reader will find contradictory conclusions. As a framework to examine the results from the eleven retrospective and prospective studies in this book (Chapters 1–11) we use the International Classification of Functioning, Disability and Health (ICF). For a discussion of ICF and hearing impairment, see Stephens and Danermark (2005). However, we are not able to cover all the relevant parameters that this classification system includes. The main reason for this is lack of data.

Table 23.1 shows the components that are related to having a FHHI. However, it is important to bear in mind that this table will give only a hint of the empirical relationships that have been discussed in this book. In order to have information on the character and magnitude of the correlation, the reader should consult the individual chapters.

The Effects of Genetic Hearing Impairment in the Family. Edited by D. Stephens and L. Jones.
Copyright © 2006 by John Wiley & Sons, Ltd.

Table 23.1 Significant relationships between FHHI and some aspects of ICF components

Components	Sub-components	Chapter(s)	Comments
Body functions and structures	Tinnitus	1	These components are
	Hearing problems/level of hearing loss	1, 2, 5	not psychological or social but they can
	Hyperacusis	1, 11	reinforce such consequences
Activities and participation	Educational achievement	3	Children
	Higher education	4, 5	
	Communication skills	3	Children
	Domestic life	3	Children
	Work	4	Want to leave work
	Type of job	5	Significant for women
Environmental factors	Role-modelling and role models	6, 9	Chapter 6: qualitative method (content
Support and relationships	Help-seeking	6, 10	analysis)
Attitudes		6	
Services, systems and policies	Sharing knowledge	7	
Personal factors	Quality of life	3	Children
	Expectation/anticipation	6	
	Acceptance, better understanding	6, 8, 9	Chapter 8, discourse analysis
	Worries about future	6	

It is important to appreciate that some studies in this book did not show any significant correlation with a FHHI, and some even contradicted the results presented in the table. For instance, no significant differences were found regarding activity limitation, participation restriction, psychological well-being, general health and well-being and use of hearing aids (in general or at work).

The role of a family history of hearing impairment is, to some extent, a story of role models. One can argue that it is strongly related to the process of social-isation. In short, the very basic idea which we would put forward – in full awareness that only a part of the story is being told – is that socialisation is a process of learning how to behave and how to act, including the mode of com-munication. This process is an ongoing one. It is not only determined by what is learned in early childhood. It continues throughout adulthood. Socialisation is a process that informs the individuals what is expected of them in various situations, but it is not seen as a stimulus–response reaction. It is an active process with reacting individuals.

In the light of the idea that socialisation is an important part of under-standing the consequences of having a family history of hearing impairment, we focus our attention on the question 'What are the factors in the family that have a significant impact on the socialisation process?' The second question will then be 'What are the long-term consequences of such socialisation?' A challenge for research on this topic is to reveal what mechanisms can result in long-term consequences and what, if any, are the counteracting mechanisms. However, there is a long way to go before we have a solid and empirical underpinned theory of family history of hearing impairment and psychosocial consequences.

It is not possible to, *a priori*, narrow down these mechanisms and we have, as mentioned earlier, only limited research so far to rely on. For instance we do not know whether the process is different between deaf and hard-of-hearing people, although there are some indications that the mode of communication in the family and the attitudes toward deafness seem to play an important part for the socialisation of deaf children (Stephens, 2005, p. 99; Chapter 4, this volume).

Given the uncertain theoretical and empirical position we can say that at the moment we are in a mode of context of discovery. Therefore Kramer et al.'s contribution (Chapter 6, this volume) is ground-breaking. Through a qualitative approach using content analysis they found six important themes in the process (see pp. 76–7 and Stephens & Kramer, 2005).

IMPACT OF FHHI

The second question was whether a family history has any impact on the individual's behaviour and activities. We can than identify a number of areas – or sub systems – where it is plausible to assume that FHHI has an impact. The areas that will be discussed briefly here are education, working life, social, and health. There might be several other areas that we do not discuss here.

EDUCATION

The choice of education is an important factor. In the beginning of the educational career, parents often heavily influence choices, but later the individuals' own wishes and goals become more and more important. However, this is a very complex process. For instance, a hard-of-hearing parent with extremely bad experiences during their own education, resulting in a very poor outcome, might not be able to give the emotional, social and intellectual support and encouragement to his/her children. The outcome could be that the child also receives a poor education. We have, to the best of our knowledge, no statistics or research that can throw some light on the relationship between having a family history of hearing impairment and choices of education among hard-of-hearing children (e.g. academic or vocational, special school or mainstream). Although the study presented in this volume by Carlsson and Danermark (Chapter 4) indicates that individuals with a family history were more likely to have a university degree than those who do not have (see p. 47). This is also supported by data in Coniavitis Gellerstedt and Danermark (Chapter 5, this volume, pp. 64–5) (see also Parving et al., 2002). Furthermore, there are indications that deaf children with at least one deaf parent have higher levels of educational achievements (see Chapter 3, this volume, p. 38) and that deaf children of deaf parents are more likely to go to schools for the deaf than deaf children of hearing parents (Stephens, 2005).

WORKING LIFE

Knowledge of hearing impairment and experiences of being hearing-impaired might influence an individual's choice of work (e.g. avoiding communication-intensive jobs), workplace (e.g. avoiding noisy environment) and awareness (e.g. using ear protection). These questions are dealt with, for instance, in Chapters 4 and 5. The overall conclusion so far is that there seems to be a weak relationship between FHHI and working condition but, due to limited numbers of subjects in the studies, these observations are very tentative (see also Dauman et al., 2000).

SOCIAL

Choice of partner, reproductive behaviour and leisure activities are all factors that might be affected by being socialised in a family with a history of hearing impairment. However, it is still an open question as to whether there is such a relationship and, if so, how it can be explained.

HEALTH

A fourth area we would put forward is the area of health. Here we treat health as a very broad concept. In the studies reported in this volume we have not been able to document any correlation between having a FHHI and self-reported health and well-being (see p. 121). From a rehabilitative perspective it is plausible to assume that individuals with knowledge of hearing impairment will have some impact on its early detection and any subsequent intervention, and that this is important for the coping process. This assumption gets some empirical support in some of the chapters in this volume (see, for example, Chapter 7).

Beside the impact on these areas there are indications that having a family history has consequences regarding emotions and identity. For instance, Polat (2003) argued that parental hearing status was one of the most important predictors of psychosocial adjustment (for a discussion, see Chapter 3 of this volume).

We can so far tentatively summarise the results in the model shown in Figure 23.1.

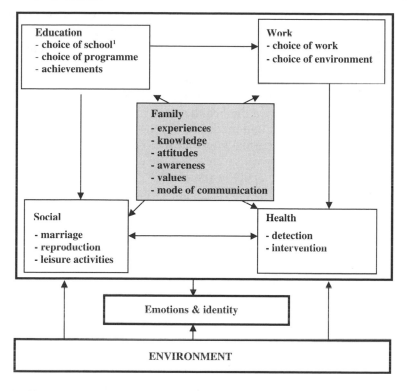

1. Choice between special schools or non-special schools.

Figure 23.1 A tentative model of FHHI and psychological and social consequences.

DECISION-MAKING IN RELATION TO HEARING PROBLEMS

It is important to have in mind, as Coniavitis Gellerstedt and Danermark write in Chapter 5:

A person's psychobiography is moulded through her/his experiences, cultural influences, group belongings etc. during the course of life and contributes to her/his attitudes and predispositions ... However, the existence of a history of hearing impairment in the family is only one of many factors having an impact on such decisions. (Chapter 5, this volume, p. 56)

As Table 23.1 shows, there are indications that having a FHHI, in some cases, plays a role and that this can be understood as a part of the socialisation process. However, there are two things we want to stress. First, our empirical knowledge is, at this stage, very uncertain and limited. All conclusions are, so far, very tentative. Second, the processes we are investigating in this book do not take place in a societal vacuum. There are important aetiological and environmental processes that will have an impact on what we can expect regarding people's decision-making in relation to their hearing problems. In the following sections we shall consider some of these processes; changes in some aetiological factors (e.g. more and more non-hereditary causes are eliminated); the demographic changes in the society (e.g. increase in life expectancy); developments in the health sector (especially the greater importance of genetics in health and medicine in relation to hearing impairment); the technical (e.g. better hearing aids) and socio-economic development (e.g. increasing cleavages and privatisation); and the changing ethnic and religious patterns (e.g. increasing diversity in society).

AETIOLOGICAL CHANGES

Dafydd Stephens

Over the past century there have been significant changes in the breakdown of causes of hearing impairment and, almost certainly, of its prevalence in the population as a whole. These stem from three main causes: the better medical and public health control of diseases, particularly infectious diseases, increased longevity and major population movements.

Infectious diseases

Among hearing-impaired children, control of infectious diseases, particularly in the more developed countries, has resulted in a major reduction in the prevalence of chronic otitis media as a principal cause of hearing loss in children. It remains, however, a major problem in less-developed countries. At the same time, developments in immunisation have led to a marked reduction in measles, mumps and rubella, all previously significant causative agents of hearing impairment in children, with the widespread introduction of the MMR vaccine. In the past few years there have been further developments with the introduction of vaccines for various causes of meningitis, and already the introduction of immunisation for haemophilus meningitis has had an impact on its prevalence.

   In the opposite direction, within certain populations, particularly in less developed countries, the appearance and spread of HIV/AIDS infection has predisposed infected individuals to a range of infectious conditions including otitis media and syphilis as well as having some direct neuropathic effects on the auditory system.

Other medical developments

The other major area in terms of a change in the cause of hearing impairment in children is in terms of the management of severe jaundice, particularly caused by rhesus incompatibility. Approaches resulting in an earlier diagnosis of the developing problem and its treatment with exchange transfusion and phototherapy, have resulted in its virtual disappearance as a major cause of congenital deafness in children over the past fifty years.

Noise

At present there are various changes taking place in different parts of the world. In the more developed world, much of the damaging occupational noise exposure has been reduced by a combination of hearing protection programmes and a closure or automation of many of the traditional heavy industries. This is not, however, true of the less developed world, where health and safety considerations have a less prominent position. Acoustic trauma with hearing loss arising from exposure to gunfire and explosions remains a worldwide problem, although less so in many of the more developed countries in which military conscription has been abolished and hearing protection implemented. Finally social noise from live and recorded music is a significant problem for many young people. While attitudes to and awareness of the impact of such noise exposure may vary from country to country, e.g. more concern and awareness in Sweden, less in the USA (Erlandsson & Widén, 2005), this is likely to remain a problem for some time, particularly in those with a genetic susceptibility to noise.

POPULATION CHANGES

Under this heading, the marked increase in life expectancy, particularly in the more developed countries, and major population movements both have a significant impact. While the medical advances have tended to reduce the prevalence of non-genetic causes of hearing impairment, these have the effect of increasing the proportion of hearing impairment due to genetic factors within the resulting populations.

In this respect, economic migration from a restricted area of the less developed world into other parts of the world while the population, at the same time, retains traditional beliefs and behavioural patterns, has led to young people seeking partners from a restricted pool of individuals, in some cases the extended family. This is potentiated by other complex factors such as economic deprivation in some migrant communities. Under such circumstances, recessive conditions, including those resulting in profound congenital hearing impairment, become more prevalent. In the past this has been associated with certain Jewish communities in Europe and the Middle East and, more recently, with South Asian populations who have moved to Europe. This has resulted in a higher prevalence of congenital hearing impairment in these populations than in the indigenous populations of the countries to which they have migrated. First-generation migrants tended to be without impairments as only the fitter and economically active groups of people would travel to seek employment in other countries. This has changed with the increasing numbers of second- and third-generation families originating from outside Europe.

Increased longevity can also be expected to have a major impact on the breakdown of causes of hearing impairment in the population as a whole, given that the likelihood of having impaired hearing increases markedly with age, particularly over the age of fifty years. Davis (1997) has published estimates of increasing numbers based on population projections from the United Nations for the period 1995–2025. Within these figures, the number of people with hearing impairment (over 25 dB in their better hearing ear) worldwide is projected as increasing from 441 million in 1995 to 915 million in 2025. Likewise, the number with profound hearing impairment (>95 dB) is predicted to increase from 9 million to 17 million. While the largest increases are predicted for the less developed world, where the figures may be somewhat questionable in the light of the HIV epidemic, even in the more developed world an increase of some 50% in numbers over this time period is predicted.

Given the altering balance of aetiological factors outlined above, the bulk of this change is likely to be in genetic hearing impairment which is currently estimated as accounting for some 50–70% of permanent childhood hearing impairment and some 50% of adult late-onset hearing impairment. Therefore, we give a short account of this aspect of hearing impairment.

HEREDITARY HEARING IMPAIRMENT

Per-Inge Carlsson

Hearing impairment is a common sensory deficit, affecting about 15% of the Caucasian populations. Approximately one in 1000 newborn children suffers from congenital severe or profound hearing impairment. In developed countries, more than 50% of these children have a hearing impairment caused by mutations in a single gene (Morton, 1991). The inheritance pattern of severe–profound childhood hearing impairment is autosomal recessive in approximately 77% of cases, autosomal dominant in 22% and X-linked in 1–4% (Reardon et al., 2004). Genetic factors account for some 50% of hearing impairment of later onset (Gates et al., 1999). Nearly all studies looking at hearing impairment of later onset have shown a dominant inheritance pattern. Epidemiological studies indicate that over 100 genes are involved into non-syndromal hearing impairment (Van Camp & Smith, 2005). Hereditary hearing impairment is subdivided into syndromal hearing impairment (1/3), associated with additional clinical abnormalities, and non-syndromal hearing impairment (2/3), without additional clinical abnormalities.

Until recently, the aetiology of most hearing impairment was uncertain, although it was frequently assumed to be due to genetic causes. In 1994, Guilford et al. (1994) identified a non-syndromal recessive deafness locus, DFNB1, on chromosome 13q12. Three years later, Kelsell et al. (1997) showed that deafness at this locus was due to a mutation in GJB2, encoding the protein Connexin 26.

Over 100 genes for non-syndromal hearing impairment have been localised in the human genome, and to date about half of these have been identified (Van Camp & Smith, 2005). It is to be expected that a large number of additional genes will be identified over the next decade. For each gene, identified so far, various disease-causing mutations have been described, revealing significant genotype–phenotype heterogeneity. Strachan and Read (2004) recently discussed three major problems regarding the issue: (1) mutations in different genes cause indistinguishable phenotypes; (2) different mutations in the same gene cause different phenotypes; (3) the same mutation in the same gene causes different phenotypes in different patients.

Despite the enormous heterogeneity of hereditary hearing impairment, it is now feasible to test for some mutations in the clinical situation. One is the 35delG of the Cx26 gene. The high prevalence of the mutation, particularly in southern Europe, makes it worth testing even when only a single hearing-impaired person is present in a family. For example, if a deaf newborn child is found to be homozygous for the Cx26 35delG mutation, we can provide the parents with a correct diagnosis and, thus, appropriate genetic counselling. The prognosis is also known in that the hearing impairment caused by the Cx26 35delG mutation is non-syndromal, meaning that there are probably no other disabilities present. Other mutations of importance to test in the clinical situation are those involved in syndromal hearing impairment, e.g. Usher and Pendred syndromes.

An important question is how far we can predefine which gene to test for. With syndromal hearing impairment, this is quite often possible. With non-syndromal hearing impairment, Mazzoli et al. (2004) have described the difficulties in predicting which of many candidate genes to suspect from the audiogram and other phenotypic features. Furthermore, the cost of genetic testing is falling constantly, and new gene chip technology allows thousands of tests to be carried out in a single operation on one DNA sample. Hence, it is likely that within the next ten years it will become possible to request the laboratory to trawl through the commoner genetic causes of hearing impairment in a patient at a reasonable cost. Negative results will not help us, but the positive identification of a mutated gene makes a correct diagnosis and prognosis possible in many cases.

Finally, we must remember that molecular techniques developed during the past 20 years have not only resulted in the detection of new genes and mutations at the DNA level. The identification of genes with important functions in the inner ear has contributed much to the understanding of the complex process of hearing. The finding of additional genes in the future will hopefully lead to the development of therapies to prevent or even cure certain forms of HI.

TECHNOLOGICAL CHANGES

Lesley Jones

Technology has fundamentally altered everyday lives throughout Late Modern societies in the West. These include those of people with impairments, who are increasingly dependent on technologies for their economic development. Information technology, in particular, has improved access for hearing-impaired people to communication with texting on mobile phones and webcams, both of which affect work and leisure. It offers inclusion in cultural life through subtitling on video, film and DVDs in a way which has previously been denied to this group of people. However, technologies are never culturally or socially neutral and are also capable of solidifying social bias as in access to their use through employment, education and cost. Some technologies, for example intercom entry phones in work and residential settings, rely on auditory sensory ability and therefore discriminate against hearing-impaired people. An information divide exists between different groups in society, often based around literacy and education as well as on ownership or access to the means of connection.

On a purely pragmatic level, the use of environmental aids (assistive listening devices) in the home and workplace, together with visual information systems in travel centres and healthcare, has made life easier for many people with hearing impairments, both genetic and acquired. Independence has been achieved for many young hearing-impaired people, resulting in them integrating more into mainstream society and less into Deaf Clubs with other Deaf young people.

In terms of medical technology, benefits have been offered through amplification by hearing aids, the hope of correction of profound hearing impairments with cochlear implants, and amelioration, as in surgery for otosclerosis, as well as auditory brainstem implants (for the dominant genetic condition NF2). Elsewhere (Prosser, 2006), it has been suggested that the identification of specific genetic disorders could result in the use of different programming and processing strategies with digital signal processing hearing aids. Furthermore, many of the best results of cochlear implantation in adults occur in individuals with late-onset dominant genetic hearing impairments.

Surgery has been controversial, as has the use of genetic testing and gene therapy. The media's portrayal of Bionic Ears and the elimination of the Deaf gene have not helped to put technology's relationship to hearing impairment into focus, particularly within the Deaf community.

SOCIO-ECONOMIC CHANGES

Closely related to the demographic and immigration developments are the changes in socio-economic status among the population. As the population get older, they tend to have lower incomes. It is also well known that most immigrant groups have a lower disposable income than individuals born in the country. The general socio-economic trend in Europe is that there was an increase of the disposable income in the EU countries during the 1970s and 1980s. In the beginning of 1980s there was a turning point and, for some, there was a decrease in disposable income but, at the same time, there was a continuing increase for a large proportion of the population. There were, in some countries, substantial decreases in income for the lowest decile group. This resulted in an increase of dispersion of disposable income. In some countries this came to a peak in the beginning of this century. Among the 15 member countries of the EU in 2001, Greece had the lowest income per capita income and Luxembourg the highest. Among the countries with the largest income dispersion of disposable income we find Portugal and among those with the smallest income dispersion is Sweden (Eurostat). An important factor in this development is the unemployment level. Employment is a major determinant of economic and social inclusion. Compared with the performance of the mid and late 1990s, the economic growth during the first three years of the 21st century has almost halved, and employment growth came to a standstill by the beginning of 2003 (European Commission, 2004, p. 12). Furthermore, employment opportunities are closely related to educational attainment.

Along with these trends there has, in some of those countries where the public sector has financed much of the cost for rehabilitation for hearing impairment, been a trend to 'privatise' this service, i.e. people have to pay the costs for individual rehabilitation from their own means. Since some people can afford this while some cannot, this is an impetus for enlargement of the cleavages among people with hearing impairment.

The trends we have highlighted regarding the socio-economic development (standstill in employment growth, increased dispersion of disposable income, and privatisation of the hearing rehabilitation process) will have an impact on the psychological and social consequences of hearing impairment. For the more affluent part of the population, these developments, along with the technological developments described above, the consequences will be positive. But there is a great risk that many of these factors, taken together, will have severe consequences for a significant proportion of hearing-impaired people. There is thus an important need for future research to investigate the outcome of these processes in terms of the standard of living of this large part of the population.

CONCLUSIONS

Finally, in this book we have focused on the relevance of having a FHHI. Although the ambiguity in the results is obvious, we have tried to highlight the relationships we have found which are theoretically and empirically justified. An agenda for future research on psychological and social consequences of hearing impairment has to further investigate the role of the socialisation process in a family with a history of hearing impairment compared with the process in a family without one. However, such an agenda must also take into account the developments in aetiology and genetics, the demographic and socio-economic changes and the greater cultural diversity we are witnessing in contemporary society.

REFERENCES

Dauman R, Daubech Q, Gavilan I et al. (2000) Long term outcome of childhood hearing deficiency. *Journal of Speech and Hearing Disorders* 52: 53–62.

Davis A (1997) Epidemiology. In D Stephens (ed). *Scott Brown's Otolaryngology*, 6th edn. Oxford: Butterworth-Heinemann, Vol. 2, 3, 1–38.

Erlandsson SE, Widén SE (2005) Attitudes towards noise and hearing protection among young individuals in Sweden and USA. 7th EFAS Congress, Göteborg, Sweden, June 2005.

European Commission (2004) *The Social Situation in the European Union 2004.*

Gates GA, Couropmitree NN, Myers RH (1999) Genetic associations in age-related hearing thresholds. *Archives of Otolaryngology* 125: 654–9.

Guilford P et al. (1994) A nonsyndromic form of neurosensory, recessive deafness maps to the pericentromeric region of chromosome13q. *Nature Genetics* 6: 24–8.

Kelsell PM et al. (1997) Connexin 26 mutations in hereditary non-syndromic sensorineural deafness. *Nature* 387: 80–3.

Mazzoli M, Newton V, Murgia A, Bitner-Glindzics M, Gasparini P, Read A et al. (2004) Guidelines and recommendations for testing of Cx 26 mutations and interpretations of results. *International Journal of Pediatric Otolaryngology* 68: 1397–8.

Morton NE (1991) Genetic epidemiology of hearing loss. *Annals of the New York Academy of Sciences* 630: 16–31.

Parving A, Christensen B, Stephens SDG (2002) Genetic hearing impairment and psychosocial consequences. *Journal of Audiological Medicine* 11: 161–9.

Polat F (2003) Factors affecting psychosocial adjustment of deaf students. *Journal of Deaf Studies and Deaf Education* 8: 325–39.

Prosser S (2006) Understanding the phenotype (basic concepts in audiology). In A Martini, D Stephens, A Read (eds) *Genes, Hearing and Deafness*. London, Dunitz (in press).

Reardon W, Toriello HV, Downs CA (2004) Epidemiology, etiology, genetic patterns and genetic counselling. In HV Toriello, W Reardon, RJ Gorlin (eds) *Hereditary Hearing Loss and Its Syndromes*, 2nd edn. New York: Oxford University Press, pp. 8–16.

Stephens D (2005) The impact of hearing impairment in children. In D Stephens, L Jones (eds) *The Impact of Genetic Hearing Impairment*. London: Whurr, pp. 73–105.

Stephens D, Danermark B (2005) The international classification of functioning, disability and health as a conceptual framework for the impact of genetic hearing impairment. In D Stephens, L Jones (eds) *The Impact of Genetic Hearing Impairment*. London: Whurr, pp. 54–67.

Stephens D, Jones L eds. (2005) (eds) *The Impact of Genetic Hearing Impairment.* London: Whurr.

Stephens D, Kramer S (2005) The impact of a family history of hearing problems on those with hearing difficulties themselves: an exploratory study. *International Journal of Audiology* 44: 206–12.

Strachan T, Read AP (2004) *Human Molecular Genetics,* 3rd edn. London: Garland (Chapter 16).

Van Camp G, Smith R (2005) Hereditary Hearing Loss Homepage. Antwerp: University of Antwerp. http://webhost.ua.ac.be/hhh/

Index

acquired hearing loss 25
activity limitations 55, 118, 123, 212
aetiology 25, 29, 43–4, 132–3, 140, 299,
    302, 348, 352
Allah 310
asylum seekers/refugees 308
anxiety 72, 95, 117–9, 121, 123–4, 136–7,
    188, 218, 221
audiology 43–4, 71, 291

background noise 176, 219
barriers 132–3, 285, 287
biobank UK
blindness 72
British Sign Language 30, 33, 222, 233,
    259, 261, 285–6

causes of deafness 260, 272
  environmental 260
  genetic 260
  unknown 29–30
childhood 18, 25, 43, 56, 58, 61–2, 67,
    208, 262, 342, 348
childhood/adolescence 58–60, 67
children 4, 25–6, 29–41, 43, 45–9, 53, 59,
    72, 75, 77–8, 83, 85–6, 93, 188, 211,
    214, 216–18, 220, 229–31, 233–4,
    241–2, 249, 257, 259–65, 267–8,
    270–7, 286–7, 290, 297, 306, 309, 312,
    319–20, 322–3, 325–9, 336, 342–4,
    346–8
children of deaf parents 30, 38, 41, 242,
    268, 275, 344
children of hearing parents 30, 41, 242,
    344
chromosomes 285, 290

cochlear implant 30–1, 33, 237, 241, 260,
    335, 337, 350
  implantation 33, 208, 350
cognitive difficulty 135
  disorder 136
  disturbance 138
  development 261, 271
  therapies 311
conductive hearing loss 118, 237, 245
Connexin 26 gene 260, 262–3, 273, 275,
    349
CT scan 319, 321

deafblindness 72
deaf activists
  community 251, 257–9, 261, 263–5,
    267–9, 271, 273–6, 286–7, 291, 293,
    350
  culture 257–8, 261, 264, 274, 276–7
  nation 264, 293
  partners/spouses 35
  people 35, 246, 250, 257–61, 264–9,
    271, 273, 275–7, 285–6, 289–92
  parents 29–31, 36–8, 40–1, 43, 241–2,
    267–8, 272 7, 309, 344
  siblings 30, 36–7, 40
deafened 217, 250, 258, 264, 319–23
deafness 30, 32, 35–6, 40, 44, 49, 93, 98,
    108, 135–8, 141, 154, 192–3, 207–8,
    211, 213, 221–2, 227, 234–5, 238–42,
    257–8, 260–5, 270–7, 286–7, 289, 291,
    297–8, 300, 302, 306, 309, 315, 319,
    325, 335, 343, 347–9
  cure for 141, 239–40, 242, 272
deaf awareness 274
  training 266, 276–7

The Effects of Genetic Hearing Impairment in the Family. Edited by D. Stephens and L. Jones.
Copyright © 2006 by John Wiley & Sons, Ltd.